Hypoglycemia: A Clinical Approach

Hypoglycemia: A Clinical Approach

Editor: Ethlyn Bishop

hayle medical

New York

Hayle Medical,
750 Third Avenue, 9th Floor,
New York, NY 10017, USA

Visit us on the World Wide Web at:
www.haylemedical.com

ISBN 978-1-64647-560-5 (Hardback)

Cataloging-in-publication Data

Hypoglycemia : a clinical approach / edited by Ethlyn Bishop.
p. cm.
Includes bibliographical references and index.
ISBN 978-1-64647-560-5
1. Hypoglycemia. 2. Hypoglycemia--Treatment. 3. Diabetes--Complications.
4. Hypoglycemia--Diagnosis. 5. Hypoglycemic agents--Side effects. I. Bishop, Ethlyn.
RC662.2 .H97 2023
616.466--dc23

Contents

Preface

Glucose is the primary source of energy in body. Hypoglycemia is a condition which occurs when the blood sugar (glucose) level falls lower than normal. It can cause headaches, fatigue, clumsiness, difficulty in speaking, disorientation, a racing heart, sweating, shakiness, nervousness, hunger, loss of consciousness, seizures, or death. Medications used to treat diabetes, such as insulin, sulfonylureas, and biguanides, are the most common cause of hypoglycemia. People with diabetes who have eaten less than usual, exercised recently, or have consumed alcohol are at higher risk for this medical condition. Medical problems like sepsis, kidney failure, liver disease, hormone insufficiency, malignancies such as insulinomas or non-B cell tumours, inborn metabolic abnormalities, numerous drugs, and alcohol can all lead to hypoglycemia. This book presents new insights into the causes and consequences of hypoglycemia. It consists of contributions made by international experts. Those in search of information to further their knowledge will be greatly assisted by this book.

The researches compiled throughout the book are authentic and of high quality, combining several disciplines and from very diverse regions from around the world. Drawing on the contributions of many researchers from diverse countries, the book's objective is to provide the readers with the latest achievements in the area of research. This book will surely be a source of knowledge to all interested and researching the field.

In the end, I would like to express my deep sense of gratitude to all the authors for meeting the set deadlines in completing and submitting their research chapters. I would also like to thank the publisher for the support offered to us throughout the course of the book. Finally, I extend my sincere thanks to my family for being a constant source of inspiration and encouragement.

Editor

Part 1

Section A

1

Development of Mulberry Leaf Extract for Suppressing Postprandial Blood Glucose Elevation

Toshiyuki Kimura
National Agricultural Research Center for Tohoku Region
Japan

1. Introduction

Epidemiological evidence indicates that postprandial hyperglycemia is an independent risk factor for cardiovascular disease (Bonora & Muggeo, 2001). Improving postprandial glycemic control is considered a target for decreasing the morbidity and mortality due to cardiovascular disease in prediabetic and diabetic individuals. Recently, clinical trials such as the STOP-NIDDM Trial and Victory Study demonstrated that α-glucosidase inhibitors (αGIs) reduced the progression from impaired glucose tolerance (IGT) to type 2 diabetes (Chiasson et al., 2002, 2003; Kawamori et al., 2009). Therefore, considerable attention has been paid to αGIs as preventive and therapeutic agents for type 2 diabetes and its complications. Some food consumed on a daily basis also contains αGIs and may therefore be effective for attenuating increase in postprandial blood glucose levels. Therefore, introducing αGIs into the diet may prevent diabetes.

In Asian countries, mulberry leaves are a known traditional medicine for preventing diabetes. According to a prior study, mulberry leaves have a potent αGI activity because of 1-deoxynojirimycin (DNJ), a glucose analog. In this chapter, we describe a method for determining DNJ in mulberry leaves; we also describe development of food-grade DNJ-enriched mulberry leaf extract (ME). Furthermore, we review the efficacy of this extract for postprandial glycemic control through human trials aimed at investigating use of mulberry leaves as food to prevent diabetes.

2. Development of ME

2.1 Diabetes mellitus

Diabetes mellitus is a chronic metabolic disorder characterized by high blood glucose levels. Type 2 diabetes, defined as noninsulin-dependent diabetes mellitus (NIDDM), is the most common form that affects 90–95 percent of all adults who develop diabetes. Type 2 diabetes is a lifestyle disease caused by reduced insulin production or impaired insulin response in target organs. It is associated with genetic background, obesity, unhealthy dietary habits, and physical inactivity. Hyperglycemia-induced oxidative stress causes serious diabetic complications such as diabetic retinopathy, nephropathy, and neuropathy, leading to decreased quality of life. The International Diabetes Federation (IDF) estimates that 285 million people around the world have diabetes; this total is expected to rise to 438 million within 20 years. Each year, a further 7 million people develop diabetes (IDF Diabetes Atlas fourth edition committee, 2009).

Type 2 diabetes increases morbidity and mortality as a result of serious macrovascular complications such as cardiovascular disease (Krolewski et al., 1987; Kannel & McGee, 1979). Recent epidemiological studies suggest that postprandial hyperglycemia is an independent risk factor for cardiovascular disease that has a greater effect on the development of this disease than fasting hyperglycemia (Ceriello, 1998; Hanefeld et al., 1996). Therefore, postprandial glycemic control is essential for effective reduction in the risk of cardiovascular disease. Carbohydrates comprise about 50% of our daily intake of calories. Carbohydrates ingested as food are digested to disaccharides by salivary and pancreatic amylases. The disaccharides are then hydrolyzed to monosaccharides by α-glucoside at the small intestine brush border and absorbed into the blood. α-Glucosidase is involved in this final step of carbohydrate digestion prior to absorption. αGIs retard the digestion and absorption of carbohydrates in the small intestinal lumen and therefore reduce the increase in blood glucose concentrations after a carbohydrate load. Acarbose, miglitol, and voglibose are α-glucosidase inhibitory agents used widely in clinical practice. These αGIs decrease both postprandial hyperglycemia and hyperinsulinemia but do not induce hypoglycemia and have a good safety profile, although their gastrointestinal adverse effects may limit long-term compliance to therapy. Long-term intervention trials of αGIs in patients with type 2 diabetes and IGT have been conducted. Recent placebo-controlled, prospective trials, including the STOP-NIDDM Trial and Victory Study, demonstrated that αGI intake before each meal reduces the risk of type 2 diabetes in patients with IGT (Chiasson et al., 2002, 2003; Kawamori et al., 2009). Therefore, improvement in postprandial hyperglycemia by αGI leads to prevention of diabetes and provides the basis for studies on the use of naturally occurring αGIs in plant foods.

2.2 Mulberry

Mulberry is a tree belonging to the genus *Morus* of the family Moraceae (Fig. 1). It is distributed over a wide area of tropical, subtropical, and temperate zones in Asia, Europe, North America, South America, and Africa. There are at least 24 species of mulberry with more than 100 known cultivars (Koidzumi, 1917). Historically, the trees have been planted for sericulture in east, central, and southern Asia. On the basis of folklore remedies, the leaves have also been used as a Chinese herbal tea, especially for diabetes. In the modern era, health benefits from mulberry products have been verified scientifically, with mulberry shown to have potent α-glucosidase inhibitory activity mainly because of azasugars. This has led to proposals that dietary mulberry intake is beneficial for attenuating postprandial hyperglycemia, thereby preventing diabetes. Several animal studies have been conducted to date. Nojima and co-workers showed that administration of mulberry leaf extract restored impaired glucose metabolism and hyperglycemic conditions in streptozotocin-induced diabetic mice (Nojima et al., 1998; Kimura et al., 1995). At present, various mulberry food products, including teas, powders, and tablets, are commercially available in Japan and many other countries. Although these products have apparent antidiabetic effects, their efficacy in humans requires further study.

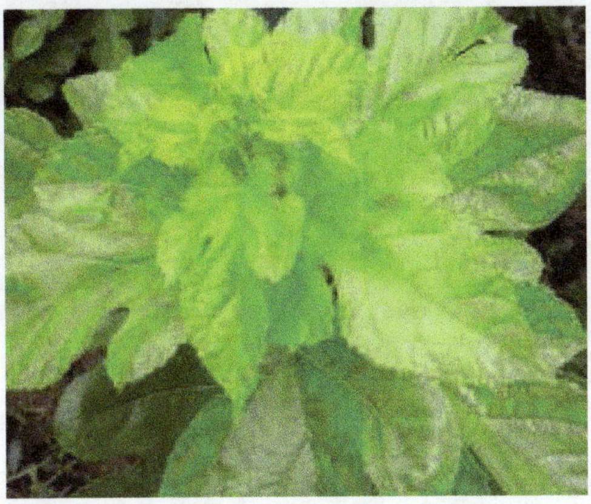

Fig. 1. Mulberry (*Morus alba* L.)

2.3 Azasugars in mulberry

Azasugars are alkaloids that mimic the structures of monosaccharides. In azasugars, the oxygen atom in the ring of these sugars is replaced by nitrogen. The first azasugar, the antibiotic nojirimycin, was discovered in 1966 in *Streptomyces* microorganisms (Inoue et al., 1966). Since then, more than 100 azasugars have been isolated from plants and microorganisms. DNJ is a 5-amino-1,5-dideoxy-D-glucopyranose or D-glucose analog (Fig. 2). Initially, DNJ was chemically synthesized by reduction of nojirimycin (Inoue et al., 1967) ; later, naturally occurring DNJ was isolated from the roots of mulberry trees and called moranoline (Yagi et al., 1976). DNJ has also been produced by microorganisms such as *Bacillus* and *Streptomyces* (Schmidt et al., 1979; Murao & Miyata, 1980; Ezure et al., 1985). Mulberry leaves are relatively rich in azasugars such as DNJ, fagomine, N-methyl-DNJ, and 2-O-R-D-galactopyranosyl-DNJ. DNJ is the dominant alkaloid, accounting for 50% of mulberry azasugars (Asano et al., 2001).

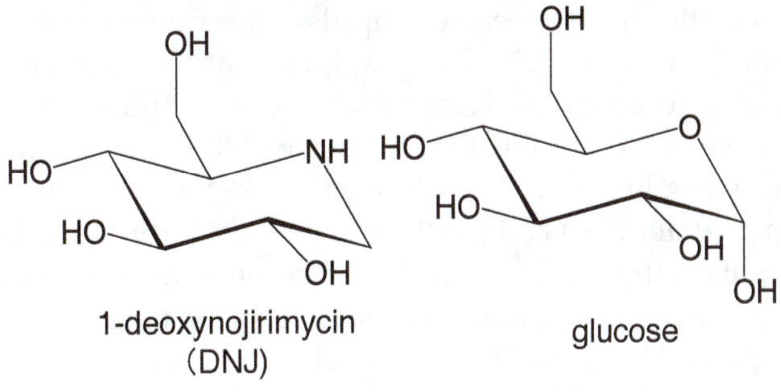

Fig. 2. Chemical structure of DNJ and glucose

Azasugars have α-glucosidase inhibitory properties because of their ability to competitively bind to the active sites of glucosidases by mimicking the corresponding natural substrates (Fig. 3). The αGI clinical agents described above are all azasugars developed from natural occurring azasugars (Junge et al., 1996). Among the naturally occurring azasugars, DNJ shows potent α-glucosidase inhibitory activity. Consequently, miglitol was developed as a lead compound from DNJ.

Based on this background, the relationship between the concentration of DNJ and the antidiabetic effect of mulberry food has attracted considerable attention. For this reason, mulberry food containing DNJ needs to be prepared.

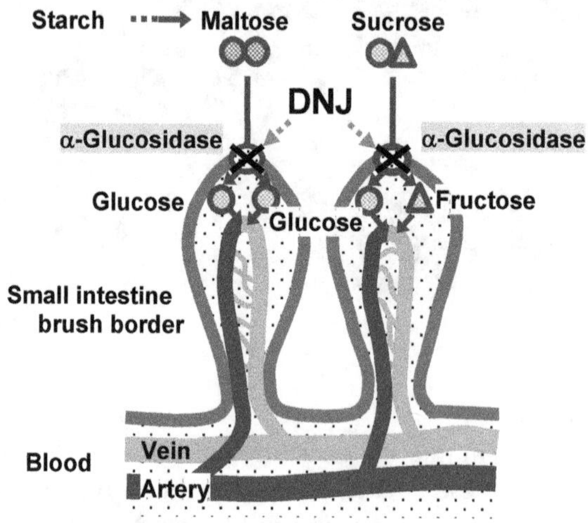

Fig. 3. Possible mechanism of DNJ in the digestive tract

2.4 Methods for determining DNJ in mulberry

Determination of DNJ levels in mulberry has been difficult because of the high polarity of DNJ and the absence of a chromophore in the molecule. Therefore, DNJ is too hydrophilic to be retained by widely used reverse-phase chromatography columns, and it cannot be detected with common ultraviolet or fluorescence detectors. Ligand-exchange and aminopropyl columns are commonly used for HPLC determination of relatively polar compounds such as carbohydrates and water-soluble vitamins (Sharpless et al., 2000). However, even these columns do not achieve reasonable retention of DNJ, and for this reason, several other methods have been developed for determining DNJ in mulberry.

Kimura et al. reported a method that used hydrophilic interaction liquid chromatography (HILIC) coupled with an evaporative light-scattering detector (ELSD) (Kimura et al., 2004); This method is known as the HILIC-ELSD method. HILIC has been developed as an efficient tool for analyzing highly hydrophilic compounds, and its analytical application to carbohydrates (Alpert et al., 1994) and peptides (Alpert et al., 1990) has been reported. The retention ability of the HILIC column basically depends on the hydrophilicity of the analytes, and if the compound has amino groups, its retention time is increased (Tolstikov & Fiehn, 2002). Therefore, a HILIC column is preferable for efficient separation of azasugars. ELSD is the universal detector that responds to nonvolatile compounds and directly detects analytes lacking chromophores.

Kim et al. (2003) reported the procedures for deriving DNJ using 9-fluorenylmethoxycarbonyl chloride, which targets secondary amino groups in DNJ, followed by reverse-phase HPLC using a fluorescence detector.

Furthermore, several other methods, such as HILIC-MS/MS (Nakagawa et al., 2010) and anion-exchange chromatography with pulsed amperometric detection methods (Yoshihashi et al., 2010), have been developed for measuring DNJ levels.

2.5 Development of ME

Since the putative effective dose of more than 10 mg DNJ per individual weighing 60 kg cannot be generally provided by commercially available mulberry leaf products because of their low DNJ content, the development of DNJ-enriched products is highly desired. Therefore, to produce nutraceutical ME, the concentrations of DNJ in mulberry leaves from different cultivars, harvest seasons, and leaf locations were examined. DNJ concentrations differed according to cultivars, with *M. alba* L. var. Tsuruta and Hayatesakari having a high DNJ content. The harvest season and region of mulberry leaves were also closely related to the DNJ content, with young mulberry leaves from the top part of the branches in the summer having the highest DNJ concentration. After optimization of harvesting and processing, ME was produced containing 1.5 % DNJ. This powder contained DNJ at concentrations approximately 15 times higher than general mulberry products (Figs. 4, 5; Kimura et al., 2007).

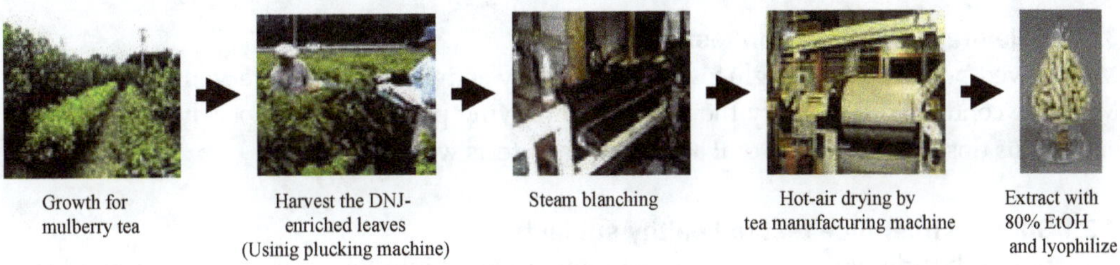
Growth for mulberry tea
Harvest the DNJ-enriched leaves (Usinig plucking machine)
Steam blanching
Hot-air drying by tea manufacturing machine
Extract with 80% EtOH and lyophilize

Fig. 4. Improved production process for DNJ-enriched mulberry extract (ME) (modified from Ref. Kimura, 2010; used with permission)

Young mulberry leaves from the top part of the branches in August contained the highest amount of DNJ. For harvesting, a method involving a plucking machine was considered an effective way for collecting young leaves. For blanching, steam treatment was used to prevent leaching of DNJ. For the drying process, hot air was employed, and the dried leaves were then disintegrated and added to a mixture of ethanol and water (20:80, v:v). After filtration, the extract was concentrated and lyophilized to a powder.

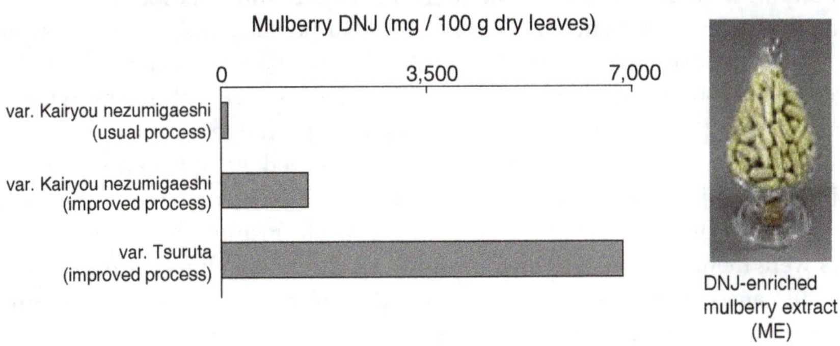

Fig. 5. DNJ concentrations in mulberry products produced by different processes (modified from Ref. Kimura, 2010; used with permission)

In the traditional process, widely cultivated leaves (*M. alba* L. var. Kairyou nezumigaeshi) were collected from whole branches and dried using hot air. In the improved process, the

DNJ content in the extract (*M. alba* L. var. Kairyou nezumigaeshi) was 15 times higher than that in the traditional mulberry product. If mulberry leaves containing high levels of DNJ (e.g., *M. alba* L. var. Tsuruta) were used, products with considerably greater DNJ concentrations could be produced.

3. Evaluation of ME

3.1 *In vitro* α-glucosidase inhibitory activity

The rat intestinal α-glucosidase inhibitory activity of ME was measured with *p*-nitrophenyl-α-D-glucopyranoside as the substrate (Yamaki & Mori, 2006). ME showed potent α-glucosidase inhibitory activity, which was approximately the same as the activity of the DNJ content in ME. This implied that the α-glucosidase inhibitory activity of ME was attributable to DNJ.

3.2 Single oral administration test

ME showed potent *in vitro* α-glucosidase inhibitory activity. Human intervention trials with ME were conducted. To clarify the effect of improving postprandial hyperglycemia and the efficacious dose of ME, single oral administration tests were performed.

3.2.1 Sucrose tolerance test in healthy subjects

Twenty-four healthy volunteers were randomly divided into four groups of six individuals. After fasting overnight, the individuals in each group received either 0 (placebo), 0.4, 0.8, or 1.2 g ME (corresponding to 0, 6, 12, or 18 mg DNJ, respectively), followed by 50 g sucrose dissolved in 100 mL water. Blood samples were collected before and 30, 60, 90, 120, 150, and 180 min after DNJ or sucrose administration. Plasma glucose and insulin levels were then measured. The results showed that oral administration of 0.8 and 1.2 g ME significantly suppressed the elevation of postprandial blood glucose and secretion of insulin (Kimura et al., 2007).

3.2.2 Carbohydrate tolerance test in subjects with borderline diabetes

To examine the diabetes preventative effect of ME in a practical daily meal, a carbohydrate tolerance test was performed in subjects with borderline diabetes. The study design was a randomized, double-blind, four-period, crossover trial. Twelve volunteers with impaired glucose metabolism [fasting plasma glucose (FPG) in the range of 100–140 mg/dL] were enrolled in the study. In each trial, all the subjects consumed 200 g boiled white rice 15 min after ME ingestion. Blood samples were drawn before ME ingestion and 30, 60, 90, and 120 min after starting the meal. Plasma glucose, plasma insulin, and other biochemical parameters were then measured. Similar to the study described above, administration of 0.8 and 1.2 g ME caused significant suppression and peak time delay of postprandial blood glucose and secretion of insulin (Fig. 6; Asai et al., 2011).

3.3 Long-term supplementation trial

Elevation of postprandial blood glucose levels and secretion of insulin were suppressed significantly at a dose of more than 0.8 g ME. To assess the safety and effects of long-term ingestion, a long-term supplementation trial was then conducted.

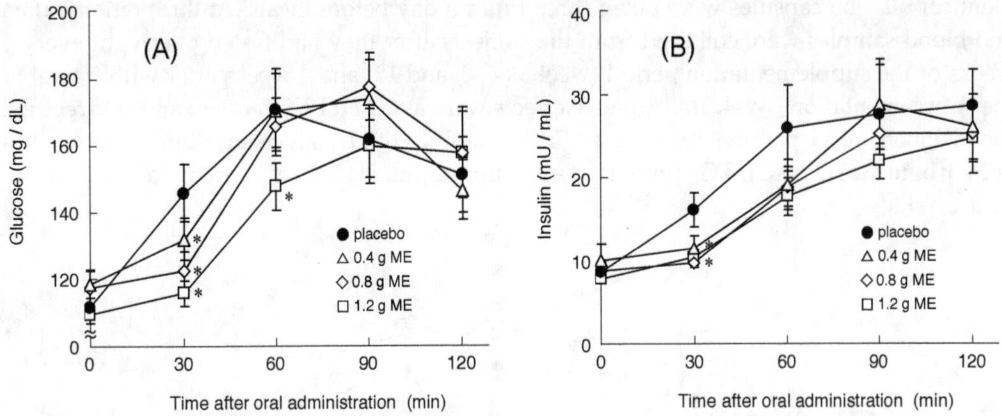

After fasting for 12 h, the subjects with borderline diabetes were orally administered either 0 (placebo), 0.4, 0.8, or 1.2 g ME (0, 6, 12, or 18 mg DNJ, respectively), followed by 200 g boiled rice. Blood samples were collected prior to intake and 30, 60, 90, and 120 min after rice intake. The plasma glucose and insulin levels were then determined. Data represent the mean ± S.E.M. (n = 10). *$P < 0.05$ vs. placebo.

Fig. 6. Effects of a single oral administration of ME on plasma glucose (A) and insulin (B) levels (from Ref. Asai et al., 2011; used with permission)

3.3.1 Thirty-eight–day supplementation trial in healthy subjects

Twelve healthy volunteers were enrolled in the study. Based on the results of the above described single oral administration test, the ME dose was set at 1.2 g before every meal. The subjects were randomly divided into two groups; they received either 0 (placebo) or 1.2 g ME before every meal for 38 days (0 or 3.6 g/day, corresponding to 0 and 54 mg DNJ/day, respectively). Fasting blood samples were collected on days 0, 24, and 38 of ME powder administration. Blood biochemical parameters such as FPG, insulin, glycated hemoglobin (HbA1c), triglyceride (TG), total cholesterol (Tcho), HDL cholesterol (HDL-C), adiponectin, high-molecular-weight adiponectin (HMW adiponectin), and lipoprotein lipase (LPL) were measured. The results showed no significant differences in any of the biochemical parameters between the placebo group and the group ingesting the test food either before, during, or after the study. The daily intake of the ME powder did not cause hypoglycemia or abnormal lipid profiles (i.e., high cholesterol). According to previous reports, long-term ingestion of αGI (acarbose, tochi extract) reduced FAG, HbA1C, TG, and Tcho levels in the subjects (Fujita et al., 2003; Hillerbrand et al., 1979), changes which may contribute to diabetes prevention and improvement. The results of our study showed no such effects, which could be attributable to the short administration period. The major side effects of αGI involve the gastrointestinal system (Harano et al., 2002). However, no subjects in our study complained of negative gastrointestinal system-related side effects such as abdominal distension, abdominal pain, retching, or flatulence (Kimura et al., 2008).

3.3.2 Twelve-week supplementation trial in subjects with borderline diabetes

Next, we conducted a 12-week randomized, double-blind, placebo-controlled trial, followed by a 4-week posttreatment observation in subjects with borderline diabetes. Seventy-six subjects with FPG in the range of 110–140 mg/dL were recruited and randomized to receive either mulberry leaf extract or placebo. During the 12-week trial, ME (18 mg DNJ) or identical placebo capsules were taken three times a day before meals. Anthropometric data and blood samples were collected from the subjects after they had fasted overnight every 4 weeks of the supplementation period (week 0, 4, 8, and 12) and 4 weeks after withdrawal of the supplementation (week 16). Adverse effects were assessed by interview and self-reports. Blood biochemical parameters such as FPG, insulin, HbA1c, glycated albumin (GA), 1,5-anhydroglucitol (1,5AG), TG, Tcho, HDL-C, adiponectin, HMW adiponectin, and LPL were measured.

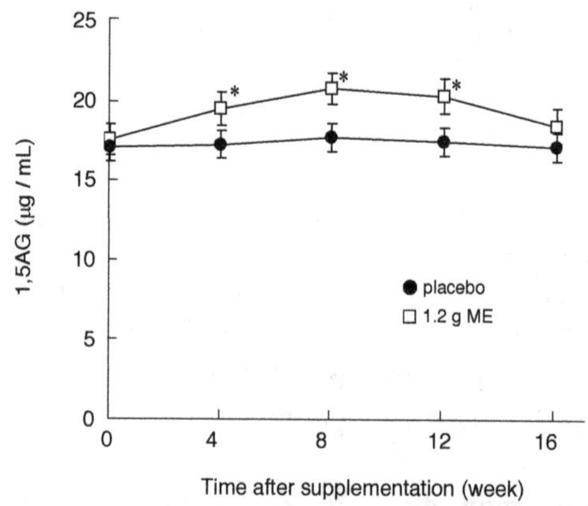

Changes in the concentration of 1,5AG during the 12-week supplementation with either ME (18 mg DNJ, thrice daily) or placebo followed by a 4-week observation without supplementation Data are expressed as the mean ± S.E.M. (n = 33 in the extract group, n = 32 in the placebo group). $^{*}P < 0.05$ vs. placebo.

Fig. 7. Effects of 12-week supplementation of ME on plasma 1,5AG levels (modified from Ref. Asai et al., 2011; used with permission)

The results showed that there were no significant differences between the ME and placebo groups in baseline values or values during the study for the glycemic control parameters (FPG, insulin, HbA1c, GA), anthropometric measurements, or serum lipid profiles. Among the glycemic control parameters, there were significant differences between the two groups with regard to the change in serum 1,5AG concentration over the study period. The 1,5AG concentration of the ME group increased gradually from baseline through to weeks 4, 8, and 12 and was higher than that in the placebo group at weeks 4, 8 and 12. The increase in 1,5AG concentration in the ME group returned to the baseline level after the 4-week posttreatment observation period (i.e., at week 16) (Fig. 7). The serum 1,5AG concentration is maintained at a constant level under euglycemic conditions; however, it decreases as a result of competitive inhibition of renal tubular reabsorption caused by glycosuria under hyperglycemic conditions (Akanuma et al., 1988; Yamanouchi et al., 1990). Serum 1,5AG concentrations therefore sensitively respond to blood glucose fluctuations within a few days (Yamanouchi et al., 1992, 1996; Dungan et al., 206). Hence, the increased 1,5AG concentration we observed may reflect a continuous reduction in postprandial hyperglycemic spikes over the 12-week supplementation period. The increase in the 1,5AG concentration returned to baseline levels after the 4-week withdrawal of ME supplementation. On the other hand, no significant differences in FPG, HbA1c, or GA concentrations were observed between the groups. While the 1,5AG concentration responded to glycemic fluctuations within a few days, the HbA1c and GA concentrations reflected time-averaged glycemia in the previous 2–3 months and 2–3 weeks, respectively. In contrast to this result, meta-analysis of αGI drug trials in patients with type 2 diabetes showed that FPG and HbA1c concentrations were reduced by acarbose and miglitol (Van Der Laar et al., 2005). Because the subjects in these trials had diabetes, their baseline HbA1c and FPG concentrations were considerably higher than those of subjects in the present trial. Moreover, these earlier trials were conducted for considerably longer durations.

Gastrointestinal symptoms such as abdominal distension, diarrhea, and flatulence are the most frequent adverse effects of αGI agents. No such adverse effects were observed through the study period (Asai et al., 2011).

4. Conclusion

Increasing evidence strongly supports the efficiency of interventions such as diet and exercise for preventing or delaying the onset of diabetes in prediabetic individuals. Pharmacological approaches are another effective strategy for achieving these objectives.

Mulberry leaves have been used in folk medicine for treating diabetes since ancient times. Three decades ago, DNJ, a potent αGI, was found in mulberry leaves. Since this discovery, DNJ has been considered to be responsible for the antidiabetic effect of mulberry leaves. However, there is only limited information on the efficacy and effective dose of DNJ in humans. Recently, food-grade mulberry leaf extract with a defined DNJ concentration (1.5%) has been developed. Human studies involving ingestion of the extract prior to meals showed suppression of postprandial hyperglycemia and hyperinsulinemia. In addition, studies on long-term supplementation of the extract at reasonable doses showed an improvement in postprandial glycemic control. Hypoglycemia; abnormal lipid profiles; gastrointestinal system-related side effects such as abdominal distension, abdominal pain, retching, or flatulence; or any other adverse effects have also not been observed. Therefore, DNJ in mulberry leaves appears to be a promising therapy for preventing or delaying the onset of diabetes, especially in prediabetic or mildly diabetic individuals.

As described above, we have gathered favorable evidence for the efficacy of ME. However, in terms of safety, there is insufficient evidence because of a lack of history of mulberry as a food for humans. Further safety evaluation on the absorption, distribution, metabolism, and excretion of mulberry DNJ is therefore required before the plant can be deployed as a functional food.

5. Acknowledgements

I would like to give sincere thanks to Professor Miyazawa whose comments and suggestions were innumerably valuable throughout my work. Special thanks also go to Associate Professor Nakagawa whose meticulous comments were an enormous help to me.

6. References

Akanuma, Y.; Morita, M. & Fukuzawa, N. Urinary excretion of 1,5-anhydro-D-glucitol accompanying glucose excretion in diabetic patients. *Diabetologia*, Vol. 31, (1988), pp. 831–835, ISSN 0012-186X

Alpert, A. J. Hydrophilic-interaction chromatography for the separation of peptides, nucleic acids and other polar compounds. *Journal of Chromatography,* Vol. 499, (1990), pp. 177-196, ISSN 0021-9673

Alpert, A. J.; Shukla, M.; Shukla, AK.; Zieske, LR.; Yuen, SW.; Ferguson, MA. J.; Mehlert, A.; Pauly, M. & Orlando, R. Hydrophilic-interaction chromatography of complex carbohydrates. *Journal of Chromatography A,* Vol. 676, (1994), pp. 191-202, ISSN 0021-9673

Asai, A.; Nakagawa, K.; Higuchi, O.; Kimura, T.; Kojima, Y.; Kariya, J.; Miyazawa, T. & Oikawa, S. Effect of mulberry leaf extract with enriched 1-deoxynojirimycin content on postprandial glycemic control in subjects with impaired glucose metabolism. *Journal of Diabetes Investigation,* in press, (2011), ISSN 2040-1116

Asano, N.; Yamashita, T.; Yasuda, K.; Ikeda, K.; Kizu, H.; Kameda, Y.; Kato, A.; Nash, R. J.; Lee, H. S. & Ryu, K. S. Polyhydroxylated alkaloids isolated from mulberry trees (*Morus alba* L.) and silkworms (*Bombyx mori* L.). *Journal of Agricultural and Food Chemistry.* Vol. 49, (2001), pp. 4208-4213, ISSN 0021-8561

Bonora, E. & Muggeo, M. Postprandial blood glucose as a risk factor for cardiovascular disease in Type II diabetes: the epidemiological evidence. *Diabetologia,* Vol. 44, (2001), pp. 2107–2114, ISSN 0012-186X

Ceriello, A. The emerging role of post-prandial hyperglycemic spikes in the pathogenesis of diabetic complications. *Diabetic Medicine,* Vol. 15, (1998), pp. 188-193, ISSN 1939-327X

Chiasson, JL.; Josse. RG. & Gomis, R. Acarbose for prevention of type 2 diabetes mellitus: the STOP-NIDDM randomized trial. *The Lancet,* Vol. 359, (2002), pp. 2072–2077, ISSN 0140-6736

Chiasson, JL.; Josse RG. & Gomis, R. Acarbose treatment and the risk of cardiovascular disease and hypertension in patients with impaired glucose tolerance: the STOP-NIDDM trial. *The Journal of the American Medical Association,* Vol. 290, (2003), pp. 486–494, ISSN 0098-7484

Dungan, KM.; Buse, JB. & Largay, J. 1,5-Anhydroglucitol and postprandial hyperglycemia as measured by continuous glucose monitoring system in moderately controlled patients with diabetes. *Diabetes Care,* Vol. 29, (2006), pp. 1214–1219, ISSN 0149-5992

Ezure, Y.; Murao, S.; Miyazaki, K. & Kawamata, M. Molanoline (1-deoxynojirimycin) fermentation and its improvement. *Agricultural and biological chemistry,* 49, (1985), pp. 1119-1125, ISSN 0002-1369

Fujita, H.; Yamagami, T. & Ohshima, K. Long-term ingestion of Touchi-extract, an α-glucosidase inhibitor, by borderline and mild type-2 diabetic subjects is safe and significantly reduces blood glucose levels. *Nutrition Research,* Vol. 23, (2003), pp. 713–722, ISSN 0271-5317

Hanefeld, M.; Fischer, S.; Julius, U.; Schulze, J.; Schwanebeck, U.; Shmechel, H.; Ziegelasch HJ. & Lindner, J. Risk factors for myocardial infarction and death in newly detected NIDDM: the Diabetes Intervention Study, 11-year follow-up. *Diabetologia,* Vol. 39, (1996), pp. 1577-1583, ISSN 0012-186X

Harano, Y.; Suzuki, M.; Koyama, Y.; Kanda, M.; Yasuda, S.; Suzuki, K. & Takamizawa, I. Multifactorial insulin resistance and clinical impact in hypertension and cardiovascular disease. *Journal of Diabetes and its Complications,* Vol. 16, (2002), pp. 19- 23, ISSN 1056-8727

Hillerbrand, I.; Boehm, K.; Frank, G.; Fink, H. & Berchtoid, P. The effects of the α-glucosidase inhibitor BAY g5421 (acarbose) on meal stimulated elevations of circulating glucose, insulin and triglyceride levels in man, *Research in Experimental Medicine*, Vol. 175, (1979), pp. 81–86, ISSN 0300-9130

IDF Diabetes Atlas fourth edition committee. (2009), Prevalence estimates of diabetes mellitus (DM) 2010 and 2030and, In: *Diabetes Atlas*, Available from http://www.diabetesatlas.org/

Inoue, S.; Tsuruoka, T. & Niida, T. The structure of nojirimycin, a piperidinose sugar antibiotic. *The Journal of Antibiotics*, Vol. 19, (1966), pp. 288-292, ISSN 0021-8820

Inoue, S.; Tsuruoka, T.; Ito, T. & Niida, T. Structure and synthesis of nojirimycin. *Tetrahedron*, Vol. 23, (1967), pp. 2125-2144.

Junge, B.; Matzke, M. & Stltefuss, J. (1996) Chemistry and structureactivity relationships of glucosidase inhibitors. In *Handbook of experimental pharmacology*, Kuhlmann, J.; Puls, W., (Eds.), Vol. 119, pp. 411-482, Springer-Verlag, ISBN 3-540-58990-2, New York, USA

Kannel, W. & McGee, D. Diabetes and cardiovascular risk factors: the Framingham Study. *Circulation Journal*, Vol. 59, (1979), pp. 8-13, ISSN 1346-9843

Kawamori, R.; Tajima, N.; Iwamoto, Y.; Kashiwagi, A.; Shimamoto, K. & Kaku, K. on behalf of the Voglibose Ph-3 Study Group Voglibose for prevention of type 2 diabetes mellitus: a randomised, double-blind trial in Japanese individuals with impaired glucose tolerance. *The Lancet*, Vol. 373, No. 9675, (May 2009), pp. 1607- 1614, ISSN 0140-6736

Kim, JW.; Kim, S.-U.; Lee, HS.; Kim, I.; Ahn, MY. & Ryu, KS. Determination of 1-deoxynojirimycin in Morus alba L. leaves by derivatization with 9-fluorenylmethyl chloroformate followed by reversed-phase high-performance liquid chromatography. *Journal of Chromatography A*, Vol. 1002, (2003), pp. 93-99, ISSN 0021-9673

Kimura, M.; Chen, F.-J.; Nakashima, N.; Kimura, I.; Asano, N. & Koya, S. Antihyperglycemic effects of N-containing sugars derived from mulberry leaves in streptozotocin-induced diabetic mice. *Journal of Traditional Medicines*, Vol. 12, (1995), pp. 214-219

Kimura, T.; Nakagawa, K.; Saito, Y.; Yamagishi, K.; Suzuki, M.; Yamaki, K.; Shinmoto, H. & Miyazawa, T. Determination of 1-deoxynojirimycin in mulberry leaves using hydrophilic interaction chromatography with evaporative light scattering detection. *Journal of Agricultural and Food Chemistry*, Vol. 52, (2004), pp. 1415-1418, ISSN 0021-8561

Kimura, T.; Nakagawa, K. & Kubota, H. Food-grade mulberry powder enriched with 1-deoxynojirimycin suppresses the elevation of postprandial blood glucose in humans. *Journal of Agricultural and Food Chemistry*, Vol. 55, (2007), pp. 5869–5874, ISSN 0021-8561

Kimura, T.; Nakagawa, K.; Kubota, H.; Kojima, Y.; Yamagishi, K.; Oikawa, S. & Miyazawa, T. Long term effect of DNJ-enriched mulberry leaf product. *Journal of Clinical Biochemistry and Nutrition*, Supple, Vol. 43, (June 2008), pp. 1–3, ISSN 0912-0009

Kimura, T. Development of mulberry leaf product with a-glucosidase inhibitor for the prevention of type2 diabetes mellitus. *Nippon Shokuhin Kagaku KogakuKaishi*, Vol. 57, No. 2, (2010), pp. 57-62 (in Japanese), ISSN 1341-027X

Koidzumi, G. (1917). Taxonomical discussion on *Morus* plants. *Bull. Imp. Sericult. Exp. Stat.*, Vol. 3, pp. 1-62. (in Japanese)

Krolewski, AS.; Kosinski, EJ.; Warram, JH.; Leland, OS.; Busick, EJ.; Asmal, AC.; Rand, LI.; Christlieb, AR.; Bradley, RF. & Kahn, CR. Magnitude and determinants of coronary artery disease in juvenile-onset, insulin-dependent diabetes mellitus. *American Journal of Cardiology*, Vol. 59, No. 8, (April 1987), pp. 750-755, ISSN 0002-9149

Murao, S. & Miyata, S. Isolation and characterization of a new trehalase inhibitor, S-GI. *Agricultural and biological chemistry*, Vol. 44, (1980), pp. 219-221, ISSN 0002-1369

Nakagawa, K.; Ogawa, K.; Higuchi, O.; Kimura, T.; Miyazawa, T. & Hori, M. Determination of iminosugars in mulberry leaves and silkworms using hydrophilic interaction chromatography–tandem mass spectrometry. *Analytical Biochemistry*, Vol. 404, (2010), pp. 217–222, ISSN 0003-2697

Nojima, H.; Kimura, I.; Chen, F.-J.; Sugihara, Y.; Haruno, M.; Kato, A. & Asano, N. Antihyperglycemic effects of N-containing sugars from *Xanthocercis zambesiaca, Morus bombycis*, Aglaonema treubii, and Castanospermum australe in streptozotocindiabetic mice. *Journal of Natural Products*, Vol. 61, (1998), pp.397-400, ISSN 0974-5211

Schmidt, DD.; Frommer, W.; Muller, L.;& Truscheit, E. Glucosidase inhibitors from bacilli. *Naturwissenshaften*, Vol. 66, (1979), pp. 584-585, ISSN 0028-1042

Sharpless, KE.; Margolis, S. & Thomas, JB. Determination of vitamins in food-matrix standard reference materials. *Journal of Chromatography A*, Vol. 881, (2000), pp. 171-181, ISSN 0021-9673

Tolstikov, VV. & Fiehn, O. Analysis of highly polar compounds of plant origin: combination of hydrophilic interaction chromatography and electrospray ion trap mass spectrometry. *Analytical Biochemistry*, Vol. 301, (2002), pp. 298-307, ISSN 0003-2697

Yagi, M.; Kouno, T.; Aoyagi, Y. & Murai, H. The structure of Moraoline, a piperidine alkaloid from *Morus* species. *Nippon Nougei Kagaku Kaishi*, Vol. 50, (1976), pp. 571-572 (in Japanese), ISSN 0002-1407

Yamaki, K. & Mori, Y. Evaluation of α-glucosidase Inhibitory activity in colored foods : a trial using slope factors of regression curves. *Nippon Shokuhin Kagaku Kogaku Kaishi*, Vol. 53, No. 4, (2006), pp. 229-231 (in Japanese), ISSN 1341-027X

Yamanouchi, T.; Akaoka, I. & Akanuma, Y. Mechanism for acute reduction of 1, 5-anhydroglucitol in rats treated with diabetogenic agents. *American Journal of Physiology*, Vol. 258, (1990), pp. E423–E427, ISSN 1522-1466

Yamanouchi, T.; Moromizato, H. & Shinohara, T. Estimation of plasma glucose fluctuation with a combination test of hemoglobin A1c and 1,5-anhydroglucitol. *Metabolism*, Vol. 41, (1992), pp. 862–867, ISSN 1744-6651

Yamanouchi, T.; Ogata, N. & Tagaya, T. Clinical usefulness of serum 1, 5-anhydroglucitol in monitoring glycaemic control. *The Lancet*, Vol. 347, (1996), pp. 1514–1518, ISSN 0140-6736

Yoshihashi, T.; Do, HT.; Tungtrakul, P.; Boonbumrung, S. & Yamaki, K. Simple, selective, and rapid quantification of 1-deoxynojirimycin in mulberry leaf products by high-performance anion-exchange chromatography with pulsed amperometric detection. *Journal of Food Science*, Vol. 75, No. 3, (April 2010), pp. 246-50, ISSN 0022-1147

Van Der Laar, FA.; Lucassen, PL.& Akkermans, RP. a-Glucosidase inhibitors for patients with type 2 diabetes: results from a Cochrane systematic review and meta-analysis. *Diabetes Care*, Vol. 28, (2005), pp. 154–163, ISSN 0149-5992

2

A New Therapy of Type 2 Diabetes: DPP-4 Inhibitors

Tatjana Ábel
National Health Center
Hungary

1. Introduction

Type 2 diabetes is a progressive disease which is significantly spreading all over the world. It is characterized by developing insulin resistance, impairment of the pancreatic beta cells and an impaired suppression of glucagon production of the pancreatic alpha cells (Figure 1) (DeFronzo 2009). When choosing a therapy for it, several aspects should be taken into consideration, e.g. is a patient obese or has he/she a normal body weight; is he/she elderly;

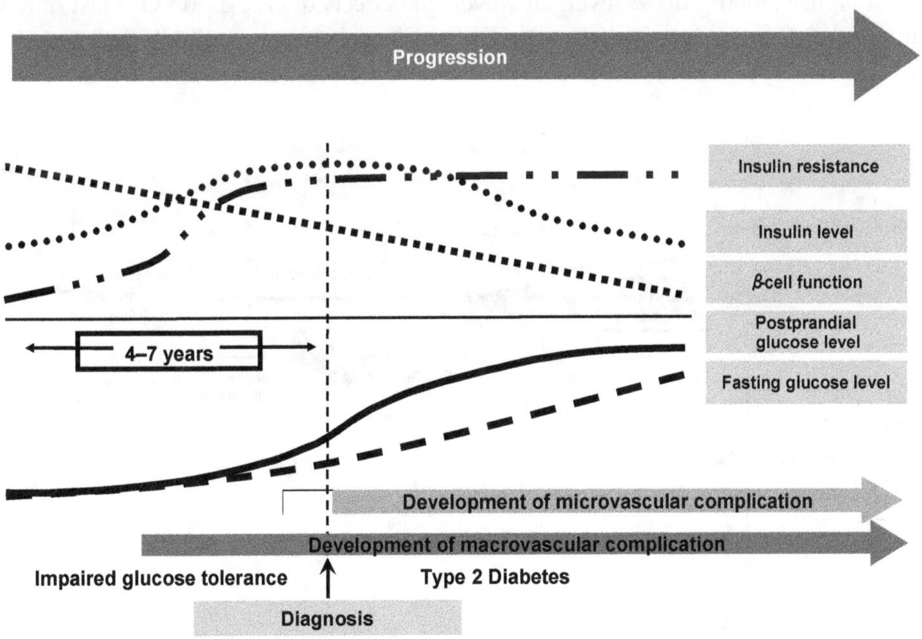

Fig. 1. Type 2 diabetes features

how long has his/her diabetes been known; were there any side effects caused by his/her previous antidiabetic medication, and are there any complications present (e.g. nephropathy). A good glycemic control reduces the rates of diabetes-associated microvascular and possibly macrovascular complications. Reduction of the associated risk factors, including those related to excessive weight, high blood pressure and dyslipidemia are also necessary to meaningfully decrease cardiovascular risk. Agents that can improve glycemia with weight neutrality could offer an additional benefit to overweight patients with type 2 diabetes. Many new drugs are currently in development for the treatment of diabetes, including products with a new mechanism of action such as dipeptidyl peptidase-4 (DPP-4) inhibitors.

2. Mechanisms of DPP-4 inhibitor action

Up to now the treatment of type 2 diabetes has been limited primarily to elevation of insulin production, increase of insulin sensitivity, reduction of glucose absorption and replacement of insulin. In the recent years, however, DPP-4 inhibitors (gliptins) emerged. These belong to a novel group of medicines which exert their action by increasing incretin levels (Drucker, Sherman et al. 2010). Incretins include glucagon-like peptide 1 (GLP-1) and glucose-dependent insulinotropic polypeptide (GIP) which are produced in the intestine and contribute to the physiological regulation of glucose homeostasis (Thornberry and Gallwitz 2009) (Figure 2). Active endogenous GLP-1 and GIP concentrations increase two- to threefold following a meal. Active GLP-1 and GIP increase the production and release of insulin by pancreatic beta cells. Approximately 60% of the postprandial insulin release is promoted by these two hormones. In addition, GLP-1 also reduces the secretion of glucagon by pancreatic alpha cells, resulting in a decreased hepatic glucose production. These effects are glucose-dependent; GLP-1 stimulates insulin secretion and reduces glucagon production only at a higher blood glucose level. However, the effects of GLP-1 and GIP last only for a few minutes as they are inactivated due to DPP-4 (Thornberry and Gallwitz 2009).

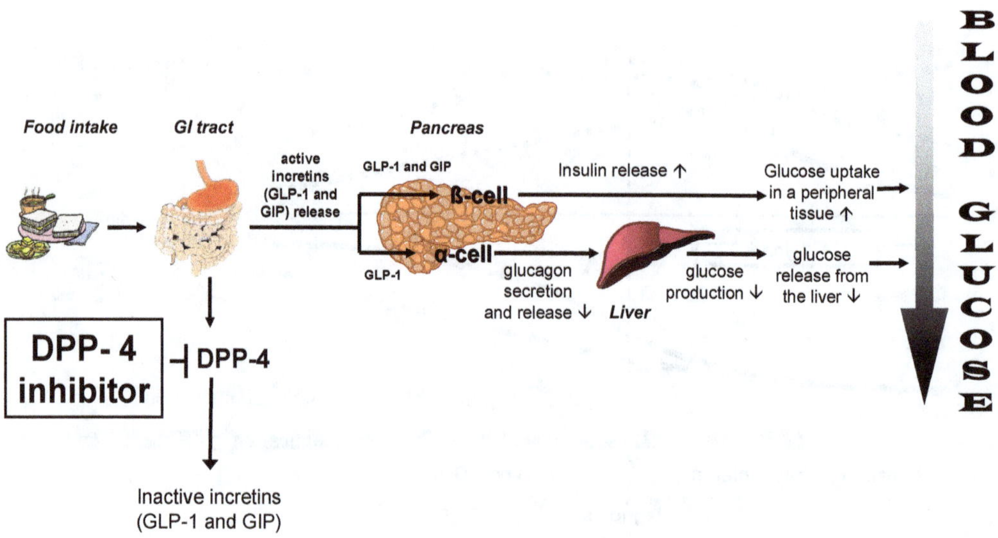

DPP-4 = dipeptidyl peptidase-4; GI = gastrointestinal; GIP = glucose-dependent insulinotropic polypeptide; GLP-1 = glucagon-like peptide-1;

Fig. 2. Mechanisms of DPP-4 inhibitor action.

The promising therapeutic potential of GLP-1 as a pharmacologycal tool for treating type 2 diabetes has been discovered in the 1990s. By inhibiting DPP-4, the gliptins increase insulin production and release as well as reduce glucagon levels in a glucose-dependent way, resulting in a decrease of fasting and postprandial glycemia, as well as HbA1c levels (Nauck, Vilsboll et al. 2009). Further, it has the ability to restore the blunted first phase insulin secretion in type 2 diabetes. Also in this respect, their mechanism of action differs from that of the sulfonylureas which stimulate insulin secretion also at low levels of blood glucose and may lead to hypoglycemia.

Fix combinations of sitagliptin and then vildagliptin with metformin have also been launched; these affect pathogenic factors of type 2 diabetes at more target points: they reduce the extent of insulin resistance, regulate insulin secretion in a glucose-dependent way, reduce glucagon secretion and also decrease hepatic glucose production (Nauck, Vilsboll et al. 2009). Their effects are additive, levels of active GLP-1 are increased not only by DPP-4 inhibitors but by metformin as well (Cho and Kieffer 2011).

3. Clinical and experimental evidence with the DPP-4 inhibitors

The oral antidiabetic drugs (OADs) used before the emergence of DPP-4 inhibitors may cause significant side effects including e.g. gastrointestinal symptoms, weight gain, cardiac heart failure, myocardial infarction, bone fractures and hypoglycemia and they do not reverse the progressive decline in beta cell function. Among others this led to the development of newer OADs, the DPP-4 inhibitors.

As a first step, according to the consensus statement of the European Diabetes Association for the Study of Diabetes (EASD) and the American Diabetes Association (ADA), in patients with no metabolic upset, lifestyle changes and metformin are recommended (Nathan, Buse et al. 2009). If no sufficient metabolic control can be attained by this way (HbA1c > 7%), or the patient should not receive metformin (it is not tolerated or it is contraindicated), addition of an oral antidiabetic of second choice is recommended. Although DPP-4 inhibitors are mentioned as second-line drugs among the less validated therapies, this seems to have to be changed due to the increasing amount of study results published in relation to them.

The use of sitagliptin, the first oral DPP-4 inhibitor was approved by the Food and Drug Administration (FDA) and the European Medicines Agency (EMA) in 2006 and in 2007 respectively (Gerich 2010). Sitagliptin can be given in monotherapy or in combination with metformin, sulfonylurea, thiazolidinediones, or as a triple combination with metformin and sulfonylurea or metformin and thiazolidinediones both in the USA and Europe. In the recent years a fix combination of sitagliptin/metformin has also been available. Concomitant administration of sitagliptin with insulin has been approved by FDA and EMA in 2010.

Saxagliptin can be used in combination with other OADs (metformin, sulfonylurea, thiazolidinediones) both in the USA and in Europe in 2007 (Gerich 2010).

Marketing of vildagliptin was not approved by the FDA due to dermal lesions and renal impairment observed in animal studies. In Europe, based on the approval of EMA in 2008, vildagliptin can be given with metformin, sulfonylurea or thiazolidinediones. A fix combination of vildagliptin/metformin has also been marketed.

3.1 Clinical efficacy

As far the results have shown no difference between DPP-4 inhibitors in the reduction of HbA1c values. Both in monotherapy and in combination (with metformin, sulfonylurea, thiazolidinediones, or insulin) they effectively reduce HbA1c levels (by 0.6% to 1.1%) (Ahrén 2011). This effect has proven to be dependent of diabetes duration and baseline HbA1c values as well. Greater reductions in HbA1c are seen in subjects with higher baseline levels and they are more effective in patients with shorter diabetes duration (< 3 years). A survey summarized the results of 18 publications and 3 presentations where elderly (≥ 65 years) patients with type 2 diabetes received DPP-4 inhibitor (sitagliptin, saxagliptin, vildagliptin, or alogliptin) treatment in monotherapy or in combination (metformin, glimepiride, glibenclamide, thiazolidinediones or insulin) (Schwartz 2010). No significant difference was found in the HbA1c level reducing effect of DPP-4 therapy in elderly and in younger patients.

Although the DPP-4 inhibitors differ from each other in several aspects, it is not known yet whether this means any substantial difference in their e.g. long-term efficacy (Table 1).

Inhibitor	Metabolism	Elimination route	Dosing	DPP-4 selectivity	DPP-4 inhibition*
Sitagliptin	not appreciably metabolized	renal (~ 80% unchanged as parent)	100mg qd	high	max ~ 97%; > 80% 24 h postdose
Saxagliptin	hepatically metabolized to active metabolite (via P_{450} 3A4/5)	renal (12-29% as parent, 21-52% as metabolite)	5mg qd	moderate	max ~ 80%; ~ 70% 24 h postdose
Vildagliptin	hydrolyzed to inactive metabolite (P_{450} enzyme independent)	renal (22% as parent, 55% as primary metabolite)	50mg bid	moderate	max ~ 95%; > 80% 12 h postdose

Table 1. Characteristics of DPP-4 inhibitors.

3.2 Hypoglycemia

Intensive glucose control increases the risk of developing hypoglycemia. In the Diabetes Control and Complications Trial (DCCT) the rate of severe hypoglycemia was 65% and 35% in the arms of intensive and conventional insulin therapy respectively (Keen 1994; The Diabetes Control and Complications Trial Research Group 1997). In the UK Diabetes Prospective Study the episodes of major hypoglycemia occurred in 0.7%, 1.4% and 1.8% in the groups receiving conventional, glibenclamide and insulin treatment respectively (Gore, McGuire 2009). Some epidemiological studies and minor prospective studies found that hypoglycemia increased cardiovascular risk (Desouza, Bolli et al. 2010). Its occurrence and a severe, even fatal outcome are not rare in patients with type 2 diabetes, primarily during the administration of insulin therapy and use of medicines which stimulate insulin secretion (sulfonylurea). Far from enough importance seems to have been attributed to hypoglycemia in the practice, although it increases the risk of accidents in certain situations, it impairs cognitive function, it may cause hemorrhage at the fundus and in the vitreous body, but it may also play a role in the development of tachycardia, hypertension and arrhythmia (Desouza, Bolli et al. 2010). Therefore it represents a not negligible risk for morbidity and mortality.

Hypoglycemia is a potential side effect of OAD, primarily sulfonylurea, therapy. As compared to metformin, sulfonylurea therapy represents an approximately threefold risk. In contrast, there has been a very low occurrence of hypoglycemia, nearly identical with that of placebo, during DPP-4 inhibitor monotherapy or its combination with metformin of thiazolidinedione (Blonde 2009). No differences were found in the risk of developing hypoglycemia between each DPP-4 inhibitor treatments (Tahrani, Piya et al. 2010) (Table 2).

DPP - 4 inhibitors	Study	Any hypoglycemia (number) investigational drug / comparator
Sitagliptin	Scott, R., Loeys, T. et al. (2008)	1/1
	Scott, R., Wu, M. et al. (2007)	12/21
	Goldstein, B. J., Feinglos, M. N. et al. (2007)	1/1
	Charbonnel, B., Karasik, A. et al. (2006)	6/5
Saxagliptin	Rosenstock, J., Sankoh, S. et al. (2008)	0/0
Vildagliptin	Schweizer, A., Couturier, A. et al. (2007)	2/1
	Bolli, G., Dotta, F. et al. (2008)	1/0
	Bosi, E., Camisasca, R. P. et al. (2007)	1/1
	Rosenstock, J., Baron, M. A. et al. (2007)	1/0

Table 2. Occurrence of hypoglycemia during DPP-4 therapy.

While the DPP-4 inhibitors and the GLP-1 increase insulin production in a glucose-dependent way, in contrast with them the sulfonylureas exert their effect via the ATP-dependent potassium channel, even at low levels of blood glucose, and therefore they make patients susceptible to hypoglycemia. Thus the incidence of hypoglycemia increases when DPP-4 inhibitors are combined with sulfonylurea. This has also been demonstrated in a metaanalysis of studies with a great number of subjects (n=10246), where sitagliptin monotherapy or its combination (with metformin, pioglitazone, sulfonylurea, sulfonylurea + metformin or metformin + rosiglitazone) was compared with placebo or other OAD (metformin, pioglitazone, sulfonylurea, sulfonylurea + metformin or metformin + rosiglitazone) treatment in patients with type 2 diabetes (Williams-Herman, Engel et al. 2010). A lower incidence of hypoglycemia (5.2%) was found in the group of sitagliptin therapy as compared to the control group (12.1%) that could be attributed primarily to sulfonylurea therapy.

3.3 Body weight

There is no increase of body weight during treatment with DPP-4 inhibitors, and even a reduction of it is possible during a combined therapy with metformin (Monami, Iacomelli et al. 2010).

The safety and tolerability of sitagliptin was investigated in patients with type 2 diabetes, who were on a stable dose of metformin for at least 8 weeks and were randomised in double-blind manner to receive either sitagliptin 100mg q.d. (n= 588) or glipizide 5mg/day (up-titrated, to a maximum dose of 20mg/day, based upon prespecified glycemic criteria) (n= 584) (Seck, Nauck et al. 2010). The analysis showed that the addition of sitagliptin to ongoing metformin monotherapy was associated with weight loss (-1.6 kg) compared with weight gain (+ 0.7 kg) with glipizide. In addition patients treated with sitagliptin compared with those treated with glipizide had a lower incidence of hypoglycemia (5% vs 34%).

The body weight neutral effect of DPP-4 inhibitors may prevail through several mechanisms which include the following (Foley and Jordan 2010):

- After a meal that is rich in fat, DPP-4 inhibitor treatment reduces the level of chylomicron apoB-48 and so it hinders intestinal triglyceride absorption.
- Postprandial catecholamine (norepinephrine) levels increase upon the administration of DPP-4 inhibitors, resulting in an increased lipolysis in the adipose tissue and fatty acid oxidation in the musculature.

3.4 Cardiovascular effects

Although it summarized the results of studies with non-cardiovascular endpoints, a metaanalysis investigating the safety of sitagliptin (100mg/day) showed no substantial differences as compared to the control group in relation to coronary artery disease (0.2 vs. 0.4 event per 100 patient-years), myocardial ischemia (0.0 vs. 0.2 event per 100 patient-years) and acute myocardial infarction (0.1 vs. 0.2 event per 100 patient-years) respectively (Williams-Herman, Engel et al. 2010).

A post hoc metaanalysis of saxagliptin's effect on major cardiovascular events (CV death, non-fatal MI, non-fatal stroke) showed no increase of CV risk in the treated patients (Wolf, Friedrich et al. 2009).

Recently, a large outcome trial with sitagliptin (A randomized placebo controlled clinical Trial to Evaluate Cardiovascular Outcomes after treatment with Sitagliptin in patients with type 2 diabetes mellitus and inadequate glycaemic control on mono or dual combination oral antihyperglycaemic therapy, TECOS) and with saxagliptin (Saxagliptin Assessment of Vascular Outcomes Recorded in patients with diabetes mellitus, SAVOR-TIMI 53) has been started.

GLP-1 receptors can be found in cardiac muscle cells and vascular endothelial cells as well (Nauck and Smith 2009; Nikolaidis, Mankad et al. 2004). The beneficial effect of GLP-1 has been demonstrated also in coronary ischemia and left ventricular failure both in animal experiments and in human studies (Nikolaidis, Mankad et al. 2004; Bose, Mocanu et al. 2005; Nikolaidis, Elahi et al. 2004). In rats, myocardial necrosis developed in a smaller area when they received GLP-1 infusion (Bose, Mocanu et al. 2005). Following intravenous infusion of GLP-1, less wall motion disorder and better left ventricular function developed in patients with and without type 2 diabetes who had undergone angioplasty after acute myocardial infarction (Nikolaidis, Mankad et al. 2004).

Based on these, a beneficial effect of DPP-4 inhibitors on cardiovascular disease may be presumed, however further long-term clinical studies with a high number of patients are required for an exact elucidation.

3.5 Other side effects and potential for drug-drug interactions

Based on the results so far, DPP-4 inhibitors seem to have no group-specific side effects (Nauck and Smith 2009; Hollander and Kushner 2010). An occurrence of slightly increased upper respiratory symptoms was not confirmed by a metaanalysis investigating the safety of sitagliptin therapy on a high number of subjects (29 placebo-controlled and 11 active comparison studies) (Williams-Herman, Round et al. 2008). Also a similar result was obtained in a study investigating the safety of vildagliptin (Ligueros-Saylan, Schweizer et al. 2010).

DPP-4 inhibitors are eliminated mostly through the kidneys, so that the question has emerged whether they can be used in patients with impaired renal function (Table 1). The results so far show that sitagliptin was tolerated well also in patients with mild, moderate and severe renal failure (including those on dialysis) (Bergman, Cote et al. 2007). Currently DPP-4 inhibitors are approved in patients with mild renal impairment (creatinine clearance [C_{Cr}] ≥ 50 mL/min) both in Europe and in the USA. However, in patients with moderately (C_{Cr} ≥30 to < 50 mL/min) and severely (C_{Cr} < 30 mL/min) impaired renal function / end stage renal disease (ESRD) in Europe it is not approved, while in the USA sitagliptin and saxagliptin can be given in a reduced dose (Deacon 2011).

In patients with mild and moderate liver disease, of the DPP-4 inhibitors solely sitagliptin has been approved with no restrictions. Monitoring of transaminase levels is required before and during saxagliptin therapy (Deacon 2011). If transaminase levels exceed three times the upper limit of normal, the therapy should be discontinued. At present, vildagliptin should not be given to patients with mild to moderate hepatic impairment. Neither DPP-4 inhibitor is approved in patients with severely impaired hepatic function.

Results show that DPP-4 inhibitors cause no more interactions with other OADs (metformin, pioglitazone, glyburide) or simvastatin. Only saxagliptin is metabolized via the CYP3A4/5 system; therefore a reduction of saxagliptin dose (2.5mg qd) is recommended when it is administered concomitantly with a strong CYP3A4/5 inhibitor (e.g. ketoconazole) (Table 1).

3.6 ß-cell funcion

Typically, islet function has already declined by approximately 50% by the time patients are diagnosed with type 2 diabetes mellitus (Wajchenberg 2007). Reduced pancreatic beta cell mass, largely because of accelerated apoptosis, seems to account for, at least in part, the impaired islet cell function (Butler, Janson et al. 2003). In vitro, neither sulfonylureas, nor metformin protect beta cell from apoptosis (Maedler, Carr et al. 2005; Kefas, Cai et al. 2004) .

Studies in diabetic animals showed beneficial effects of GLP-1 on pancreatic beta cells (Farilla, Hui et al. 2002; Mu, Petrov et al. 2009; Gallwitz and Häring 2010) (Figure 3). GLP-1 stimulates beta cell proliferation and differentiation while it hinders beta cell apoptosis both in vitro and in animal studies. DPP-4 inhibitors increased the number of insulin-positive beta-cells in islets and the beta to alpha cell ratio in different diabetic animals was normalized.

The effects of sitagliptin vs. sulfonylurea therapy were compared in mice with type 2 diabetes (Mu, Petrov et al. 2009). Sitagliptin treatment was found to have repaired the amount of beta and alpha cells and also alpha/beta cell rate to a significantly greater degree as compared to glipizide therapy. The effect of sitagliptin therapy (50mg/day) on beta cell function in patients with type 2 diabetes (n=28) taking metformin was analyzed in a double-blind randomized placebo-controlled study (Brazg, Xu et al. 2007). Beta cell function was determined with the 'C-peptide minimal model' by measuring blood glucose and C-peptide levels for 5 hours after a standardized breakfast. Sitagliptin therapy was found to have significantly improved beta cell function in comparison to the placebo group. In addition sitagliptin and vildagliptin significantly improved HOMA-B value and it also reduced the proinsulin/insulin rate.

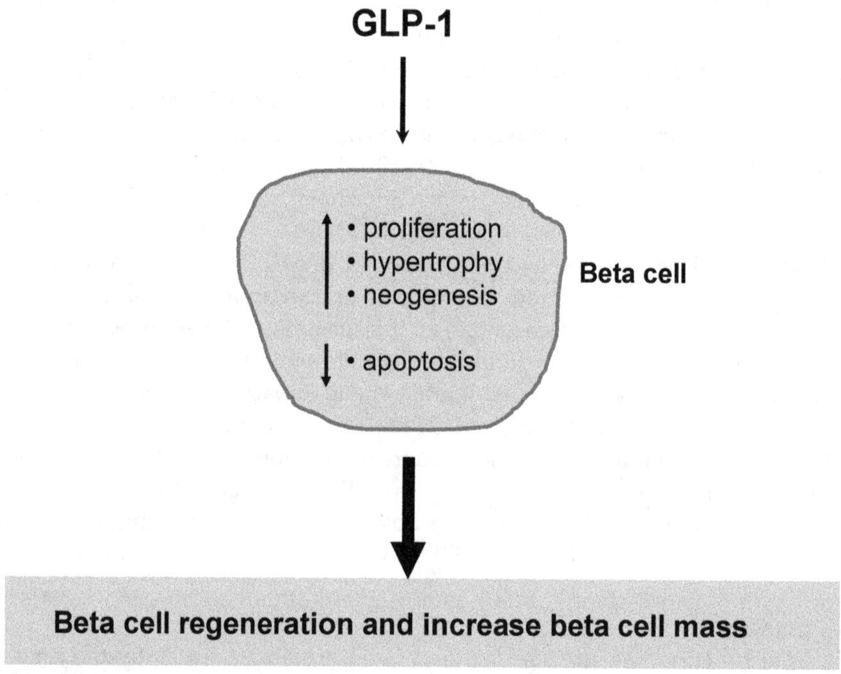

Fig. 3. Effects of GLP-1 on beta cell.

Thus, DPP-4 therapy can delay or prevent the progression of type 2 diabetes, but further studies are required in order to obtain a more exact knowledge relating to its effect on beta cells, as well as its mechanism of action.

4. Conclusion

Large intervention studies demonstrated that antihyperglycemic therapy with treatment goals aiming at normoglycemia can reduce the risk or the progression of microvascular as well as macrovascular risk.

Sulfonylureas, glinides and insulin therapy are associated with an increased risk for hypoglycemia and are also associated with weight gain. The novel incretin based therapies with DPP-4 inhibitors, both in monotherapy and in combination therapy, can effectively reduce fasting and postprandial blood glucose levels and also HbA1c value. When administered concomitantly with metformin, their GLP-1-increasing effects are additive.

Based on studies and clinical experience so far, they can be tolerated very well, and they cause no increase of body weight, hypoglycemia and gastrointestinal side effects and the potential, based on animal and in vitro studies, for preservation or enhancement of beta cell function. Their administration is particularly beneficial in overweight patients who represent the majority of patients with type 2 diabetes, as well as in elderly patients and in diabetics who are susceptible to hypoglycemia. At present, there seems to be little to distinguish between the different inhibitors in terms of their efficacy as antidiabetic agents and their safety. Long-term accumulated clinical experience will reveal whether compound-related characteristics lead to any clinically relevant differences.
In the future further gliptins (alogliptin, linagliptin, denagliptin) may be marketed, with which Phase III studies are in progress or the results have already been published.

5. References

DeFronzo, R.A. (2009) From the triumvirate to the ominosus octet: a new paradigm for the treatment of type 2 diabetes mellitus. Diabetes 58 (4): 773-795.

Drucker, D.J., Sherman, S.I. et al. (2010) Incretin-based therapies for the treatment of type 2 diabetes: evaluation of the risks and benefits. Diabetes Care 33 (2): 428-33.

Thornberry, N.A., Gallwitz, B. (2009) Mechanism of action of inhibitors of dipeptidyl-peptidase-4 (DPP-4). Best Practice & Research Clinical Endocrinology & Metabolism 23 (4): 479-86.

Nauck, M.A., Vilsboll, T. et al. (2009) Incretin-based therapies. Diabetes Care 32 (11): S223-31.

Cho, Y. M., Kieffer, T. J. (2011) New aspects of an old drug: metformin as a glucagon-like peptide 1 (GLP-1) enhancer and sensitiser. Diabetologia 54 (2): 219-22.

Nathan, D. M., Buse, J. B. et al. (2009) Medical management of hyperglycemia in type 2 diabetes: A consensus algorithm for the initiation and adjustment of therapy. Diabetes Care 32 (1): 193-203

Gerich, J. (2010) DPP-4 inhibitors: What may be the clinical differentiators? Diabetes Research and Clinical Practice 90 (2):131-140.

Ahrén, B. (2011) Are sulfonylureas less desirable than DPP-4 inhibitors as add-on to metformin in the treatment of type 2 diabetes? Curr Diab Rep 11(2): 83-90.

Schwartz, S. L. (2010) Treatment of elderly patients with type 2 diabetes mellitus: A systematic review of the benefits and risks of diapeptidyl peptidase-4 inhibitors. Tha American Journal of Geriatric Pharmacotherapy. 8 (5): 405-418.

Keen, H. (1994) The Diabetes Control and Complications Trial (DCCT). Health Trends 26: 41-43.

The Diabetes Control and Complications Trial Research Group. (1997) Hypoglycemia in the Diabetes Control and Complications Trial. Diabetes 46: 271-186.

Gore, M. O., McGuire, D. K. (2009) The 10-year post-trial follow-up of the United Kingdom Prospective Diabetss Study (UKPDS): cardiovascular observations in context. Diab Vasc Dis Res 6: 53-55.

Desouza, C. V., Bolli, G. B. et al. (2010) Hypoglycemia, diabetes, and cardiovascular events. Diabetes Care 33(6): 1389-1394.

Blonde, L. (2009) Current antihyperglycemic treatment strategies for patients with type 2 diabetes mellitus. Cleveland Clinic Journal of Medicine 76, S4-11.

Tahrani, A. A., Piya, M. K. et al. (2010) Glycaemic control in type 2 diabetes: targets and new therapies. Pharmacology and therapeutics 125(2): 328-361.

Scott, R., Loeys T. et al. (2008) Efficacy and safety of sitagliptin when added to ongoing metformin therapy in patients with type 2 diabetes. Diabetes Obes Metab 10: 959-69.

Scott, R. Wu, M. et al. (2007) Efficacy and tolerability of the dipeptidyl peptidaese-4 inhibitor sitagliptin as monotherapy over 12 weeks in patients with type 2 diabetes. Int J Clin Pract 61: 171-80.

Goldstein, B. J., Feinglos, M. N. et al. (2007) Effect of initial combination therapy with sitagliptin, a dipeptidyl peptidase-4 inhibitor, and metformin on glycemic control in patients with type 2 diabetes. Diabetes Care 30: 1979-87.

Charbonnel, B., Karasik, A. et al. (2006) Efficacy and safety of the dipeptidyl peptidase-4 inhibitor sitagliptin added to ongoing metformin therapy in patients with type 2 diabetes inadequately controlled with metformin alone. Diabetes Care 29: 2638-43.

Rosenstock, J., Sankoh, S. et al. (2008) Glucose-lowering activity of dipeptidyl peptidase-4 inhibitor saxagliptin in drug- naive patients with type 2 diabetes. Diabetes Obes Metab 10: 376-86.

Schweizer, A., Couturier, A. et al. (2007) Comparison between vildagliptin and metformin to sustain reductions in HbA(1c) over 1 year in drug-naive patients with type 2 diabetes. Diabet Med 24: 955-61.

Bolli, G., Dotta, F. et al. (2008) Efficacy and tolerability of vildagliptin vs pioglitazone when added to metformin: a 24-week, randomized, double blind study. Diabetes Obes Metab 10: 82-90.

Bosi, E., Camisasca, R. P. et al. (2007) Effects of vildagliptin on glucose control over 24 weeks in patients with type 2 diabetes inadequately controlled with metformin. Diabetes Care 30: 890-5.

Rosenstock, J., Baron, M. A. et al. (2007) Comparison of vildagliptin and rosiglitazone monoterapy in patients with type 2 diabetes: a 24 week, double blind, randomized trial. Diabetes Care 30: 217-23.

Williams-Herman, D., Engel, S. S. et al. (2010) Safety and tolerability of sitagliptin in clinical studies: a pooled analysis of data from 10,246 patients with type 2 diabetes. BMC Endocrine Disorders 10 (7): 1-21.

Monami, M., Iacomelli, I. et al. (2010) Dipeptydil peptidase-4 inhibitors in type 2 diabetes: a meta-analysis of randomized clinical trials. Nutrition, Metabolism and Cardiovascular Diseases 20: 224-235.

Seck, T, Nauck, M et al. (2010) Safety and efficacy of treatment with sitagliptin or glipizide in patients with type 2 diabetes inadequately controlled on metformin: a 2-year study. Int J Clin Pract 64 (5): 562-576.

Foley, J. E., Jordan, J. (2010) Weight neutrality with the DPP-4 inhibitor, vildagliptin: mechanistic basis and clinical experience. Vascular Health and Risk Management 6: 541-548.

Wolf, R., Frederich, R. et al. (2009) Evaluation of CV risk in saxagliptin clinical trials. Diabetes, 58 (Suppl 1): 8-LB.

Nauck, M., Smith, U. (2009) Incretin-based therapy: How do incretin mimetics and DPP- 4 inhibitors fit into treatment algorithms for type 2 diabetic patients? Best Practice & Research Clinical Endocrinology & Metabolism 23: 513-23.

Nikolaidis, L. A., Mankad, S. et al. (2004) Effects of glucagon-like peptid-1 in patients with acute myocardial infarction and left ventricular dysfunction after successful reperfusion, Circulation 109: 962-5.

Bose, A. K., Mocanu, M. M. et al. (2005) Glucagon-like peptid 1 can directly protect the heart against ischemia/reperfusion injury. Diabetes 54: 146-51.

Nikolaidis, L.A., Elahi, D. et al. (2004) Recombinant glucagon-like peptide-1 increases myocardial glucose uptake and improves left ventricular performance in conscious dogs with pacing-induced dilated cardiomyopathy. Circulation 110: 955-61.

Hollander, P. A., Kushner, P. (2010) Type 2 diabetes comorbidities and treatment challenges: rationale for DPP-4 inhibitors. (2010) Posgraduate Medicine 122 (3):71-80

Williams-Herman, D., Round, E. et al. (2008) Safety and tolerability of sitagliptin in patients with type 2 diabetes: a pooled analysis. BMC Endocrine Disorders 8, 14-29.

Ligueros-Saylan, M., Foley, J. E. et al. (2010) An assessment of adverse effects of vildagliptin versus comparators on the liver, the pancreas, the immune system, the skin and in patients with impaired renal function from a large pooled database of phase II and III clinical trials. Diabetes, Obesity and Metabolism 12 (6): 495-509.

Bergman, A. J., Cote, J. et al. (2007) Effect of renal insufficiency on the pharmacokinetics of sitagliptin, a dipeptidyl peptidase-4 inhibitor. Diabetes Care 30: 1862-1864.

Deacon, C. F. (2011) Dipeptidyl peptidase-4 inhibitors in the treatment of type 2 diabetes: a comparative review. Diabetes, Obesity and Metabolism 13: 7-18.

Wajchenberg, B. L. (2007) Beta-cell failure in diabetes and presentation by clinical treatment. Endocr Rev 28: 187-2018.

Butler A. E., Janson, J et al. (2003) Beta-cell deficit and increased beta-cell apoptosis in humans with type 2 diabetes. Diabetes 52: 102-10.

Maedler, K., Carr, R. D. et al. (2005) Sulfonylurea induced beta-cell apoptosis in cultured human islets. J Clin Endocrinol Metab 90: 501-6.

Kefas, B. A., Cai, Y. et al. (2004) Metformin-induced stimulation of AMP-activated protein kinase in beta-cells impairs their glucose responsiveness and can lead to apoptosis. Biochem Pharmacol 68: 409-16.

Farilla, L., Hui, H. et al. (2002) Glucagon-like peptide-1 promotes islet cell growth and inhibits apoptosis in Zucker diabetic rats. Endocrinology 143: 4397-4408.

Mu, J., Petrov, A. et al. (2009) Inhibition of DPP-4 with sitagliptin improves glycemic control and restores islet cell mass and function in a rodent model of type 2 diabetes. European Journal of Pharmacology 623: 148-154.

Gallwitz, B., Häring H. U. (2010) Future perspectives for insulinotropic agents in the treatment of type 2 diabetes-DPP-4 inhibitors and sulphonylureas. Diabetes, Obesity and Metabolism 12: 1-11.

Brazg, R., Xu, L. et al. (2007) Effect of adding sitagliptin, a dipeptidyl peptidase-4 inhibitor, to metformin on 24-h glycemic control and ß-cell function in patients with type 2 diabetes. Diabetes, Obesity and Metabolism 9: 186-193.

3

Pathogenetic Mechanisms of Exercise-Associated Hypoglycemia: Permanent and Reversible Counterregulatory Failure

Pietro Galassetti
University of California, Irvine
United States of America

1. Introduction

These are times when health awareness has become part of everyday life to an extent that may have never been true before. We see health related articles and advertisement numerous times every day on newspapers, TV programs, and of course the internet and all related forms of novel electronic media. We are told repeatedly what is best for us, what we should or should not do, why we have been wrong in the past and how we can improve in the future. Unfortunately, these messages often comes to us in a very confusing and inconsistent manner, making it very hard to filter out what is backed by sound, proven scientific principles, and what is just the "in" new trend that may fade away in a few weeks or months. Among the many messages that are more systematically thrown at us, however, is that we should definitely try to incorporate at least some form of exercise in our daily routine. This is nothing new in general, as going back in history, looking at most ancient civilizations, from the Chinese to the Romans or Greeks, they all seemed to value and implement forms of structured physical exercise. And in fact in our society, if one were to ask anybody, even people who are not health professionals, whether they think that exercise is "good" for you, in the overwhelming majority of cases they would respond that yes, of course it is. And if you were to be more specific, and ask if exercise were "good" for people with diabetes, they would also most likely answer "yes, of course it is going to be good for them". And common sense indicate that would be right. Now, if you were to ask why exercise is "good", both for the general population and for patients with diabetes, you would probably get a variety of responses, (mostly "I am not sure"), with some mixture of truth, speculation and traditional lore. In reality, even among exercise and metabolism professionals, as well as health care professionals, a complete answer to this question is still far from clear. We certainly do know that a number of positive things happen if people exercise regularly, and we have in past decades rather quantified what these beneficial effects are, but we still not know in detail why they occur.

Nevertheless, abundant empirical evidence indicates that, while we may not be sure about the underlying mechanisms, a lot of positive health effects are associated with regular exercise, and are especially important for patients with T1DM (Berenson *et al.* 1998; Hannon *et al.* 2005; Laaksonen *et al.* 2000; Lakka *et al.* 1994; Larson *et al.* 2006). In these patients, in fact, exercise is advocated as a necessary preventive measure against their increased risk of vascular-related diseases, protecting against both micro- and macro-vascular complications such as diabetic retinopathy, nephropathy, neuropathy, and cardio- and cerebro-vascular diseases (Anonymous 1993b; Anonymous 2002; Diabetes Control and Complications Trial/Epidemiology of Diabetes Interventions and Complications (DCCT/EDIC) Study Research Group. 2005; Hambrecht *et al.* 2000; The Diabetes Control and Complications Trial/Epidemiology of Diabetes Interventions and Complications Research Group 2000; White *et al.* 2001). Exercise also improves insulin sensitivity (Pedersen *et al.* 1980), helps to control body weight, and exerts positive intracellular molecular effects such as activation of the peroxisome proliferator-activated receptors (PPARs) target genes, coding for anti-inflammatory cytokines and other novel protective candidate targets, and enhancing cellular metabolism and insulin sensing pathways (Nieman *et al.* 2005b; Smith & Muscat 2005; Teran-Garcia *et al.* 2005). In children, there is also the added issue of regulation of physiological growth and development. It is therefore in fact now very well established that during their schools years, children must perform multiple bouts of moderate to vigorous exercise every day, in order to achieve proper development of their musculoskeletal and cardiovascular systems, as well as an appropriate psychomotor and behavioral equilibrium. Different authors have suggested different amounts of minimum necessary duration of daily physical activity, but in general the recommendation of at least 60 minutes of exercise per day is considered appropriate, and supported by a recent revision of several hundred scientific articles published on the topic (Strong *et al.* 2005).

As we stated above, despite this broad consensus on the vague concept that "exercise is good", many of the detailed biochemical mechanisms by which exercise actually induces its health effects remain incompletely elucidated. This is due in part to the simple fact that the number of interwoven mechanisms that are trigger by exercise is enormous, and probably included several additional still un-identified components. Among the most typical responses to exercise are those aimed at maintaining constant circulating level of glucose, and at making sure that sufficient amounts of energy substrates, such as glucose and lipids, are made available to the exercising muscle, whose metabolic need may have increased by several fold. These responses are collectively defined as counterregulatory responses, and include secretion of hormones such as catecholamines, cortisol, glucagon, growth hormone (GH), with stimulation of both hepatic glycogenolysis and gluconeogenesis, as well as lipolysis. In addition to its glucoregulatory effects, GH is also part of the GH→ insulin-like growth factor I (GH→IGF-I) axis (Nemet *et al.* 2002), which modulates growth and development, and ins therefore especially relevant for subjects of pediatric age. Another series of adaptive response to exercise includes the production of reactive oxygen species, (ROS), the causing agents of oxidative stress, that can be acutely increased by strenuous exercise, as well as mitigated by appropriate antioxidant mechanisms (Nikolaidis *et al.* 2007; Urso & Clarkson 2003). Also, exercise can exert a strong effect on immunologic and inflammatory status, by inducing substantial changes in circulating concentrations of leukocytes (WBC), as well as their level of secretion of cytokines, chemokines, colony-stimulating factors, adhesion molecules and other inflammatory markers (Cryer 1993; Galassetti *et al.* 2006a). Inflammatory and oxidative stress pathways, as well as other critical homeostatic pathways, are also stimulated by exercise at the level of gene expression; in fact hundreds of genes in all subtypes of WBCs (Nemet *et al.* 2004), skeletal muscle (Nieman *et al.* 2005a) and other tissues undergo either up-or down-regulation, as well as post-translational epigenetic regulation especially during physical exertions of considerable intensity (Cooper *et al.* 2004). This chapter is focused on hypoglycemia and exercise, and therefore, among the many adaptive response listed above, counterregulatory functions are the most relevant. However, this broader context of multiple, simultaneous and coordinated adaptive response to exercise had been presented to make the point that hypoglycemic counterregulation does not occur as an isolated set of events, but together with the stimulation or suppression of numerous other systems with which it interacts and by which it can be regulated. Along this line of thought, it is important to remember that in diabetes management, one must constantly evaluate the reciprocal balance of all components of glycemic responses; as specifically related to exercise, it is necessary to determine if all physiological exercise response are preserved, and if alterations are present, whether these are permanent or reversible, and what factors may have affected them (Cooper *et al.* 2007). It is in fact now amply established that many components the comprehensive exercise response to exercise may indeed become altered. Several glucoregulatory responses to exercise can become attenuated permanently (for instance when diabetic autonomic neuropathy develops, typically after years of poor glycemic control), or acutely and reversibly, which may occur even in well controlled patients, in whom diabetic tissue complications have not yet developed.

In this chapter we will therefore review in detail the key known physiologic molecular mechanisms that during exercise maintain glucose homeostasis, and how their potential alterations in T1DM may result in increased incidence of hypoglycemia both during the performance of physical activity, in the first several hours after exercise cessation, and during the following night or even several days.

2. Glucose homeostasis during exercise of varying intensity in type 1 diabtes

The concentration of glucose in plasma is one of the most tightly controlled variables in overall human homeostasis. The range of values within which plasma glucose levels physiologically fluctuate is in fact very narrow, and any changes below or above this range are rapidly corrected by a series of extremely effective adaptive mechanisms. A number of sensors for glucose concentrations are in fact located at critical sites, both within the central nervous system (hypothalamus)(Biggers *et al.* 1989) and in peripheral tissues (walls of the portal vein to detect differences in arterial vs. venous blood, pancreatic islets to directly affect beta- and alpha cells' output of insulin an glucagon, respectively, etc.)(Cherrington 1994; Donovan *et al.* 1994; Hamilton-Wessler *et al.* 1994; Pagliassotti *et al.* 1991). As soon as changes in glucose levels are perceived, corrective actions are immediately undertaken. With increasing glucose concentration insulin is released and counterregulatory hormone secretion is suppressed. I glucose levels are dropping, hormones such as cortisol, glucagon, epinephrine, norepinephrine and growth hormone are released, rapidly activating glycogenolysis an gluconeogenesis in the liver and, to a lesser extent, in other tissues such as the kidney and some areas of the gut. Exercise imposes an additional layer of stress upon these mechanisms, by causing very rapid changes in the skeletal muscle requirement of energy substrates (both carbohydrates and lipids) paralleled by acute increases in insulin sensitivity.

As in T1DM the very hallmark of the disease is an impairment of insulin availability, not surprisingly, in these patients major disruptions of this complex equilibrium are often present. The number of possible events that may occur during exercise in T1DM is actually very broad, but fundamentally most glycemic alterations derive from the combination, in variable proportions, of two main homeostatic situations. First, T1DM patients are often unable to avoid hypoglycemia during exercise performance of in the hours following exercise cessation. This seems to happen more often if the exercise challenge was moderate in intensity but long in duration. Second, at the opposite end of the glycemic spectrum, when patients perfume very intense, albeit brief exercise formats, they can experience acute hyperglycemia, typically beginning during exercise and further increasing afterwards.

A healthy person of average body size, in resting conditions and at least 2-3 hours after the last meal, (i.e. not actively absorbing carbohydrates), "burns" every minute about 2 mg of glucose per Kg of body weight. This is referred to as glucose rate of disposal, or glucose Rd, and is a measure of all the glucose that at any given time is taken up cumulatively by all cells in the body. In these conditions, the movement of glucose into human cells is mediated by baseline systemic insulin concentration ranging between ~ 5 and 10 □U/ml.

If glucose were gradually take up from the bloodstream without replacement, glycemia would progressively decreases over time; this is prevented, however, by endogenous glucose sources, which simultaneously release into the bloodstream an amount of glucose exactly matching the amount that is being taken up. This occurs via breakdown of existing glycogen stores (glycogenolysis) and *de novo* synthesis of glucose molecules (gluconeogenesis). Interestingly, while the body's greatest glycogen stores are contained in the skeletal muscle, muscle glycogen cannot be used to sustain systemic glycemia, as muscle does not express glucose-6-phospahtae, an enzyme necessary to "free" glucose molecules before they are released into the bloodstream. Muscle glycogen can therefore only be used for energy production within the muscle cell. For exercise to be sustained for prolonged periods of time, it must be at a "sub-maximal" level, i.e. at a workload below the anaerobic (or lactate) threshold (normally occurring at 50-60% of individual maximal aerobic capacity). With this type of exercise, glucose Rd typically increases by two- or three- fold, due to the increased metabolic needs of contracting skeletal muscle. This increase in uptake, however, results in only minimal or no decrease in glycemia by the combined effects of two key mechanisms: a) a quick compensatory increase in endogenous glucose production, and b) a parallel decrease in the amount of insulin secreted by the pancreatic beta cells, which is induce by an acute increase in autonomic nervous system efferent stimulation of the pancreas through alpha-adrenergic fibers. This reduction in insulin levels is critical, because during exercise not only insulin sensitivity is markedly enhanced, resulting in increased glucose disposal for the same concentration of insulin, but the is also a simultaneous activation of non-insulin dependent glucose transport across the sarcolemmal membrane, mediated by the increase intracellular calcium release associated with exercise. As a result, if baseline insulin levels do not decrease, the amount of glucose transported into the skeletal muscle cells would actually be excessive, and glycemia in the bloodstream would drop.

It is then evident how this situation can become problematic in T1DM subjects, who can't any longer regulate endogenous insulin release. Preventing the onset of hypoglycemia during exercise then becomes a matter of how accurately patients can reproduce the physiological profile of insulin secretion. If they are using an insulin-infusion pump, they can try and decrease, or even completely stop insulin infusion (many prefer to do so even if this may result in mild hyperglycemia). Conversely, subjects who administer insulin via multiple insulin injections cannot reduce their baseline insulin level, and may find themselves in a state of relative hyperinsulinemia. In fact, sometimes even the opposite may occur, i.e. they may experience an acute increase in insulin release. This may happen if the last insulin injection before exercise was performed close to a muscle mass likely to be mobilized during exercise, such as the side of the thigh; part of the injected fluid, in fact, may occasionally be trapped in a subcutaneous pocket, and be acutely released into the bloodstream when exercise in started, which is practically equivalent to a small additional insulin shot. The added amount of insulin will then not only cause an exaggerated uptake of glucose by the skeletal muscle, but will also suppress endogenous glucose production. These two effects combined markedly enhance the likelihood of the development of an acute hypoglycemic episode.

Conversely, if the type of exercise is very intense, i.e. well above the anaerobic threshold and closer to individual maximal aerobic capacity, a series of drastically different adaptive event are likely to take place. This type of exercise can only be sustained for a much shorter time - rarely more than 20 to 30 min-, and induces a very strong whole-body activation of adrenergic efferents. The main purpose of this response is to generate a sufficiently strong up-regulation of cardiovascular function to match the now extremely increased systemic metabolic needs. The increase in endogenous glucose production resulting from this level of adrenergic activation actually exceeds required by peripheral tissues, resulting in a state transient hyperglycemia of moderate magnitude (typically under 140 mg/dl), which spontaneously subsides shortly after exercise ends, in response to a prompt insulin response (in fact, in the immediate post-exercise state the combination of this insulin secretion with increased insulin sensitivity often induce brief, mild hypoglycemia). In T1DM the initial hypoglycemic response is similar, but at exercise cessation, as the diabetic cannot produce the expected insulin response, the magnitude of hyperglycemia often continues to increase, sometimes up to very elevated levels.

Exercise in real life is almost never exclusively moderate and prolonged, or brief and intense, but most commonly a combination of the two in various proportions. The actual glycemic fluctuations that can be experience in the presence of any given specific exercise format, therefore, could fall anywhere across this broad range. In fact, moderate and intense exercise, performed within the same exercise session, could exert opposite hypo- and hyper-glycemic effects that could, to some effect, cancel each other out. Used in a controlled manner, this principle could conceptually result in optimal glycemic control without additional interventions, and its use has indeed be explored in a series of controlled studies on a group of diabetic Australian youth (Bussau *et al.* 2007a).

3. Altered counterregulatory mechanisms in t1dm

Unfortunately even in T1DM patients who manage to administer themselves an ideal amount of exogenous insulin, and indeed reproduce as closely as possible the physiological profile of endogenous insulin secretion, a variable degree of counterregulatory impairment may still occur, although the underlying mechanisms to date are not understood in full (Tansey *et al.* 2006a). Evidence derived from several studies indicates that the exercise response of major counterregulatory hormones is in general decreased in T1DM when compared to healthy controls (Galassetti *et al.* 2006b; Tansey *et al.* 2006b; Wanke *et al.* 1996).

The issue of counterregulation is very complex, and extends to a number of conditions other than exercise. Of these, the best studied is hypoglycemia itself. The possible blunting of counterregulatory response to exercise, in fact, is very similar to what occurs when counterregulatory responses to hypoglycemia (occurring independent of exercise) become impaired (Bjorgaas *et al.* 1997; Hoffman *et al.* 1991), (the response to hypoglycemia also include associated neurogenic symptoms-hunger, sense of anxiety, sweating, palpitations) caused by the sympathoadrenal effects of epinephrine (Hoffman *et al.* 1991).

This parallelism between altered adaptation to exercise and hypoglycemia is important, as most involved hormones and autonomic pathways are shared by the two conditions. A notable exception, however, is glucagon. Patients with T1DM, in fact, within the first two years after having been diagnosed with the disease, become completely unable to secrete glucagon during a hypoglycemic episode (this was demonstrated by Dr. Gerich and co-authors in a classic study appeared in the journal Science in 1973, (Gerich *et al.* 1973) and confirmed in numerous subsequent studies in both adult and pediatric patients, in which hypoglycemia of varying depth, duration and onset kinetics was induced, always with glucagon concentrations remaining unchanged as compared to baseline values (Ross *et al.* 2005). Interestingly, it appears that pancreatic α-cells in these patients are not unable to secrete glucagon (in fact basal levels are normal), but rather are incapable of increasing glucagon secretion when hypoglycemia is induced artificially via elevated levels of exogenous insulin, which is by far the most common way in which hypoglycemia occurs in T1DM. In animal models of T1DM, however, it was observed that if hypoglycemia was induced by other means, (i.e. via administration of agents such as AICAR and phlorizin, (Banarer *et al.* 2002; McCrimmon *et al.* 2002), the glucagon response was restored. Similarly, and pertinent to the focus of this chapter, the □-cells of patients with T1DM retain the full ability to secrete glucagon in response to other stimuli, including physical exercise (Marliss & Vranic 2002).

Before we further advance in our discussion of altered adaptive mechanisms to exercise, we should now clearly delineate the distinction between those alterations in counterregulatory responses to exercise in diabetes that are permanent (irreversible) and those that are transient (reversible). This is not just and academic distinction, but has a series of obvious practical implications that affect the way a patient may approach exercise. Permanently lost responses, in fact will require alternative ways to substitute lost mechanisms; dealing with reversible alterations, on the other hand, will instead imply focusing on prevention of the causes inducing the temporary impairment.

The two counterregulatory hormones that are commonly defined as the "first line" intervention against hypoglycemia are epinephrine and glucagon; quantitatively, they account for large majority of counterregulatory function during the first hour or so hypoglycemia or exercise have started. In T1DM, with long lasting, poorly controlled diabetes, the characteristic tissue complications of the disease start appearing, including diabetic neuropathy. As part of this condition, the catecholamine response to stress is gradually attenuated until, in the most advanced stages of the disease, may become completely suppressed (Cryer *et al.* 2003) (it should be noted that these complications are not a mandatory part of being diabetic, but can be virtually completely prevented with continuous optimal glycemic control) (Karavanaki & Baum 2003).

If autonomic neuropathy becomes established, however, it is typically irreversible. This means that among other related alterations, the epinephrine response to stress is lost; this essentially leaves the burden of counterregulation at the beginning of a stress event to glucagon alone. If the stress is a hypoglycemic episode, however, as stated above the glucagon response is lost, and very little resistance is offered against the rapid onset of hypoglycemic episode. May of these patients in fact suffer form repeated severe hypoglycemia, often leading to serious accidents if occurring during driving or the operation of heavy machinery, with sometimes catastrophic consequences. If the stress is exercise, on the other hand, the glucagon response is still preserved, producing at least some of the expected counterregulation. This, at least, provided that one of the mechanisms inducing temporary blunting of counterregulatory response is not also present.

Independent of the presence of autonomic dysfunction, in fact, all major counterregulatory responses to stress may undergo a variable degree of reversible attenuation. In general, this occurs according to this general paradigm: a certain stimulus occurs, that is able to blunt the activity of the hypothalamus-pituitary-adrenal axis (that coordinates counterregulation), and for the following hours to days, if counterregulation is needed in response to an episode of stress (hypoglycemia, exercise or other), it can only occur to a reduced degree, or not at all.

Prior Blunting Stimulus → **↓ Responses to Subsequent Stress**

The best studied set of blunting stimulus/subsequent stress if repeated hypoglycemia, in which indeed hypoglycemia acts as both prior stimulus and subsequent stress. Therefore in this case the above paradigm can be re-written as:

Prior Hypoglycemia → **↓ Responses to Subsequent Hypoglycemia**

The scenario is unfortunately very common in T1DM, in which, even after a long period of optimal glycemic control, a hypoglycemic episode may be triggered by excessive insulin administration, insufficient carbohydrate ingestion, acute increase in insulin sensitivity, etc. Once this first episode occurs (during which counterregulatory responses may be normal)

For a number of hours to days the subject will be more susceptible to developing an additional hypoglycemic episode. This condition is now describe as Hypoglycemia-Associated Autonomic Failure (HAAF), and often results in more and more episodes of hypoglycemia, in which each episode acts as the blunting stimulus for the next, de facto starting a vicious cycle out of which it is very difficult for the patients to break. Paradoxically, this happens most commonly in those patients who put the greatest effort into tightly controlling their glycemia. By testing glycemia many times a day, and aggressively adjusting their insulin administration regimen in order to prevent any possible hyperglycemic episode, they in fact often inadvertently expose themselves repeatedly to situations of relative hyperinsulinemia, favoring the onset of hypoglycemia of variable depth and duration. It is unfortunately well documented that in these patients the incidence of hypoglycemic episodes is markedly higher that in patients with worse glycemic control(Amiel *et al.* 1987; Simonson *et al.* 1985). Now, as stated above, both hypoglycemia and exercise elicit similar responses; a logical development of this axiom should therefore be that these two situations could also reciprocally act as blunting stimuli. For instance, if an episode of hypoglycemia preceded an exercise challenge, the above paradigm could be hypothetically become:

Prior Hypoglycemia	→	**↓ Responses to Subsequent Exercise**

As it turns out, this was directly demonstrated in a recent study on sixteen young adults with T1DM (eight males and eight females) (Galassetti *et al.* 2003). These subjects participated in an experimental protocol that included biking on a stationary cycle for one hour and a half. If this exercise challenge was performed after several days of very tight glycemic control, i.e. with no episodes of hypoglycemia occurring, all response to exercise (including the expected increase in glucagon and epinephrine, cortisol, GH, endogenous glucose production and mobilization of free fatty acids), were the same as measured in age-matched, healthy control subjects. If, however, prolonged hypoglycemia was artificially induced on the day before the exercise challenge (four hours of glycemia at ~ 50 mg/dl, divided in two 2-hour blocks, morning and afternoon), the glucagon response to exercise was abolished, the epinephrine response was reduced by 50%, and other counterregulatory hormones, as well as tracer-determined endogenous glucose production and lipolysis, were all significantly reduced by 40-60%. Interestingly, while healthy subjects, unlike T1DM, \don't ever experience hypoglycemia of this depth in normal life, when exposed to the same experimental protocol they displayed an identical pattern of blunted exercise responses (Davis *et al.* 2000b). An important notion to keep in mind is also that this blunting effect is not an all-or-nothing phenomenon, but occurs in a dose-dependent fashion with respect to the depth of the antecedent hypoglycemic episode. This was well exemplified in a separate set of experiments, similar to those described above, in which again a group of patients with T1DM performed a standard 90 min cycling exercise after having been exposed to hypoglycemia for four hours on the previous day. This time, however, each subjects performed the study several times, with several weeks between study visits, and each time was exposed to hypoglycemia of different depth (50 mg/dl, 60 mg/dl, 7- mg/dl or no hypoglycemia). Not surprisingly, the deeper the antecedent hypoglycemia, the more blunted were the responses to subsequent exercise. Considering the glucagon response, for instance, the milder prior hypoglycemia (70 mg/dl) induced a suppression of ~ 35%, prior hypoglycemia of 60 mg/dl a suppression of ~ 60%, and prior hypoglycemia of 50 mg/dL an almost complete suppression of > 95% (Galassetti *et al.* 2001a). A progressively smaller blunting effect on subsequent exercise responses, in addition to a smaller prior stimulus, can be observed as time passes after t he blunting has occurred. In the studies, reported above, prior hypoglycemia occurred ~18-20 before the exercise challenge during which blunted responses were measured. To date no definitive data have been published reporting the exact duration of this blunting effects; however, general consensus exists that within a few days to a week following the antecedent stimulus, provided that no additional blunting stimuli occur, the full ability to mount physiological counterregulatory responses is re-gained. Preventing these recurrent blunting stimuli, however, is no minor challenge in every-day diabetes management. Recurrent, often profound episodes of hypoglycemia are unfortunately very common, and this paradoxically seems to occur even more often in subjects who are very aggressive in their attempts to obtain close to perfect glycemic control (Anonymous 1993a). A final piece of the puzzled is generated by the fact that exercise itself may act as an antecedent blunting stimulus. Going back to our initial paradigm, we can then derive two more combinations:

Prior Exercise → **↓ Responses to Subsequent Hypoglycemia**

Prior Exercise → **↓ Responses to Subsequent Exercise**

Both these possibilities have been documented to actually occur. An exercise bout performed in the morning, for instance, was shown to reduces a wide range of adaptive response to a second bout of exercise performed in the afternoon of the same day (while counterregulatory responses were attenuated, in this study hypoglycemia was not actually allowed to occur, to prevent its confounding effect on data interpretation) (Galassetti *et al.* 2001a). Further, in at least one study prior exercise of different intensity was shown to reduce next-day responses to hypoglycemia, again in a dose dependent manner (Sandoval *et al.* 2004). While a somewhat similar protocol form a different laboratory failed to reproduced the same effect (McGregor *et al.* 2001), possibly due to differences in the intensity of the exercise format used during experiments, an increased incidence of hypoglycemia in the hours following exercise is commonly reported by T1DM patients. This is especially true if exercise was of long duration and/or high intensity, after which insulin sensitivity is markedly increased and redistribution of circulating carbohydrate is shifted toward preferential replenishment muscle glycogen stores, that become depleted during the exercise activity (Borghouts & Keizer 2000).

Further, counterregulatory responses to hypoglycemia, even in standard physiological conditions, become attenuated during sleep (Jones *et al.* 1998); therefore, not surprisingly, a second peak of incidence of hypoglycemia has been described occurs during the nights that follow intense physical activity (Anonymous 2007; Kaufman *et al.* 2002; Tsalikian *et al.* 2005a), with the highest incidence occurring between midnight and 4 am. (McMahon *et al.* 2007).

A separate of issues to be taken into consideration is that male and female patients may responds differently to the same blunting stimulus. Gender differences, often very pronounced, are very common in many aspects of human physiology, and the coordinated adaptive response to stress is no exception(Diamond *et al.* 1993). In particular, the hormonal response to stresses activating the hypothalamo-pituitary-adrenal axis are in general much more pronounced in males than in females. This is true for hypoglycemia as well as exercise which, as we stated in detail above, share many of their adaptive responses. This concept was recently confirmed in group of young healthy adults of both genders, who performed 90 minutes of submaximal cycling exercise. In this group, all hormonal and metabolic responses to the exercise challenge were significantly lower, after normalization for individual exercise intensity, in women as compared to men (Davis *et al.* 2000a). When a blunting stimulus occurs prior to exercise or hypoglycemia, the extent of the blunting on counterregulatory responses is much greater in men (who had a greater response to begin with, and in whom some of the counterregulatory hormones can be suppressed by 80-95%), while in women a much milder, 20-40% blunting occurs (Galassetti *et al.* 2001b). Therefore, in a blunted state responses in males and females become much more similar. In T1DM, the same pattern is preserved, with men displaying greater responses to exercise than women in conditions of standard glycemic control, and again greater blunting of responses after appropriate stimulus in male patients(Galassetti *et al.* 2004).

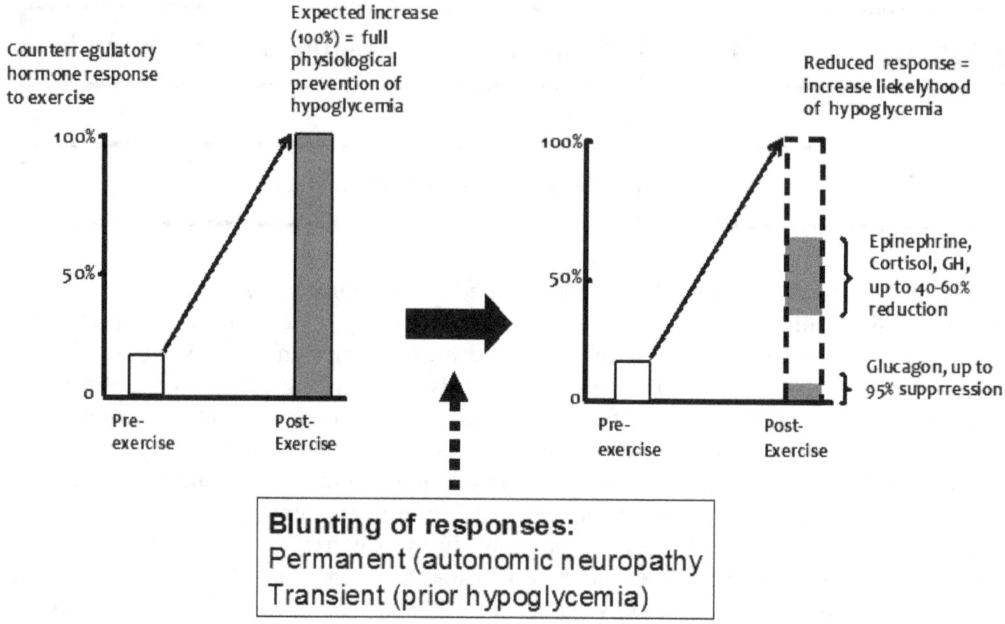

Fig. 1. Schematic representation of counterregulatory events occurring during exercise in healthy subjects and in patients with type 1 diabetes. Counterregulatory responses, including increased secretion of glucagon, epinephrine, norepinephrine, cortisol and growth hormone, display a typical amplitude, exemplified on the left hand-side panel by a 100% response (this general concept can in fact be extrapolated to a number of additional responses not directly related to glucose homeostasis, such as production of the appropriate balance of pro- and anti-inflammatory mediators, or of growth factors; the physiological, full manifestation f the possible, expected health of exercise only occurs when these responses are 100% activated). In the right hand-side panel, conversely, is exemplified the presence of multiple, simultaneous failures of sever involved counterregulatory hormones. Depending of the degree of suppression of these responses, a variable impairment will also occur in endogenous glucose production, which these hormones regulate, and therefore glucose availability will become acutely inadequate to match the increase metabolic needs of the exercising muscle, resulting in the likely onset of a hypoglycemic episode.

Translated in practical terms, this complex interaction between exercise and hypoglycemia means that the more frequent the hypoglycemia, the more likely that subsequent slight hyperinsulinemia (or bouts of exercise) will result in additional hypoglycemia, and so on (Tsalikian *et al.* 2005b). Due to the variety and instability of these several factors, exercise-associated hypoglycemia is often difficult to manage clinically. One of the most basic approaches is trying to optimize circulating insulin. Patients on an insulin pump can reduce the basal infusion rate, in the attempt to reproduce the physiological 40-50% insulin drop occurring in non-diabetic subjects (many T1DM subjects in fact are even more aggressive than that, and completely stop insulin infusion. Absolute recommendation as to the magnitude and duration of insulin reduction/suspension are impossible to generate, as every subjects will react differently, and within the same subject, different strategies will have to be implemented for exercise of different duration and intensity. Further, none of the currently available sets of practical guidelines incorporates the effects of prior stimuli described above. Therefore, often, even in the same subjects exercising in seemingly identical conditions in two different days, in one occasion glycemic control may be perfect, and in the next hypoglycemia may occur. A combination of insulin reduction and ingestion of carbohydrate snacks may be the best overall approach, but again the exact type and amount of ingested carbohydrate, as well as the fractioning and timing of the ingestion, is the objects of considerable controversy, and personal, careful experience seems to still yield the best results. Carbohydrate ingestion is the only tool available for patients utilizing multiple insulin injection, who derive their basal insulin rate from long-acting insulin preparation, and for whom therefore rapid reduction in insulin concentrations during exercise is not possible. Finally, as briefly mentioned above, a new approach has been proposed recently by members of the research group lead by Dr TW Jones, who have attempted to use the intrinsic characteristics of exercise itself to counterbalance its hypoglycemic effects. The principle is simple: to utilize the hyperglycemic effect of brief, intense exercise, to offset the opposite effect of prolonged, moderate exercise. In two studies performed in well controlled T1DM subjects, these authors have introduced a very brief (only 10 seconds) all-out sprint either before or at the end of a prolonged, moderate exercise session. When the sprint was performed before the training session, it decrease the magnitude of glycemic decline only for the first 45 min after exercise; when it was performed at the end, it reduced glycemic decline for several hours after exercise (Bussau *et al.* 2007b; Guelfi *et al.* 2007). The beauty of this approach, if its broader applicability to diabetes management will be confirmed by larger follow-up studies, is that it utilizes only physiological tools, it takes very little time and is easily implemetable any time exercise is performed. More in-depth description of hypoglycemic prevention techniques, in relation to physical exercise, can be found in several excellent recent publications, such as the Clinical Practice Consensus Guidelines of the International Society for Pediatric and Adolescent Diabetes (Robertson K *et al.* 2009).

4. Conclusion

Recent research advances, summarizing the efforts of a large number of laboratories across the globe, demonstrate the high (sometimes incomprehensibly so) complexity of the many interwoven molecular mechanisms that translate exercise into a long-term positive health status. Most likely, our still incomplete understanding of these many mechanisms derives from the fact that they are often activated simultaneously, can partially replace each other in function, and can markedly influence the reciprocal effects. Complex as they may be, some of them have been relatively well elucidated in physiological conditions. Specific alterations in some of these mechanisms, however, appear to be present in subjects with T1DM, potentially reducing the overall benefits of exercise. Among these, alterations in the mechanisms regulating the glycemic homeostasis are especially important, as this alteration may result in exercise-associated hypoglycemia, one of the acute complications of diabetes that patients fear the most. Exercise-associated hypoglycemia may be caused by permanent counterregulatory impairment, as can be seen for instance in the failure to secrete catecholamines when diabetic autonomic neuropathy has become established. More commonly, however, it is observed as the result of acute and reversible blunting of adaptive responses, caused by the occurrence of some prior events, such as prior hypoglycemia, intense exercise or even intense emotional stress. The latter category of events is therefore preventable with the avoidance of these prior stimuli, rendering the control of hypoglycemia, or the identification of the most appropriate exercise formats, a priority in every-day diabetes management. The issue of optimization of exercise regimens is indeed not a simple one, as many different formats (with varying type of activity, duration, intensity and repetition patterns) may not be similarly applicable to all subjects. Finally, it is absolutely necessary to gain a definitive, thorough understanding of all molecular complexities underlying exercise adaptations; in no other way will we be able to conclusively provide the conceptual foundation on which evidence-based exercise guidelines can be systemically developed. As a very final thought, I would like to address here a question that is very often asked after I give a talk on some of the topics discussed above. Considering that the multiple possible alterations in the exercise response that are observed in patients with T1DM, and their implications regarding the overall health effects of exercise in general and on increased incidence of hypoglycemia in particular, I am in fact often asked something along the lines of: "Should then T1DM patients avoid exercise?". I would like to make absolutely clear that the answer is no, they should not avoid exercise. In fact, with all the limitations related to their altered metabolism, they should still try to exercise as much as possible. The possibility that in several situations the potential health effects of exercise may be somewhat reduced, does not take away from the fact that some beneficial effects are still there, and these normally by far outweigh the decision of not exercising. It is up to us, who work in this field, to keep elucidating all possible ways in which the discrepancy between possible and actually achieved beneficial effects of exercise in these patients can be gradually narrowed and hopefully, in the not too distant future, completely eliminated.

5. Acknowledgements

Several of the studies included in this review were performed by the author at the UCI Institute for Clinical and Translational Science, whose nursing, technical, and administrative staff members are thankfully acknowledged for their outstanding research support. This is truly a wonderful research environment that fosters not only the performance of outstanding science, but also the training a new generations of clinical scientists.

The author would also like to acknowledge the outstanding editorial support of Ms Rebecca Flore and Ms Diana Vigil, who have helped to remarkably improve the overall appearance of this manuscript.

Financial support for some of the above experiments was provided through JDRF grant # 11-2003-332, and NIH grants K23 RR-018661, PO1 HD-048721, MO1 RR00827, K24 DK085223, and UL 1RR031985.

6. References

Anonymous (1993b) The effect of intensive treatment of diabetes on the development and progression of long-term complications in insulin-dependent diabetes mellitus. The Diabetes Control and Complications Trial Research Group. *N.Engl.J Med*, 329, 977-986.

Anonymous (2002) Effect of intensive therapy on the microvascular complications of type 1 diabetes mellitus. *JAMA*, 287, 2563-2569.

Anonymous (1993a) The effect of intensive treatment of diabetes on the development and progression of long-term complications in insulin-dependent diabetes mellitus. The Diabetes Control and Complications Trial Research Group. *N.Engl.J Med*, 329, 977-986.

Anonymous (2007) Impaired overnight counterregulatory hormone responses to spontaneous hypoglycemia in children with type 1 diabetes. *Pediatr Diabetes*, 8, 199-205.

Amiel, S. A., Tamborlane, W. V., Simonson, D. C. & Sherwin, R. S. (1987) Defective glucose counterregulation after strict control of insulin-dependent diabetes mellitus. *N.Engl.J.Med.*, 316, 1376-1383.

Banarer, S., McGregor, V. P. & Cryer, P. E. (2002) Intraislet hyperinsulinemia prevents the glucagon response to hypoglycemia despite an intact autonomic response. *Diabetes*, 51, 958-965.

Berenson, G. S., Srinivasan, S. R., Bao, W., Newman, W. P., III, Tracy, R. E. & Wattigney, W. A. (1998) Association between multiple cardiovascular risk factors and atherosclerosis in children and young adults. The Bogalusa Heart Study. *N.Engl.J Med*, 338, 1650-1656.

Biggers, D. W., Myers, S. R., Neal, D. W., Stinson, R., Cooper, N. B., Jaspan, J. B., Williams, P. E., Cherrington, A. D. & Frizzell, R. T. Role of brain in counterregulation of insulin-induced hypoglycemia in dogs. Diabetes 38[1], 7-16. 1989. Ref Type: Journal (Full)

Bjorgaas, M., Vik, T., Sand, T., Birkeland, K., Sager, G., Vea, H. & Jorde, R. (1997) Counterregulatory hormone and symptom responses to hypoglycemia in diabetic children. *Diabet.Med.*, 14, 433-441.

Borghouts, L. B. & Keizer, H. A. (2000) Exercise and insulin sensitivity: a review. *Int.J.Sports Med.*, 20, 1-12.

Bussau, V. A., Ferreira, L. D., Jones, T. W. & Fournier, P. A. (2007a) A 10-s sprint performed prior to moderate-intensity exercise prevents early post-exercise fall in glycaemia in individuals with type 1 diabetes. *Diabetologia*, 50, 1815-1818.

Bussau, V. A., Ferreira, L. D., Jones, T. W. & Fournier, P. A. (2007b) A 10-s sprint performed prior to moderate-intensity exercise prevents early post-exercise fall in glycaemia in individuals with type 1 diabetes. *Diabetologia*, 50, 1815-1818.

Cherrington, A. D. The acute regulation of hepatic glucose production. Pagliassotti, M. J., Davis, S. N., and Cherrington, A. D. [Chapter 2], 19-43. 1994. R.G.Landes Company. The role of the liver in maintaining glucose homeostasis. Ref Type: Serial (Book,Monograph)

Cooper, D. M., Nemet, D. & Galassetti, P. (2004) Exercise, stress, and inflammation in the growing child: from the bench to the playground. *Curr.Opin.Pediatr.*, 16, 286-292.

Cooper, D. M., Radom-Aizik, S., Schwindt, C. & Zaldivar, F., Jr. (2007) Dangerous exercise: lessons learned from dysregulated inflammatory responses to physical activity. *J Appl Physiol*, 103, 700-709.

Cryer, P. E. (1993) Glucose counterregulation: prevention and correction of hypoglycemia in humans. *Am J Physiol*, 264, E149-E155.

Cryer, P. E., Davis, S. N. & Shamoon, H. (2003) Hypoglycemia in diabetes. *Diabetes Care*, 26, 1902-1912.

Davis, S. N., Galassetti, P., Wasserman, D. H. & Tate, D. (2000a) Effect of gender on neuroendocrine and metabolic counterregulatory responses to exercise in normal man. *J.Clin.Endocrinol.Metab.*, 85, 224-230.

Davis, S. N., Galassetti, P., Wasserman, D. H. & Tate, D. (2000b) Effects of antecedent hypoglycemia on subsequent counterregulatory responses to exercise. *Diabetes*, 49, 73-81.

Diabetes Control and Complications Trial/Epidemiology of Diabetes Interventions and Complications (DCCT/EDIC) Study Research Group. (2005) Intensive diabetes treatment and cardiovascular disease in patients with type 1 diabetes. *N.Engl.J Med*, 353, 2643-2653.

Diamond, M. P., Jones, T., Caprio, S., Hallarman, L., Diamond, M. C., Addabbo, M., Tamborlane, W. V. & Sherwin, R. S. (1993) Gender influences conterregulatory hormone responses to hypoglycemia. *Metabolism*, 42, 1568-1572.

Donovan, C. M., Hamilton-Wessler, M., Halter, J. B. & Bergman, R. N. (1994) Primacy of liver glucosensors in the sympathetic response to progressive hypoglycemia. *Proc.Natl.Acad.Sci.USA*, 91, 2863-2867.

Galassetti, P., Mann, S., Tate, D., Neill, R. A., Wasserman, D. H. & Davis, S. N. (2001a) Effect of morning exercise on counterregulatory responses to subsequent, afternoon exercise. *J.Appl.Physiol.*, 91, 91-99.

Galassetti, P., Tate, D., Neill, R. A., Morrey, S., Wasserman, D. H. & Davis, S. N. (2003) Effect of antecedent hypoglycemia on counterregulatory responses to subsequent euglycemic exercise in Type 1 Diabetes. *Diabetes*, 52, 1761-1769.

Galassetti, P., Neill, R. A., Tate, D., Ertl, A. C., Wasserman, D. H. & Davis, S. N. (2001b) Sexual dimorphism in counterregulatory responses to hypoglycemia after antecedent exercise. *J.Clin.Endocrinol.Metab.*, 86, 3516-3524.

Galassetti, P., Tate, D., Neill, R. A., Morrey, S., Wasserman, D. H. & Davis, S. N. (2004) Effect of sex on counterregulatory responses to exercise after antecedent hypoglycemia in type 1 diabetes. *Am.J.Physiol Endocrinol.Metab*, 287, E16-E24.

Galassetti, P. R., Iwanaga, K., Crisostomo, M., Zaldivar, F. P., Larson, J. & Pescatello, A. (2006a) Inflammatory cytokine, growth factor and counterregulatory responses to exercise in children with type 1 diabetes and healthy controls. *Pediatr Diabetes*, 7, 16-24.

Galassetti, P. R., Iwanaga, K., Crisostomo, M., Zaldivar, F. P., Larson, J. & Pescatello, A. (2006b) Inflammatory cytokine, growth factor and counterregulatory responses to exercise in children with type 1 diabetes and healthy controls. *Pediatr Diabetes*, 7, 16-24.

Gerich, J. E., Langlois, M., Noacco, C., Karam, J. & Forsham, P. H. (1973) Lack of a glucagon response to hypoglycemia in diabetes: evidence for an intrinsic pancreatic alpha-cell defect. *Science*, 182, 171-173.

Guelfi, K. J., Ratnam, N., Smythe, G. A., Jones, T. W. & Fournier, P. A. (2007) Effect of intermittent high-intensity compared with continuous moderate exercise on glucose production and utilization in individuals with type 1 diabetes. *Am J Physiol Endocrinol Metab*, 292, E865-E870.

Hambrecht, R., Wolf, A., Gielen, S., Linke, A., Hofer, J., Erbs, S., Schoene, N. & Schuler, G. (2000) Effect of exercise on coronary endothelial function in patients with coronary artery disease. *N Engl J Med*, 342, 454-460.

Hamilton-Wessler, M., Bergman, R. N., Halter, J. B., Watanabe, M. & Donovan, C. M. (1994) The role of liver glucosensors in the integrated sympathetic response induced by deep hypoglycemia in dogs. *Diabetes*, 43, 1052-1060.

Hannon, T. S., Rao, G. & Arslanian, S. A. (2005) Childhood obesity and type 2 diabetes mellitus. *Pediatrics*, 116, 473-480.

Hoffman, R. P., Singer-Granick, C., Drash, A. L. & Becker, D. J. (1991) Plasma catecholamine responses to hypoglycemia in children and adolescents with IDDM. *Diabetes Care*, 14, 81-88.

Jones, T. W., Porter, P., Sherwin, R. S., Davis, E. A., O'Leary, P., Frazer, F., Byrne, G., Stick, S. & Tamborlane, W. V. (1998) Decreased epinephrine response to hypoglycemia during sleep. *N.Engl.J.Med.*, 338, 1657-1662.

Karavanaki, K. & Baum, J. D. (2003) Coexistence of impaired indices of autonomic neuropathy and diabetic nephropathy in a cohort of children with type 1 diabetes mellitus. *J Pediatr Endocrinol Metab*, 16, 79-90.

Kaufman, F. R., Austin, J., Neinstein, A., Jeng, L., Halvorson, M., Devoe, D. J. & Pitukcheewanont, P. (2002) Nocturnal hypoglycemia detected with the Continuous Glucose Monitoring System in pediatric patients with type 1 diabetes. *J Pediatr*, 141, 625-630.

Laaksonen, D. E., Atalay, M., Niskanen, L. K., Mustonen, J., Sen, C. K., Lakka, T. A. & Uusitupa, M. I. (2000) Aerobic exercise and the lipid profile in type 1 diabetic men: a randomized controlled trial. *Med Sci Sports Exerc.*, 32, 1541-1548.

Lakka, T. A., Venalainen, J. M., Rauramaa, R., Salonen, R., Tuomilehto, J. & Salonen, J. T. (1994) Relation of leisure-time physical activity and cardiorespiratory fitness to the risk of acute myocardial infarction. *N.Engl.J Med*, 330, 1549-1554.

Larson, E. B., Wang, L., Bowen, J. D., McCormick, W. C., Teri, L., Crane, P. & Kukull, W. (2006) Exercise is associated with reduced risk for incident dementia among persons 65 years of age and older. *Ann.Intern.Med*, 144, 73-81.

Marliss, E. B. & Vranic, M. (2002) Intense exercise has unique effects on both insulin release and its roles in glucoregulation: implications for diabetes. *Diabetes*, 51 Suppl 1, S271-S283.

McCrimmon, R. J., Evans, M. L., Jacob, R. J., Fan, X., Zhu, Y., Shulman, G. I. & Sherwin, R. S. (2002) AICAR and phlorizin reverse the hypoglycemia-specific defect in glucagon secretion in the diabetic BB rat. *Am J Physiol Endocrinol Metab*, 283, E1076-E1083.

McGregor, V. P., Greiwe, J. S., Banarer, S. & Cryer, P. (2001) Limited impact of vigorous exercise on defenses against hypoglycemia: relavence to hypoglycemia-associated autonomic failure. *Diabetes*, 40, A138.

McMahon, S. K., Ferreira, L. D., Ratnam, N., Davey, R. J., Youngs, L. M., Davis, E. A., Fournier, P. A. & Jones, T. W. (2007) Glucose requirements to maintain euglycemia after moderate-intensity afternoon exercise in adolescents with type 1 diabetes are increased in a biphasic manner. *J Clin Endocrinol Metab*, 92, 963-968.

Nemet, D., Connolly, P. H., Pontello-Pescatello, A. M., Rose-Gottron, C., Larson, J. K., Galassetti, P. & Cooper, D. M. (2004) Negative energy balance plays a major role in the IGF-I response to exercise training. *J.Appl.Physiol*, 96, 276-282.

Nemet, D., Oh, Y., Kim, H.-S., Hill, M. A. & Cooper, D. M. (2002) The effect of intense exercise on inflammatory cytokines and growth mediators in adolescent boys. *Pediatrics*, 110, 681-689.

Nieman, D. C., Davis, J. M., Henson, D. A., Gross, S. J., Dumke, C. L., Utter, A. C., Vinci, D. M., Carson, J. A., Brown, A., McAnulty, S. R., McAnulty, L. S. & Triplett, N. T. (2005a) Muscle cytokine mRNA changes after 2.5 h of cycling: influence of carbohydrate. *Med Sci Sports Exerc*, 37, 1283-1290.

Nieman, D. C., Davis, J. M., Henson, D. A., Gross, S. J., Dumke, C. L., Utter, A. C., Vinci, D. M., Carson, J. A., Brown, A., McAnulty, S. R., McAnulty, L. S. & Triplett, N. T. (2005b) Muscle cytokine mRNA changes after 2.5 h of cycling: influence of carbohydrate. *Med Sci Sports Exerc*, 37, 1283-1290.

Nikolaidis, M. G., Kyparos, A., Hadziioannou, M., Panou, N., Samaras, L., Jamurtas, A. Z. & Kouretas, D. (2007) Acute exercise markedly increases blood oxidative stress in boys and girls. *Appl Physiol Nutr Metab*, 32, 197-205.

Pagliassotti, M. J., Myers, S. R., Moore, M. C., Neal, D. W. & Cherrington, A. D. (1991) Magnitude of negative arterial-portal glucose gradient alters net hepatic glucose balance in conscious dogs. *Diabetes*, 40, 1659-1668.

Pedersen, O., Beck-Nielsen, H. & Heding, L. (1980) Increased insulin receptors after exercise in patients with insulin-dependent diabetes mellitus. *N Engl J Med*, 302, 886-892.

Robertson K, Adolfsson P, Scheiner G, Hanas R & Riddell MC (2009) Exercise in children and adolescents with diabetes. *Pediatr Diabetes*, 10, 154-168.

Ross, L. A., Warren, R. E., Kelnar, C. J. & Frier, B. M. (2005) Pubertal stage and hypoglycaemia counterregulation in type 1 diabetes. *Arch Dis Child,* 90, 190-194.

Sandoval, D. A., Guy, D. L., Richardson, M. A., Ertl, A. C. & Davis, S. N. (2004) Effects of low and moderate antecedent exercise on counterregulatory responses to subsequent hypoglycemia in type 1 diabetes. *Diabetes,* 53, 1798-1806.

Simonson, D. C., Tamborlane, W. V., DeFronzo, R. A. & Sherwin, R. S. (1985) Intensive insulin therapy reduces counterregulatory hormone responses to hypoglycemia in patients with Type I diabetes. *Ann.Intern.Med.,* 103, 184-190.

Smith, A. G. & Muscat, G. E. (2005) Skeletal muscle and nuclear hormone receptors: implications for cardiovascular and metabolic disease. *Int J Biochem.Cell Biol,* 37, 2047-2063.

Strong, W. B., Malina, R. M., Blimkie, C. J., Daniels, S. R., Dishman, R. K., Gutin, B., Hergenroeder, A. C., Must, A., Nixon, P. A., Pivarnik, J. M., Rowland, T., Trost, S. & Trudeau, F. (2005) Evidence based physical activity for school-age youth. *J.Pediatr.,* 146, 732-737.

Tansey, M. J., Tsalikian, E., Beck, R. W., Mauras, N., Buckingham, B. A., Weinzimer, S. A., Janz, K. F., Kollman, C., Xing, D., Ruedy, K. J., Steffes, M. W., Borland, T. M., Singh, R. J. & Tamborlane, W. V. (2006a) The effects of aerobic exercise on glucose and counterregulatory hormone concentrations in children with type 1 diabetes. *Diabetes Care,* 29, 20-25.

Tansey, M. J., Tsalikian, E., Beck, R. W., Mauras, N., Buckingham, B. A., Weinzimer, S. A., Janz, K. F., Kollman, C., Xing, D., Ruedy, K. J., Steffes, M. W., Borland, T. M., Singh, R. J. & Tamborlane, W. V. (2006b) The effects of aerobic exercise on glucose and counterregulatory hormone concentrations in children with type 1 diabetes. *Diabetes Care,* 29, 20-25.

Teran-Garcia, M., Rankinen, T., Koza, R. A., Rao, D. C. & Bouchard, C. (2005) Endurance training-induced changes in insulin sensitivity and gene expression. *Am J Physiol Endocrinol Metab,* 288, E1168-E1178.

The Diabetes Control and Complications Trial/Epidemiology of Diabetes Interventions and Complications Research Group (2000) Retinopathy and nephropathy in patients with type 1 diabetes four years after a trial of intensive therapy. *N.Engl.J Med,* 342, 381-389.

Tsalikian, E., Mauras, N., Beck, R. W., Tamborlane, W. V., Janz, K. F., Chase, H. P., Wysocki, T., Weinzimer, S. A., Buckingham, B. A., Kollman, C., Xing, D. & Ruedy, K. J. (2005a) Impact of exercise on overnight glycemic control in children with type 1 diabetes mellitus. *J Pediatr,* 147, 528-534.

Tsalikian, E., Mauras, N., Beck, R. W., Tamborlane, W. V., Janz, K. F., Chase, H. P., Wysocki, T., Weinzimer, S. A., Buckingham, B. A., Kollman, C., Xing, D. & Ruedy, K. J. (2005b) Impact of exercise on overnight glycemic control in children with type 1 diabetes mellitus. *J Pediatr,* 147, 528-534.

Urso, M. L. & Clarkson, P. M. (2003) Oxidative stress, exercise, and antioxidant supplementation. *Toxicology,* 189, 41-54.

Wanke, T., Auinger, M., Formanek, D., Merkle, M., Lahrmann, H., Ogris, E., Zwick, H. & Irsigler, K. (1996) Defective endogenous opioid response to exercise in type I diabetic patients. *Metabolism,* 45, 137-142.

White, N. H., Cleary, P. A., Dahms, W., Goldstein, D., Malone, J., Tamborlane, W. V. & Diabetes Control and Complications Trial (DCCT)/Epidemiology of Diabetes Interventions and Complications (EDIC) Research Group. (2001) Beneficial effects of intensive therapy of diabetes during adolescence: outcomes after the conclusion of the Diabetes Control and Complications Trial (DCCT). *J.Pediatr.,* 139, 804-812.

4

Relationship Between Age and Diabetic Treatment Type on the Frequency of Hyperglycemic Episodes Monitored by Continuous Glucose Monitoring

Boby G. Thekadeth et al.*
Rosalind Franklin University of Medicine and Science
VA Med Ctr, North Chicago, IL
USA

1. Introduction

Diabetes mellitus is a chronic debilitating disease affecting over 23 million children and adults in the United States. Many of the ill effects of this disease lie in part with uncontrolled glucose levels in the body. Hypoglycemia increases the risk of cardiovascular and cerebrovascular events, progression of dementia, injurious falls, emergency department visits, and hospitalizations (Desouza, 2003; Leese, 2003; Schwartz, 2008; Whitmer, 2009).

Hypoglycemia-associated autonomic failure is another major complication that diabetic individuals go through when their glucose levels are not properly regulated. In this complication, antecedent hypoglycemia causes both defective glucose counter-regulation and hypoglycemia unawareness (by reducing autonomic and neurogenic symptom response) thus making it difficult for patients to properly sense a hypoglycemic event and thus cause further complications in the future (Cranston, 1994; Cryer, 2004; Dagogo-Jack, 1994, Fanelli, 1994).

Hyperglycemia is associated with secondary damage to many organ systems especially the kidneys, eyes, nerves and blood vessels. Hyperglycemia is associated with both macro- and microvascular complications. The macrovascular complications include increased risk of myocardial infarction as well as stroke, cerebrovascular disease, and coronary artery disease (Kannel, 1979; Lehto et al., 1996). On the microvascular level, hyperglycemia is associated with vascular damage, leakage, and edema. Such inflammation can lead to occlusion and ischemia as well as nerve damage (Kannel, 1979).

Since the Diabetes Complications and Control Trial (DCCT) established hemoglobin A1C as the gold standard of glycemic control there has been a lot of research on other factors that might better predict the risk of diabetic complications. One such factor has been glycemic variability. Large changes in glycemic levels lead to production of reactive oxygen species (ROS), which in turn accelerate the micro- and macrovascular complications of diabetes. It is

* P. Zachariah, Zeenat Parveen, Pavan Patel, Matthew Schoeck, Andrew Mazulis, Lawrence Perlmuter and Sant P.Singh
Rosalind Franklin University of Medicine and Science VA Med Ctr, North Chicago, IL USA

also possible that neglecting these variations in glycemic control could lead to misinterpretation of the risk of diabetic complications even if the mean A1C levels fall within the normal accepted range (Hirsch & Brownlee, 2005).
However, for a variety of reasons ranging from biomedical to psychosocial it is difficult to achieve optimal glycemic control (Amir et al., 1990). Continuous glucose monitoring (CGM) provides a useful method to help monitor glucose values and to provide useful feedback to more effectively control glycemic levels (Klonoff, 2005). In a multicenter clinical trial studying two groups, one using CGM and the other using self-glucose monitoring it was found that there was a significant improvement in hemoglobin A1C in patients using CGM as compared to patients using self-monitored finger stick glucose measurements after a 26 week trial (Tamborlane et al., 2008).
To further study some of these observations, in our study we used CGM over a 72 hour period to examine 84 male patients who had been diagnosed with either Type I or II diabetes. Our goal was to characterize the time the patient spent in a hypo-, hyper-, and eu-glycemic state with respect to age and the treatment type the patient received (oral medication vs. insulin).

2. Methods

Eighty-four treated adult male diabetic patients (18 oral treatment, 51 insulin only, and 15 both oral and insulin) were studied. All patients had attended a comprehensive diabetes clinic on a regular basis and had received diabetes education including diet, exercise and self-monitoring of blood glucose (SMBG) instructions.
Assessment of clinical data included age, sex distribution, and duration of diabetes, body mass index, diabetic complication (i.e. Diabetic neuropathy, retinopathy, nephropathy, cardiovascular disease and peripheral vascular disease). Pertinent laboratory data included HbAIC, plasma glucose, creatinine, liver function tests, lipid levels and microalbuminuria. The patient's home medications were also reviewed for potential effect on glucose homeostasis.
A CGMS sensor was inserted and calibrated according to the Minimed Medtronic procedure. Patients were instructed to continue with their regular lifestyle, to keep a food diary and to record event markers into the monitor e.g. insulin administration, exercise, SMBG and hypoglycemic episode. After 72 hours, the monitor was removed and the data were downloaded using Minimed Solutions Software version 2.0b.

2.1 Statistical analyses

Standard procedures were used to calculate the means, SD, SEM, hyperglycemia frequency and correlation coefficients. SMBG glucose values were paired with corresponding CGMS glucose values for linear regression analyses. Blood glucose concentration >140 mg/dL for at least 30 minutes indicated hyperglycemia. Hyperglycemic prevalence was calculated as the percentage of a specified time period spent during hyperglycemia. Changes in blood glucose > 100mg/dL within a 60-min period were defined as rapid glucose excursions.

3. Results

During the 3-day evaluation, 84 men provided a continuous measure of blood glucose levels using a CGM device[4]. The participants mean age was = 66.17 (± 11.36) years, with N=36 subjects younger than 65 and N= 48 subjects 65 and older. Of the 84 patients, 18 were on oral medications alone, 51 were on insulin alone, while 15 were on both. Table 1 provides demographic information including age, BMI, systolic blood pressure and HbA1C. The correlations among BMI, systolic BP, hemoglobin A1C and age are presented in Table 2. The analysis of the glycemic levels were divided into 3 time periods: 6 am - 6 pm (daytime), 6 pm - midnight (evening), and midnight - 6 am (early morning).

Age	$\bar{x}$ = 66.17 ± 11.36
BMI	$\bar{x}$ = 30.3 ± 5.86
Systolic Blood Pressure	$\bar{x}$ = 135.04 ± 18.9
HbA1C	$\bar{x}$ = 7.76 ± 1.62

Table 1. Demographics (N = 84)

	Age	**BMI**	**HbA1c**	**Systolic BP**
Age	1	-0.15	-0.41*	0.32*
BMI	-0.15	1	-0.11	-0.06
HbA1c	-0.41*	-0.11	1	-0.15
Systolic BP	0.32*	-0.06	-0.15	1

*p <.05; **p < .01

Table 2. Zero order correlations

Overall, a greater percentage of time was spent in hyperglycemia during the day (57.86% ± 14.59) than at night (16.11% ± 10.40), $t_{(83)} = 16.50$, $p < 0.01$. The analysis of hypoglycemic and euglycemic states showed no statistically significant difference (multiple regression analysis) between time intervals when comparing the association with age, BMI, treatment, HbA1c, or any other predictive variables. Also no significant findings were seen in the evening hours (6 pm to midnight) when examining the same variables for either age or treatment type for any glycemic state.

The effects of Age Grouping (<65 and ≥65) on the percentage time that subjects were in the hyperglycemic state during the early morning was evaluated with multiple regression analyses using covariates (BMI, systolic blood pressure, and hemoglobin A1C) that were found to be statistically significantly related to hyperglycemic events. The model outlined in Table 3 included BMI entered on the first step, systolic blood pressure entered on the second step and HemoglobinA1c (HbA1C) entered on the third step. The same analysis was done for the daytime interval. Increasing values of HbA1C were associated with a significantly greater percentage of time in the hyperglycemic state, as expected, but only during the early morning hours.

However, BMI and systolic blood pressure were not significant predictors of percentage time in the hyperglycemic state. On the other hand, subjects older than 65 years exhibited a significantly greater percentage of time in the hyperglycemic state for the daytime interval and a lower percentage of time in the hyperglycemic state for the early morning interval. The opposite pattern was found for subjects younger than 65. That is subjects younger than 65 spent a greater percentage of time in hyperglycemia during the early morning interval and a lower percentage of time in hyperglycemia during the daytime interval. The difference between the age groups for the percent time hyperglycemic during the day was significant, p = 0.02 while a borderline difference was evident during the early morning, p = 0.06. These effects are displayed in Figure 1 and Table 3. In addition, Figure 2 displays the percentage of time in the hyperglycemic state as a function of age for the early morning period (A) and for the daytime (B). The distinctive positive and negative effects of increasing age has a beneficial effect (lower percentage time in hyperglycemia) during early morning and a detrimental effect (higher percentage time in hyperglycemia) during the day. Although these effects were not significant, the results are of interest due to the fact that clinical evidence of hyperglycemic patterns can help physicians better control glycemic excursions. The reasoning behind this finding remains unexplained.

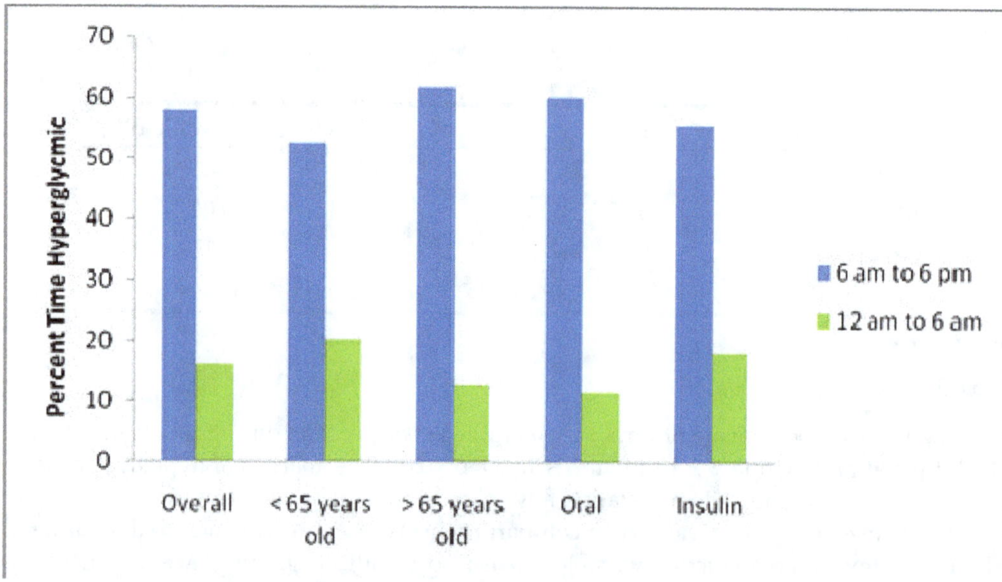

Fig. 1. Percent Time Hyperglycemic based on Age and Type of Medication (Oral, Insulin)

	% Time Hyperglycemic from 12 am to 6 am		% Time Hyperglycemic from 6 am to 6 pm	
Predictors	**Beta**	**R^2**	**Beta**	**R^2**
BMI	0.68	0.01	- 0.09	0.01
Systolic Blood Pressure	-0.15	0.02	0.05	0.00
Hemoglobin A1c	0.31	0.09*	- 0.16	0.03
Age Group	0.24	0.04 ‡	- 0.30	0.07**

Beta = Standardized Beta
*p<.05; **p< .01; ‡p < 0.06

Table 3. Multiple Linear Regressions – Relationship between Age Group and % Time Hyperglycemic

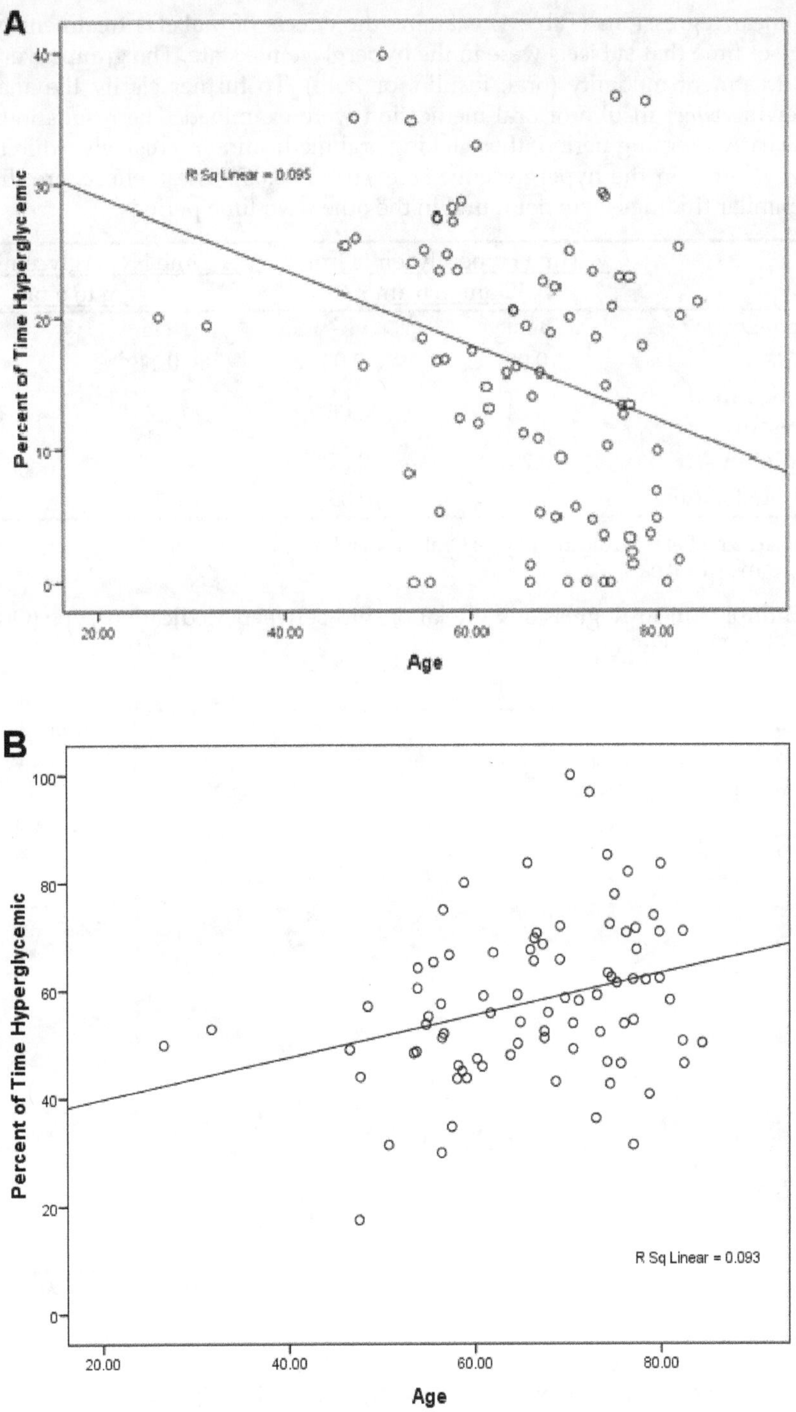

Fig. 2. Percentage of time spent in hyperglycemia as a function of age during the time interval from 12 am to 6 am (A) and from 6 am to 6 pm (B)

Multiple linear regressions (Table 4) examine the effects of diabetes treatment type on the percentage of time that subjects were in the hyperglycemic state. The groups were analyzed based on treatment modality (oral, insulin, or both). To further clarify the analyses only those receiving *either* insulin or oral medication were examined. The results indicated that during the early morning period, those taking oral medication exclusively exhibited a lower percentage of time in the hyperglycemic state (p = < 0.06). These effects are displayed in Figure 3. Similar findings were not found in the other two time periods.

	% Time Hyperglycemic from 12 am to 6 am		% Time Hyperglycemic from 6 am to 6 pm	
Predictors	**Beta**	**R^2**	**Beta**	**R^2**
BMI	-0.02	0.00	- 0.11	0.01
Systolic Blood Pressure	-0.24	0.06*	0.24	0.06*
Hemoglobin A1c	0.28	0.07*	- 0.12	0.01
Type of Medication	0.22	0.05‡	-0.13	0.02

Beta = Standardized Beta; Medication Type: Oral= 1, Insulin = 2
* p< .05; **p< .01; ‡p < 0.06

Table 4. Multiple Linear Regressions – Relationship between Medication Type (Oral, Insulin) and % Time Hyperglycemic

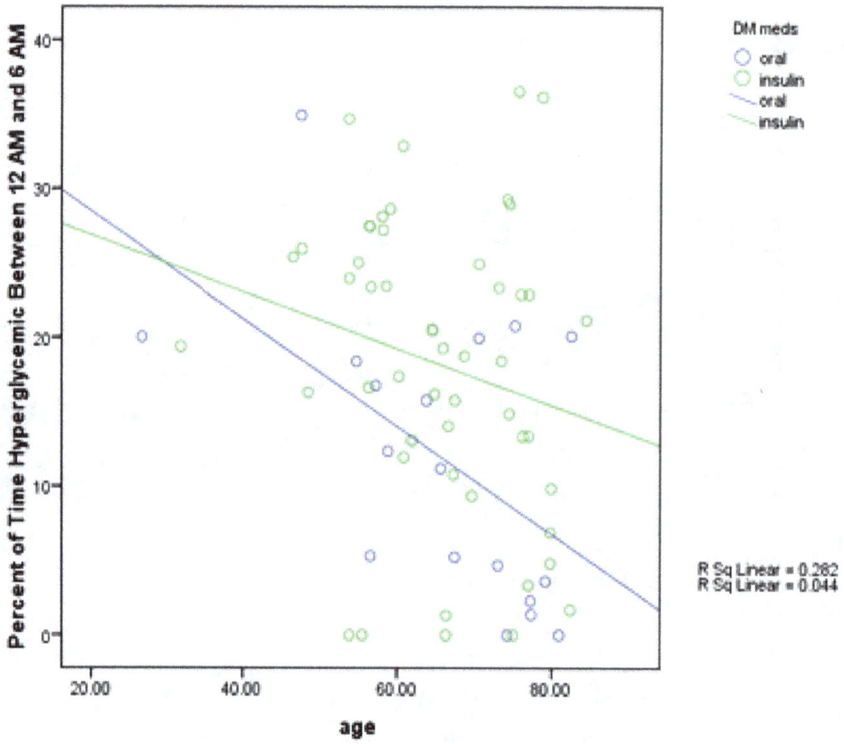

Fig. 3. Percent of time spent in hyperglycemia from 12 am to 6 am as a function of age and type of medication.

Finally to test the hypothesis that age and type of treatment may have interacting effects with respect to percentage time in the hyperglycemic state a third multiple regression was constructed (Table 5). The Interaction was not significant for either the early morning interval or for the daytime interval. Apparently, age and type of treatment have relatively independent influences on the percentage of time in the hyperglycemic state.

	% Time Hyperglycemic from 12 am to 6 am		% Time Hyperglycemic from 6 am to 6 pm	
Predictors	**Beta**	**R^2**	**Beta**	**R^2**
Hemoglobin A1c	0.31	0.09*	- 0.14	0.02
Age Group	0.23	0.04	-0.19	0.03
Medication Type	0.24	0.06*	-0.14	0.02
Age Group X Type	-0.50	0.01	- 0.47	0.01

Beta = Standardized Beta; Medication Type: Oral =1, Insulin =2

*p< .05; **p<.01

Table 5. Multiple Linear Regressions – Relationship Between the Interaction of Age X Medication Type (Oral, Insulin) and % Time Hyperglycemic

4. Conclusion

Results from this study demonstrate that both increasing age and the exclusive use of oral anti-hyperglycemic medications are associated with a lower percent of time spent in hyperglycemia during the early morning. On the other hand, as age increases, the opposite effect is exhibited during the daytime interval, namely a higher percent of time in the hyperglycemic state. In search for an explanation for these findings there is evidence from the animal literature that in older rats, glucose utilization by the brain, using autoradiography, tended to increase more slowly in the morning and decrease faster in the afternoon and evening (Wise et al., 1988). That is, glucose utilization is overall less effective during the day for older rats leading to elevated levels of blood glucose and possibly hyperglycemia during the day. Thus, glucose levels in older human subjects (≥65 years) compared to younger subjects (<65 years) appear to display a similar pattern as those found in the older rats. If the interspecies mechanism is similar, this would give some explanation to the pattern of increased percentage of diurnal hyperglycemia found in the older subjects with diabetes.

There was no interaction between age of patient and type of medication administered. Therefore, our findings showing that older people and people taking only oral medication exhibit less time spent in hyperglycemia during the early morning are two completely independent predictors of hyperglycemic episodes and do not influence each other.

Secondly, elevated HbA1c levels correlated with the percent time spent in a hyperglycemic state primarily during the early morning time interval. A study of Type II diabetics revealed that non-euglycemic states in the morning (pre-breakfast) and at night (bedtime) correlated with increased HbA1c levels. Therefore, patients whose glucose levels were not regulated well in the morning or late night tended to have poorer overall glycemic control as measured by HbA1c. Perhaps the reason why the strongest association with HbA1c was "exerted" during the night (between the bedtime and pre-breakfast measurements) was due to the inability to effectively respond to extreme glucose values while asleep. Thus in the absence of an insulin injection (or comparable treatment) to correct for the elevated blood glucose levels, these patients may have an overall higher HbA1c. This indicates the importance of normalizing glucose levels overnight so as to avoid hyper and hypoglycemic states.

Future studies are needed to help account for the mechanisms behind both the age and percent time spent in hyperglycemia as well as the use of oral medication and percent time spent in hyperglycemia. Cortisol, for example, has been shown to promote the release of large amounts of glucose into the bloodstream as well as to block the absorption of insulin and it was shown that cortisol increases with age (Larsson et al., 2009). Therefore it would be beneficial to look further into this relationship as a means of explaining some of our results. It was also shown that the amount of REM sleep is reduced by about half in late life. This loss of REM sleep has been correlated with elevated cortisol levels throughout the day (Van Cauter et al., 2000). Increased cortisol elevates insulin resistance thereby promoting hyperglycemic episodes that may be reflected in older subjects with presumptive sleep difficulties.

Among the limitations of the present study is the absence of female subjects. Also many of the Type II diabetics recruited for this study were found to be taking insulin with or without oral medication. This led to treatment overlap between the diabetic types making it difficult to justify analysis based on type of diabetes, so instead the treatment modality was compared. This analytic strategy resulted in the elimination of 15 patients due to their treatment plan using both insulin and oral medications.

In summary, this continuous glucose monitoring study presents some novel observations into the relationship between hyperglycemia, advancing age and treatment type. While hypoglycemic episodes may also cause life-threatening situations, prolonged hyperglycemic episodes throughout the night, while asleep, will promote life-threatening sequellae and reduced quality of life. Although the complications of hyperglycemia may not be as instantaneously debilitating or as acute as hypoglycemia, more research is needed to prevent these episodes (Greene et al., 1992; Morello, 2007; Resnikoff et al., 2004). By understanding the pathophysiology behind circadian fluctuations of hyperglycemic episodes, physicians may be better able to help patients reduce the frequency and duration of these occurrences and thus reduce the complications that are associated with them.

5. References

Amir, S., Rabin, C., & Galatzer, A. (1990). Cognitive and Behavioral Determinants of Compliance in Diabetics. *Health & Social Work*, 15(2), pp. (144-151).

Cranston, I. et al., 1994. Restoration of hypoglycaemia awareness in patients with long-duration insulin-dependent diabetes. *Lance*, 344(8918), pp.283-287.

Cryer, P.E., 2004. Diverse causes of hypoglycemia-associated autonomic failure in diabetes. *The New England Journal of Medicine*, 350(22), pp.2272-2279.

Dagogo-Jack, S., Rattarasarn, C. & Cryer, P.E., 1994. Reversal of hypoglycemia unawareness, but not defective glucose counterregulation, in IDDM. *Diabetes*, 43(12), pp.1426-1434.

Desouza, C. et al., 2003. Association of hypoglycemia and cardiac ischemia: a study based on continuous monitoring. Diabetes Care, 26(5), pp.1485-1489.

Fanelli, C. et al., 1994. Long-term recovery from unawareness, deficient counterregulation and lack of cognitive dysfunction during hypoglycaemia, following institution of rational, intensive insulin therapy in IDDM. Diabetologia, 37(12), p.1265-1276.

Greene D A, Sima A A, Stevens M J, Feldman E L, and Lattimer S A. (1992). Complications: Neuropathy, Pathogenetic Considerations. *Diabetes Care.* December 1992 vol. 15, pp. 1902-1925.

Hirsch, I., and M. Brownlee. (2005). "Should Minimal Blood Glucose Variability Become the Gold Standard of Glycemic Control?" *Journal of Diabetes and Its Complications*, pp. 178-181.

Kannel WB, McGee DL. (1979). Diabetes And Cardiovascular Disease: The Framingham Study. *JAMA* vol. 241, pp. 2035–2038.

Klonoff, D.C., (2005). Continuous glucose monitoring: roadmap for 21st century diabetes therapy. *Diabetes Care*, 28(5), pp.1231-1239.

Larsson, C.A., Gullberg, B., Rastam, L., Lindblad, U. (2009). Salivary Cortisol Differs With Age And Sex And Shows Inverse Associations With WHR In Swedish Women: A Cross-Sectional Study. *BMC Endocrine Disorders*, vol. 9, no. 16, pp. 16.

Leese, G.P. et al., 2003. Frequency of severe hypoglycemia requiring emergency treatment in type 1 and type 2 diabetes: a population-based study of health service resource use. *Diabetes Care*, 26(4), pp.1176-1180.

Lehto S, Ronnemaa T, Pyorala K, Laakso M. (1996). Predictors Of Stroke In Middle-Aged Patients With Non-Insulin-Dependent Diabetes. *Stroke* vol. 27 pp. (63–68).

Morello, C. (2007). Etiology And Natural History Of Diabetic Retinopathy: An Overview. *American Journal of Health-System Pharmacy*, vol. 64, pp. S3-S7.

Resnikoff S, Pascolini D, Etya'ale D et al. (2004). Global Data On Visual Impairment In The Year 2002. *Bull World Health Organ*. Vol. 82, pp. 844–851.

Schwartz, A.V. et al., 2008. Diabetes-related complications, glycemic control, and falls in older adults. *Diabetes Care*, 31(3), pp.391-396.

Tamborlane, W. V., Beck, R. W., Bode, B. W., Buckingham, B., Chase, H. P., Clemons, R., Fiallo-Scharer, R., et al. (2008). Continuous glucose monitoring and intensive treatment of type 1 diabetes. *The New England Journal of Medicine*, vol. 359, no. 14, pp. 1464-1476.

Van Cauter E, Leproult R, Plat L. (2000) Age-Related Changes In Slow Wave Sleep And REM Sleep And Relationship With Growth Hormone And Cortisol Levels In Healthy Men. *JAMA*, vol. 284, pp. 861–868

Whitmer, R.A. et al., 2009. Hypoglycemic episodes and risk of dementia in older patients with type 2 diabetes mellitus. *Jama The Journal Of The American Medical Association*, 301(15), pp.1565-1572.

Wise PM, Cohen IR, Weiland NG, London ED. (1988). Aging Alters The Circadian Rhythm Of Glucose Utilization In The Suprachiasmatic Nucleus. *Proceeding of the National Academy of Science,* vol. 85, pp. 5305-5309

Part 2

Section B

5

Neonatal Hypoglycemia - Current Concepts

Blanca Álvarez Fernández and Irene Cuadrado Pérez
University Hospital of Getafe, Madrid
Spain

1. Introduction

Hypoglycaemia is a common problem in the neonatal period, and it frequently reflects difficulties in adapting to extra uterine life. Strategies to facilitate this physiological adaptation should be enhanced. (Sem fetal neo del 2005)

Incidence is variable depending on the definition criteria used in different studies, but according to Cornblath (Cornblath et al 1993, 2000 as cited by Fernández Loranzo et al 2011) it varies from 5-7% in term newborns and from 3.2 to 14.7% in preterm infants. Respective to weight, it occurs in 8% of Large for Gestational Age (LGA) and up to 15% of Small for Gestational Age (SGA) infants.

There is still no universal consensus on how to define hypoglycaemia. Establishing a universal cut-off glucose value is difficult and considerations must be made regarding the measuring device used, type of sample (blood, serum or plasma), moment of measurement after birth, duration and degree of hypoglycaemia and characteristics of the newborn. Based on the World Health Organization (WHO) recommendations (WHO 1997 as cited by Fernández Lorenzo et al 2011) thresholds would be:

Sick newborn, (signs of illness): <2.5mmol/L or 45 mg/dL

Healthy term / preterm (feeding well): < 1.1 mmol/L or < 19.8 mg/dL

Most expert authors support the cut-off value of 36mg/dL for asymptomatic healthy newborns, rather than the WHO suggested threshold, and some authors even suggest that values down to 1.7mmol/L should be accepted in an otherwise healthy term infant (Fugelseth 2001). In a recent review on neonatal hypoglycaemia, operational thresholds of less than 40mg/dL (2.2mmol/L) during the first 24 hours and less than 50mg/dL (2.8mmol/L) thereafter are suggested (Chan 2011). Other definitions have been suggested such as using an epidemiological concept: considering hypoglycaemia when glucose levels are 2 standard deviations below the mean value for infants of the same age (which would be around 20-30mg/dL). However, this value does not seem like the optimal threshold, so this definition is rarely used in clinical practice or for study purposes.

Experts agree that the neurological disabilities associated to neonatal hypoglycaemia depend on gestational and chronological age and associated risk factors such as Hypoxic-Ischemic Encephalopathy (HIE) and that they frequently result after situations of persistent and severe hypoglycaemia (Fernández Lorenzo et al 2011). What is more, the vast majority of healthy term newborns with isolated glucose levels under the target of 45 mg/dL will have a normal neurological prognosis. (Hay et al 2009)

Recent consensus workshop (Straussman & Levitsky 2010) results reveal that there has been little progress in establishing a clear numerical definition for hypoglycaemia, but understanding of underlying pathogenic mechanisms (specially in persistent hypoglycaemias), new information in genetic causes and promising information based on neuroimaging to define neurological outcomes, help define new strategies in preventing and treating hypoglycaemia in newborns (Chan, 2011).

2. Glucose metabolism physiology in the term and preterm newborn

Glucose is the most important foetal energy substrate (mainly for brain metabolism). Foetal glucose needs are met thanks to the continuous transplacental glucose transfer, and although the necessary enzyme systems needed for gluconeogenesis develop early during pregnancy, the foetus only produces its own glucose in extreme conditions such as maternal starvation. (Gustaffson 2009). The foetal glucose level is 60-80% of that of the mother's.

In order to provide the foetus with glucose, the mother undergoes different metabolic changes throughout gestation, such as increase in hepatic glucose production. Also, during the first trimester, the mother has a higher sensitivity to insulin that leads to fat depot formation. Later on, on the third trimester, when the baby has its own fat depots, the mother metabolizes these depots via lypolisis for her own needs under the influence of specific hormone changes therefore saving glucose for foetal use only.

The foetus is exposed to high insulin concentrations, as it has a very important anabolic action. During the third trimester, insulin stimulates fat deposition and increases energetic stores in the form of glycogen.

At birth, the constant placental supply is interrupted. Healthy term infants are prepared to adapt to this new situation thanks to a series of metabolic and hormonal changes that will ensure that the newborn's glucose demands (Central Nervous System (CNS) in particular) will de adequately met in the first 48 hours, while sufficient enteral feeding is being established. It has been demonstrated that early, frequent, breastfeeding together with skin to skin contact, promote adequate transition and meet the needs of healthy full-term infants. (Wight, 2006; Achoki et al, 2010).

First, an increase in glucagon and catecholamine levels and a decrease in insulin levels occur. This induces hepatic glucose production, (which in a healthy full term baby is 4-6micrgo/kg/min, three times that of an adult). This rate of hepatic glucose production is proportional to the baby's estimated brain weight. During the first 10 hours of life, it occurs by glycogenolisis. After, it takes places via gluconeogenesis (production of glucose "de novo" from alanine, pyruvate, lactate and glycerol). To further help in neoglucogenesis, lypolisis is stimulated (to levels comparable to an adult fasting), due to an increase in TSH levels after birth, which generates glycerol and free fatty acids. These free fatty acids play an important role as they promote further neoglucogenesis, and together with ketone bodies and lactate, are used as an alternative energy substrate for the brain. (Gustaffson, 2009; Mitanchez, 2007))

After birth, an adequate balance between tissue consumption of glucose, hepatic glucose production and exogenous glucose supply is necessary to establish glucose homeostasis. Glucose levels in the newborn decrease in the first two hours, but steadily rise afterwards and thereafter remain constant. Hypoglycaemia occurs when this equilibrium fails, and is usually transient.

In the presence of persistent hypoglycaemia, three main possible scenarios must be considered: depletion of energetic storage (prematurity and intra-uterine growth restriction), increase tissue energetic consumption and foetal hyperinsulinism. (Mitanchez, 2008; Wight, 2006; Ward Platt & Desphande 2005).

Preterm and intrauterine growth restricted (IUGR) newborns have different patterns of adaptation to that of a full-term neonate: they both have limited energy depots, and they have a higher risk of impaired compensatory ketogenesis. (Ward Platt & Desphande 2005). These babies are capable of neoglucogenesis and lypolisis, with some differences and restrictions.

Preterm infants have limited energy stores plus immature metabolic pathways to ensure an adequate glucose production, that lead to a larger fall in blood glucose in the first hours after birth. Because they have limited glycogen liver storage depots (since this takes place mainly during the third trimester), glycogenolisis is limited, therefore neoglucogenesis (from glycerol, alanine and lactate) is the main pathway for glucose production. Because neoglucogenesis requires some time to begin, in the absence of adequate glycogenolisis, hypoglycaemia in these "babies is hard to" avoid if exogenous glucose is not administered (Mitanchez, 2007), although some authors suggest that though neoglucogenesis occurs at slower rates in these infants than in term newborns, it may be just sufficient to prevent hypoglycaemia in the first hours of life (Gustafsson, 2009). Lypolisis occurs. However, the depot fat in an infant born after at 28 weeks is only 2% of total body weight (7 times less than in term infants) therefore the degree of lypolisis is decreased (Gustafsson, 2009; Diderholm , 2009).

Preterm infants are therefore at higher risk for hypoglycaemia because of their limitations for adequate glucose metabolism, but also because other clinical conditions which are associated with hypoglycaemia are common in this population, such as perinatal asphyxia, hypoxia, sepsis, and hypothermia. Preterm infants are less capable of compensating these glucose alterations than term infants are, being the final goal to ensure sufficient energy substrate for the brain to use, and even moderate hypoglycaemia can lead to an adverse neurodevelopmental outcome. Enteral feeding is a stimulus for postnatal metabolic adaptation. Thus, early milk feeding should be encouraged as soon as possible when tolerated, even at a minimal level (Mitanchez, 2007).

On the other hand, preterm infants (particularly those less than 30 weeks of gestational age (GA)) frequently have impaired insulin - glucose balance, leading to hyperglycaemia during the first weeks of life. This occurs because processing of pro-insulin in the pancreatic beta-cells is deficient, therefore preterm infants are partially resistant to insulin. Exogenous insulin infusion is efficient and may be used with caution. (Mitanchez, 2008). These patterns of metabolic adaptation are further influenced by feeding practices. (Ward Platt & Desphande, 2005)

As mentioned before, compared to adequate for gestational age (AGA), infants with IUGR have smaller energy depots. Gluconeogenesis has been shown to occur effectively from glycerol in these infants (50% of glycerol is converted to glucose and this rate increases in babies who do not receive extra parenteral glucose infusion) and from pyruvate. Ketogenesis is severely limited in preterm infants. Lypolisis also occurs but is limited because it correlates with birth weight (that is: the rate of lypolisis depends on the amount of stored fat), and it is therefore reduced in IUGR babies (Gustafsson, 2009, Mitanchez, 2007).

Infants born to diabetic mothers are at risk for hypoglycaemia, due to increased levels of insulin in the baby. This increase occurs due to increased maternal glucose levels throughout the pregnancy. Despite insulin normally reducing lypolisis, this does not happen in these babies, probably as a compensation for the lower level of glucose production seen in these newborns (Gustafson, 2009).

There is limited information on metabolism in newborn LGA infants. These babies tend to have increased lypolisis rates (partly due to higher body and brain weight) and variable degrees of insulin resistance (as happens with obese children in later periods of life) (Gustafsson, 2009).

3. Defining aetiology and risk factors

When considering aetiology and risk factors in hypoglycaemia, the differentiating marker is whether it is transient (< 3-5 days) or persistent (> 5-7 days). (Fernández Lorenzo et al, 2011; Cloherty & Stark, 2009; Polin & Yoder 2007; Chan 2011).

3.1 Transient hypoglycaemia

Low endogenous glucose production or low glycogen deposits.

This occurs in situations where glucose metabolic pathways are impaired or immature such as in preterm infants, intrauterine growth retardation (IUGR) and small for gestational age (SGA) newborns and in situations of insufficient calorie intake (feeding difficulties, problems with breastfeeding or intolerance of enteral feedings etc…).

Increase in glucose use or diminished exogenous administration.

Exposure to situations with high energy consumption rates such as perinatal stress (asphyxia, sepsis, respiratory distress, hypothermia, congenital cardiopathy…). In these situations, anaerobic glycolisis occurs due to decreased tissue perfusion and low oxygen blood content. When polycythemia occurs, the higher number of red blood cells consume glucose at higher rates than normal, as would happen during and after an exanguinotransfussion procedure. An abrupt cease in intravenous glucose administration may induce transient hypoglycaemia that is normally reverted reinitiating the glucose infusion.

RISK FACTOR	MECHANISM
Preterm and Intrauterine Growth Restriction	Low glycogen deposits Restriction in fluids / energy Hormonal and enzymatic immaturity Feeding difficulties
Diabetic mother Beckwith-Wiedemann Syndrome RH haemolytic disease	Transient hyperinsulinism
Pancreatic islets dysregulation Syndrome Pancreatic islets adenoma	Persistent hyperinsulinism
Perinatal stress; asphyxia, sepsis Polycythemia, hypothermia	Low glycogen deposits Hyperinsulinism Feeding difficulties Fluid / energy restrictions
Maternal drugs: propanolol, oral antidiabetic preparations	Altered cathecolamin response
Adrenal insufficiency Hypothalamic / Hypopituitaric deficiency	Counter-regulatory hormone deficiency
Inborn errors in metabolism	Enzyme defects, altered glucogenolisis, neoglucogenesis or fatty acid oxidation.

Table 1. Risk factors and physiopathological mechanisms that cause hypoglycaemia

Transient hyperinsulinemic hypoglycaemia

There are many situations where the newborn is exposed to intra-uterine hyperinsulinism, rendering the infant prone to hypoglycaemia after birth, when that hyperinsulinism persists until pancreatic beta cells commence to work and regulate insulin secretion, but the constant transplacental glucose supply has been terminated.

Diabetic mothers (specially those needing insulin during gestation, which implies worse glucose regulation), big for gestational age neonates, erytroblastosis, misplaced umbilical arterial line (near the pancreas) or if the mother receives intrapartum Pre-par* or other beta-sympaticomimetics that interrupt glycogenolisis, tiazides, clorpropamide, anti-hyperglycaemic agents or glucose infusion rates of more that 10g/h before birth, may develop transient hyperinsulinemic hypoglycaemia. In the Beckwith-Wiedemann Syndrome (LGA newborn, macroglosia, onphalocele and visceromegaly), hypoglycaemia occurs secondary to transient hyperinsulinism due to pancreatic beta cells hypertrophy.

3.2 Persistent hypoglycaemia

When persistent hypoglycaemia occurs (that is, need for glucose infusion for more than 5-7 days, in particular when high rates are required) other clinical scenarios must be ruled out and specific diagnostic procedures must be started.

Prolonged neonatal hyperinsulinemic hypoglycaemia may occur as a result of nesidioblastosis, pancreatic adenoma or beta cell hyperplasia, that is, clinical situations that increase insulin production at the pancreatic beta cell. However, up to 30-40% of **persistent hyperinsulinism cases are congenital or genetic**, with increasing knowledge of genetic mutations in specific calcium channels that control insulin secretion. This will be further explained.

Other causes of persistent hypoglycaemia are syndrome such as **Usher Syndrome** (hearing loss and retinitis pigmentosa), **endocrine disorders** (pituitary hormone deficiencies or primary adrenocortical insufficiency) and **inborn errors of carbohydrate metabolism** (glucogenosis, hereditary fructose intolerance and galactosemia) **or amino-acid metabolism** (methylmalonic and glutaric acidemias, leucinosis (MUSD), carnitine deficiency and others…) and **defects in fatty acid beta-oxidation.**

4. Clinical manifestations of hypoglycaemia in the neonatal period

These are unspecific and may resolve within minutes-hours after normoglycaemia is restored, unless cerebral damage has occurred.

Neurological symptoms such as irritability, tremor, jitteriness, hypotonia, exaggerated Moro reflex, and weak cry may appear gradually and progress towards seizures, acute encephalopathy, lethargy and coma. Altered state of consciousness is a common finding, with alternate jitteriness and stupor (Chan, 2011).

Jitteriness is not very specific of hypoglycaemia though a frequent form of presentation, as it may be present in up to 44% of healthy term infants (Alkalay et al, 2005). In some cases, it may be pathological, resembling a brainstem release reflex (impaired function of superior cortical inhibitory structures that normally control the brainstem). As for tremor, it is also frequent in healthy term newborns, and only normally correlates to hypoglycaemia or hypocalcaemia when it persists despite suckling stimulation, rather than stopping as it does in healthy babies. As for seizures, these may present very early after hypoglycaemia

appears, but normally occur after persistently or recurrently low glucose values over at least 12 hours.
Other clinical manifestations include tachypnea, cyanosis (due to apnea, autonomic response or decreased pulmonary flow) or apnea spells. Difficulty to suck and feeding problems may also occur. Autonomic alterations are frequent, such as hypothermia or unstable temperature, pallor, profuse sweating or bradycardia (Alkalay et al, 2005).

5. Monitoring glucose levels and how to do so?

In the presence of asymptomatic newborns with any of the known risk factors (preterm, IUGR, SGA and LGA infants; newborns with diabetic mothers; perinatal stress situations; maternal drugs before or during labour, infants requiring intensive care, those with polycythemia and syndromes such as Beckwith-Wiedemann) glucose must be closely monitored. Blood glucose should also be monitored in infants receiving long duration parenteral nutrition, even when stable. Healthy asymptomatic newborns without risk factors do not need routine evaluation. **Chan 2011**
Glucose determination must be done at the first hour of life, and afterwards, depending on different guidelines (Fernańdez Lorenzo et al, 2011) every 2-4 hours for the first 8 hours of life, and every 6-8 hours for the following 24 hours of life. The main point however, is to carefully assess glucose metabolism during the more vulnerable stages of transition. Normally, if glucose levels are maintained in the first hours of life (when hypoglycaemia is most likely), they rarely fall afterwards. Nevertheless, periodic measurements (more or less frequently depending on glucose values and associated risk factors) must be performed during at least the first critical 24 hours.
Specifically, suggested controls in newborns of diabetic mothers would imply: glucose testing in the first hour of life, and afterwards, every 6-12 hours, since hypoglycaemia is most probable around the first six hours of life. These controls may be suspended after 12 hours of normal glucose values.
In preterm and SGA infants however, controls should be more frequent, every 2-4 hours depending on glucose values: are they normal, just on the limit or actually low? Do they require clinical management that must be monitored?
On the other hand, whenever a newborn presents with clinical symptoms that could be due to hypoglycaemia, particularly if the newborn has risk factors for hypoglycaemia, rapid glucose determination is imperative, as early treatment is essential to prevent brain damage. This implies having a wide scope of suspicion in any situation, as symptomatic hypoglycaemia con vary from very unspecific clinical symptoms such as discrete irritability to more alarming and obvious presentations such as seizures, and recognition is determinant.

6. Diagnosis

In order to diagnose hypoglycaemia, a cut-off value has to be established. There is still no evidence of what that numerical value is, and it probably differs amongst different babies (term, preterm, IUGR, asphyxiated, septic…) as tolerance thresholds of glucose values are probably different in each of these scenarios (sick babies are probably more susceptible to hypoglycaemia than healthy term newborns, specially if hypoglycaemia persists or is severe). Therefore, in order to diagnose hypoglycaemia, operational guidelines exist, and diagnosis is normally made in the presence of blood glucose concentration <45mg/dL (<2.5mmol/L) in the first hours - days of life. (Fugelseth, 2001). Later on, a certain degree of glucose control is expected and hypoglycaemia is diagnosed with glucose levels < 50-55 mg/dL. (Chan , 2011).

Accurate measurement of blood glucose levels in the newborn is important in order to prevent and treat hypoglycaemia effectively, therefore reducing the risk of adverse neurological outcomes. Commonly used Point of care (POC) glucose testing provides immediate results with small sample volumes. This enables treatment, when necessary, to start fast and permits the necessary modifications according to the infants´ clinical situation. These devices are perfected constantly, and yet, they still lose accuracy at the limits of both low and high glucose values (hypoglycaemia with blood glucose <2.0 mmol/l or <2.6 mmol/l and hyperglycaemia with blood glucose >10 mmol/l). Knowing these limitations is important and so strictly speaking, these devices cannot be completely relied on for an accurate diagnosis. However, as a screening tool, they are essential, and when accuracy is doubtful, laboratory confirmation is necessary. This will require intermittent blood samples and results are somewhat delayed. Less invasive and continuous methods of glucose monitoring are under development. These devices provide constant information and being increasingly used for control and care of patients with diabetes mellitus, but they are not currently in use in neonates (Beardsall, 2010). Continuous interstitial glucose monitoring has been tested on newborns thought to be at risk for hypoglycaemia, and though apparently reliable, it is still not known how to best interpret the results, and therefore more studies are needed before implementation of this technique. (Harris et al, 2010; Hay et al , 2010 as cited in Chan, 2011).

When using laboratory measurement of glucose, it is important to know what sample is used. Glucose concentration in whole blood is up to 15% lower than that in plasma and may be even lower in the presence of a high hematocrit. Once the sample has been taken, analysis should be performed rapidly, as glucose values in blood can decrease by 15 to 20 mg/dL per hour in blood samples at room temperature. (Chan, 2011).

Diagnosis of hypoglycaemia begins with determining low glucose levels in the presence or not of clinical symptoms. It should be emphasized that surveillance and intervention thresholds are not the same: when treating hypoglycaemia, the desired range for normoglycaemia should be 72-90 mg/dL (4-5 mmol/L), as opposed to the diagnostic suggested thresholds of <46mg/dL (<2.6mmol/L) (Kalhan & Peter-Wohl, 2000).

This is normally a transient problem in adaptation in a newborn with frequently recognisable risk factors or other treatable underlying causes such as sepsis, insufficient exogenous glucose administration or errors in administration. However, when hypoglycaemia is persistent (at least more than 72 hours, and specifically more than the first week of life), and high rates of iv glucose (some times up to 12 mg/kg/min) are required to maintain normal glucose levels, specific laboratory test must be begun to rule out causes of persistent hypoglycaemia in order of frequency (Chan, 2011): prolonged neonatal hyperinsulinemic hypoglycaemia, congenital hyperinsulinemic hypoglycaemia, endocrine disorders and inborn errors of metabolism.

The diagnostic algorithm requires defining ketone body production, and plasma levels of both free fatty acids and of lactic acid. With these three parameters, we can establish which diagnosis is most probable:

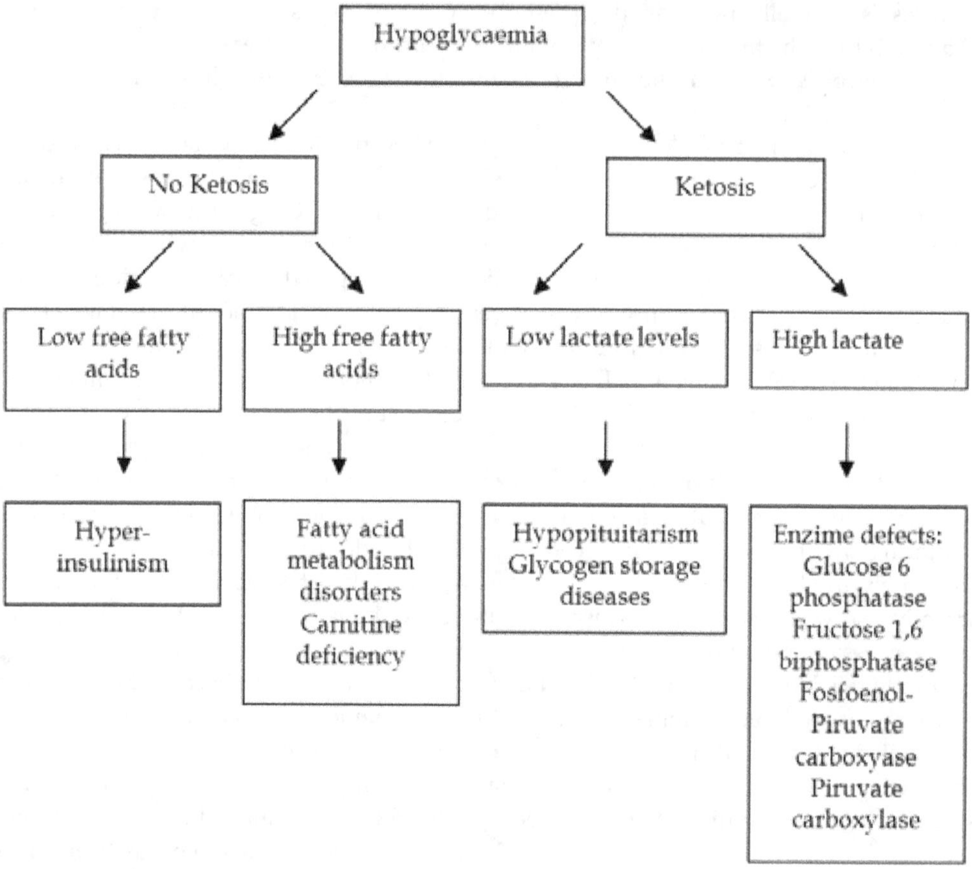

Fig. 1. Algorithm for hypoglycaemia diagnosis

Ketone body production is the normal alternative pathway to obtain energy in the absence of sufficient glucose supply. Free fatty acids are oxidized to obtain ketone bodies, which are an important energy substrate for the heart, muscle and brain. In this scenario, high levels of lactic acid suggest a defect in neoglucogenesis, whereas low lactic levels suggest glycogen storage disease or hypopituitarism.

On the other hand, in the absence of ketone body production and with low free fatty acid levels, hyperinsulinism must be suspected, as insulin inhibits glycogenolisis (turning glycogen stores into glucose), neoglucogenesis (de novo glucose production from non-carbohydrate sources such as lipids and proteins) lipolysis and therefore ketogenesis. No ketosis with high levels of free fatty acids in the setting of hypoglycaemia suggests fatty acid oxidation defects, because free fatty acids cannot be used to produce ketone bodies as an alternative energy substrate in the presence of hypoglycaemia.

First level laboratory tests:

Glycaemia / Insulinemia ratio

Ketone bodies in urine (3 beta hidroxybutiric acid)

Lactate / Piruvate ratio

Plasmatic insulin higher than 13mU/ml when plasmatic glucose is lower than 40mg/dL (that is, a glucose/insulin rate < 3:1) without ketosis and low free fatty acids is patognomonic of hyperinsulinism: excessive insulin levels despite having low glucose levels without the normal alternative energy ketone body production.

Second level laboratory tests:

Ketone bodies and organic acids in blood

Organic acids in urine

This is a first step towards diagnosing possible inborn errors in metabolism, specially specific enzyme defects found in organic acidemias.

Third level laboratory tests:

Thyroid hormones (T4, TSH)

Glucagon

Cortisol / ACTH (poner nombre entero) / Growth Hormone (GH)

Amino-acids in blood and in urine

Growth hormone and Cortisol are counter-regulatory hormones that normally rise with hypoglycaemia. If there are low levels of GH (< 7-10 ng/mL) or of cortisol (<20 microg/dL) this suggests an isolated hormone deficiency or hypopituitarism.

Glucagon basal levels are suggestive, but specifically, an increase in plasma glucose of more than 30 mg/dl after glucagon administration suggests that the hepatic glycogen stores are not depleted, which is also characteristic of hyperinsulinism.

Diagnostic criteria to define hyperinsulinism are:

Glucose < 40mg/dL

Insuline > 13 microU/mL

Glucose/insuline ratio < 3:1

Glucose intravenous needs > 6-8 mg/kg/min

Negative ketone bodies in plasma and urine (3-beta-hidroxi-butiric acid < 1mmol/L)

Low free fatty acids (< 1 mmol/L)

Cortisol > 20 microg/dL

GH > 7-10 ng/mL

Glucemic reaction to glucagon administration > 30 mg/dL (ie: positive response)

7. Persistent hypoglycaemic hyperinsulinism

When hypoglycaemia persists for more than 5 days, initial laboratory tests must commence to rule out other possible causes of persistent hypoglycaemia. In this scenario, persistent hypoglycaemic hyperinsulinism is a frequent entity and deserves a mention of its own, as it is a major cause of hypoglycaemic brain injury and mental retardation. (Kapoor et al, 2009a; 2009b).

In normal conditions, the pancreatic islet beta cells produce insulin that is secreted outside the cell via an ATP sensitive potassium channel (ATP-K). Genetic mutations that produce altered proteins that form part of different sub units of this channel explain the dysregulation of insulin secretion (that is: excess secretion even in the presence of low plasma glucose levels).

It has two main characteristics: high glucose needs to maintain normoglycaemia and responsiveness to exogenous glucagon. Hypoglycaemia occurs due to a dysregulated insulin secretion with defects in the normal counter-regulatory hormones (cortisol or GH). It is possible that there may be an increased insulin sensitivity in these patients, although this has not been proven. The excess insulin secretion leads glucose into the insulin sensitive tissues (mainly skeletal muscle, adipose tissue and liver) so hypoglycaemia occurs. On the other hand, insulin inhibits glycogenolisis (turning glycogen stores into glucose), neoglucogenesis (de novo glucose production from non-carbohydrate sources such as lipids and proteins) lipolysis and therefore ketogenesis (oxidation of fatty acids to produce alternative energy substrate ketone bodies). As was mentioned before, the normal counter-regulatory cortisol and glucagon responses are blunted, so hypoglycaemia persists. In this scenario, the brain is being deprived of any form of energy substrate, as glucose (its main energy source) is depleted in plasma, but also, alternative energy sources (ketone bodies and lactate) are characteristically low in these cases, so the risk for brain damage is increased greatly.

Understanding this is crucial, as management to prevent brain damage will differ from other underlying processes. Initially, 2.6 mmol/l was suggested as definition for hypoglycaemia based on the neurophysiological changes associated to hypoglycaemia, but these were established under conditions of non-hyperinsulinism, that is, the brain does have alternative energy fuel. Later, "operational thresholds" were suggested for different groups of neonates (Cornblath, 2000), since there is still uncertainty as to what levels of hypoglycaemia and for what duration, promote brain injury. And though many centres have accepted 2.6mmol/L as the operational threshold for hyperinsulinism, based on the complete absence of alternative energy sources for the brain in a crucial moment (intense development in the neonate and during infancy), a higher threshold of at least 3.5-6 mmol/L is necessary in order to prevent cerebral glycopenia, as the brain will be completely dependant on glucose plasma levels for an adequate glucose intake (Hussain et al, 2007).

There is great variability in terms of clinical presentation, histology, genetics and treatment response and hyperinsulinism can be classified according to three main characteristics: (Giurgea et al, 2005)

Onset of hypoglycaemia: neonatal period or later during infancy
Histological lesion: focal or diffuse
Genetic transmission: sporadic recessive or less frequently, dominant

Hyperinsulinism may be isolated or may be part of a more complex syndrome. The former tends to present early in the neonatal period and is frequently severe as compared to syndromic hyperinsulinism which commonly has later onset during infancy, with a milder presentation. Severity is evaluated considering the exogenous glucose administration rate required for normoglycaemia and the response to medical treatment which may be highly variable amongst individuals. (Cloherty & Stark, 2009; Chan, 2011; Arnoux et al, 2010).

Over the past decades, there is increasing information on the genetic aspects of hyperinsulinism. Congenital hyperinsulinism is caused by mutations in genes involved in regulation of insulin secretion. To date, seven genes involved have been identified (ABCC8, KCNJ11, GLUD1, CGK, HADH, SLC16A1 and HNF4A). These genes encode glucokinase, glutamate dehydrogenase, the mitochondrial enzyme short-chain 3-hydroxyacyl-CoA dehydrogenase plus the proteins that form the subunits of the ATP-K channel (which are the most common underlying mechanisms). Severe forms of congenital hyperinsulinism, that is, those with early neonatal presentation, are caused by mutations in these ATP-K channel subunits: ABCC8 or sulfonylurea receptor gene (SUR1) and KCNJ11 or inward-rectifying potassium channel gene (KIR6.2), both located in the 11p15.1 region. Mutations in HNF4A, GLUD1, CGK, and HADH lead to transient or persistent hyperinsulinism, whereas mutations in SLC16A1 cause exercise-induced hyperinsulinism.

In focal pancreatic islet-cells hyperplasia, mutations of the ABCC8 or the KCNJ11 genes are inherited from the father, with a loss of the maternal allele specifically in the hyperplasic islet cells. In diffuse isolated hyperinsulinism, genetic inheritance is heterogeneous and may

be recessive (ABCC8 and KCNJ11) or dominant (ABCC8, KCNJ11, GCK, GLUD1, SLC16A1, HNF4A and HADH). Syndromic hyperinsulinism is always diffuse and genetic inheritance depends on the specific syndrome. (Arnoux et al, 2010 ; Giurgea, 2005 ; Kapoor et al, 2009a)
Despite the increasing amount of genetic information already available, there are still up to 50% of the cases where no known genetic alteration can be identified.

Therefore, defining the histological forms of hyperinsulinism is particularly important as they involve different genetic mutations and inheritance but most importantly, because they have different treatment options. Focal hyperplasia consists of a focal adenomatoid hyperplasia of islet cells, while diffuse forms involve all the pancreatic beta cells of the whole pancreas. Infants suffering from ATP-K hyperinsulinism present shortly after birth with severe and persistent hypoglycaemia, and the majority do not respond to medical treatment. Up to 40-60% of the children with ATP-K hyperinsulinism have focal lesions in the pancreas and are candidates for local resection which is effective while avoiding the long-term complications of near-total pancreatectomy such as diabetes-mellitus. Diffuse hyperinsulinism however, when resistant to medical treatment (octreotide, diazoxide, calcium antagonists and continuous feeding) may require subtotal pancreatectomy.

To distinguish between focal and diffuse forms, trans-hepatic catheterisation with pancreatic venous sampling has been used, but is being replaced by [(18)F] Fluoro-L-Dopa PET scan, which is easier to perform, and is not only a diagnostic tool, but may also be used to guide laparoscopic surgery. Therefore, rapid genetic analysis combined with an understanding of these histological features (focal or diffuse disease) and the introduction of (18)F Fluoro-L-Dopa PET scan, have totally transformed the clinical approach to this complex metabolic alteration (Arnoux et al, 2010; Kapoor et al 2009).

Treatment options:	Diazoxide	Octreotide	Ca antagonist	Glucagon
Mechanism	Opens K channel Stimulates CA production	Opens K channel: inhibits insulin secretion	Inhibits Ca channel	Increases glucogenolisis & neoglucogenesis
Doses	10-15 mg/kg/day every 8h (maximum of 25mg/kg/day)	10 microg/kg/day subcutaneous every 4-6h	0.25-0.7 mg/kg/day every 8h oral	0.2 mg/kg im fast Maintenance infusion of 2-10 microg/kg/h iv
Indications & effectiveness	Fist line 20-50%	Second line 20-80%	Not enough experience	Emergency treatment and stabilization
Adverse effects	Liquid retention Hypertrichosis Hyperglycaemia Cetoacidosis Hypertension Leucopenia Trombopenia Hyperuricemia	GH, TSH and glucagon suppression Steatorrhea Cholestasis	Hypotension	Increases myocardial contractility Lowers Ca & K Lowers gastric acid and pancreatic enzymes Frequently nauseas and vomiting

Table 2. Medical treatment options in hyperinsulinemic hypoglycaemia.

Before considering possible surgical treatments (once the diagnosis of hyperinsulinism has been made), medical treatment must be started, with the goal of maintaining glucose values within a normal target range. Initially exogenous glucose administration will be required and glucagon infusion may be useful in certain emergency situations. In terms of specific medical treatment, oral diazoxide is the first line option. If the infant does not respond, somatostatin analogues and calcium antagonists may be considered. Except for ATP-K channel defects hyperinsulinism (ABCC8 and KCNJ11), most forms are sensitive to diazoxide.

In conclusion, there are two main points that sum up the management of hyperinsulinism cases: prevention of brain damage by normalizing glycaemia and screening for focal forms as they may be definitively cured after a limited pancreatectomy. (Arnoux et al, 2010).

8. Treatment for hypoglycaemia

When treating hypoglycaemia, there are two mains aspects that must be considered and that will define a different approach: first, whether the neonate is symptomatic or not and secondly, the initial glucose values. (Fernández Lorenzo et al, 2011; Chan, 2011).

8.1 Asymptomatic hypoglycaemia

When glucose levels are under 46mg/dl (2.6mmol/L) but higher than 30mg/dL, and the baby has no feeding intolerance or difficulty, breastfeeding is the first option, together with supplementation either with extracted mothers´ milk or adapted infant formula if necessary. This provides a higher glucose intake than offering plain 5% glucose solution orally. Capillary glycaemia controls are needed every 20-30 minutes after intake. If normoglycaemia has been achieved, normal feedings can be established (preferably breastfeeding ad libitum, that is, as often as the baby needs, but at least every two-three hours), and considering adding supplements of the mothers´ extracted breast milk or adapted formula if necessary).

If there are feeding difficulties or intolerance, or if glucose levels are below 30mg/dL, intravenous exogenous glucose administration must be considered. 10% glucose infusion at a rate of 5-8 mg/kg/min will be required as a starting point. As feeding tolerance recuperates, oral feedings must begin, promoting the physiological fractioned enteral feeding pattern that will better regulate insulin secretion. As glucose levels are maintained, parenteral glucose administration must be tapered until complete and exclusive fractioned enteral nutrition has been established.

In some cases, if an intravenous line is difficult to obtain, or if a baby is persistently hypoglycaemic but asymptomatic despite fractioned enteral feedings, continuous enteral feeding may be considered, which provides a continuous glucose intake, but requires adequate gastrointestinal tolerance.

8.2 Symptomatic hypoglycaemia

When hypoglycaemia persists (less than 46 mg/dL or 2.6mmmol/L) and symptoms are present, rapid glucose correction is warranted. An intravenous bolus of 10% glucose must be administered at a dose of 2ml/kg/dose (200mg/kg/dose). Higher glucose concentrations should not be used, in order to avoid the possible insulin peak secretion that may occur in response to the bolus. In the presence of seizures, higher doses of 4ml/kg/dose (400mg/kg/dose) must be considered. In any case, after bolus administration, a continuous glucose perfusion must be started to prevent rebound hypoglycaemia due to peak insulin secretion; again, around 5-8 mg/kg/min to begin with.

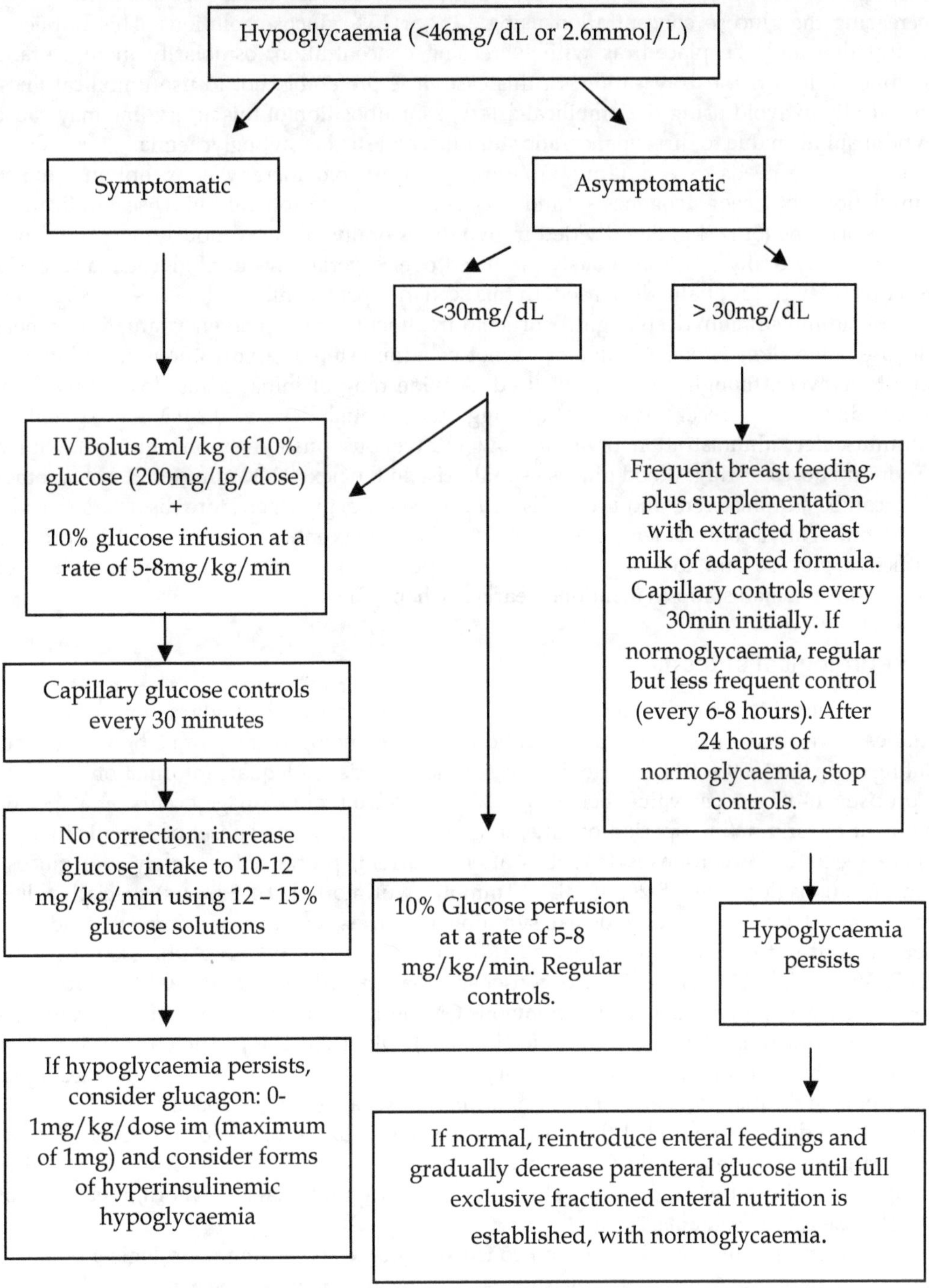

Fig. 2. Treatment algorithm for neonatal hypoglycaemia

Depending on glycaemia control afterwards, the exogenous glucose intake may be increased further either initially increasing perfusion rate (up to a maximum volume intake the baby will tolerate according to gestational age, weight and clinical status) or, more frequently, increasing the glucose concentration using 12% or 15% glucose solutions. This implies a central line must be placed, as with increasing concentration, osmolarity increases and peripheral lines risk extravasation. In this case, it is preferable not to use umbilical lines, specifically to avoid using the umbilical artery, as malposition of this artery line may cause hyperinsulinism due to direct pancreatic stimulus, and further hypoglycaemia.
When glucose needs exceed 12mg/kg/min, glucocorticoid therapy is an option,, due to stimulation of neoglucogenesis and reduction in peripheral glucose utilization. Hydrocortisone (5mg/kg/day divided in two doses orally or intravenously) or prednisone (2mg/kg/day orally or intravenously) are used over several days until glycaemia recovers and doses can be gradually decreased. In this scenario (persistently high needs of exogenous glucose administration, despite glucocorticoid treatment) or in emergency situations where glucose bolus alone is not effective or cannot be administered rapidly enough, glucagon is an alternatively, though infrequently used. A wide rang of initial bolus doses have been reported, but in a recent review, the suggested initial dose is 0.2-0.3 mg/kg (either intramuscular administration or as a slow intravenous push over one minute) with a maximum doses of 1mg. Blood glucose should rise in the next 20-30 minutes. If not, another does can be administered, and if there is still no response, glycogen store disorders must be ruled out. This is only a temporary option, while interventions are planned to provide sufficient glucose and to start diagnosis of hyperinsulinism which may prompt use of diazoxide or somatostatin as mentioned earlier (Chan, 2011).

9. Neurological outcome

There is increasing concern about neurodevelopment after hypoglycaemia and many studies have tried to establish a correlation between hypoglycaemia and brain damage, dating since the 1960´s. But, to date there is still not sufficient adequate information to define a precise cut-off glucose value, below which irreversible brain damage occurs, at a specific moment or for a defined period of time, in a given infant or in a subset of specific infants. There seems to be consensus that it is after recurrent, protracted, severely low glucose concentrations (less than 18-20mg/dL (< 1mmol/L) for more that 1-2 hours) specially when accompanied by severe neurological symptoms such as seizures or coma, that adverse neurological outcome is to be expected (Rozance & Hay,2006; Cornblath, 2000; Alkalay, 2005; Vannuci, 2001). There is also consensus that in order to define CNS injury as a consequence of hypoglycaemia, other obvious CNS lesions must be absent (such as hypoxia-ischemia, intracranial haemorrhage, infection, etc.). Other conditions such as confirmed or suspected hyperinsulinemic hypoglycaemia in the presence of seizures, for example, contribute to the diagnosis of hypoglycaemic injury (Rozance & Hay, 2006).
Because we do not know what the absolute threshold value is, operational thresholds have been suggested, where clinical guidance is compulsory, so an infant with neurological symptoms will need more urgent evaluation than an asymptomatic newborn, regardless of the glucose value (Williams, 2005).
In the preterm population, there are no conclusive studies regarding neurological outcome in case of hypoglycaemia, but they suggest that even mild but repeated hypoglycaemia could be detrimental on brain development. Retrospective data from a multicenter trial of

nutrition in premature infants found lower Bayley mental and psychomotor scores at 18 months in infants with at least five confirmed hypoglycaemia events, with a higher rate of developmental delay and cerebral palsy, but however failed to confirm these findings at 7.5 and 8 years of age (Lucas et al, 1988; Cornblath, 1999 as cited in Chan, 2011).

Considering the innate risk for adverse neurodevelopment in the preterm infant, emphasis must be put on monitoring glucose levels in these infants to avoid further possible CNS injury (Wayenberg & Pardou, 2008).

It is worth pointing out that the physiopathological mechanisms that promote injury in hypoglycaemia vary from injury mechanisms in HIE, with some areas being more sensitive to deprivation of glucose and others to deprivation of oxygen and a greater tendency towards selective neuronal necrosis in hypoglycaemic babies. Also, concurrent hypoglycaemia and HIE have worst prognosis than either condition individually, therefore extreme caution must be taken to maintain normoglycaemia in an HIE setting (Vannuci, 2001; Garg & Devaskar, 2006).

Neonatal hypoglycaemia can lead to reduced head circumference at follow-up, lower psychomotor scores, motor deficit and mental retardation. Specifically neonates with recurrent episodes had lower psychomotor scores than those with a single episode. (Lucas, 1988; Nunes, 2000; Greery, 1966 as cited in Alkalay 2005).

Hypoglycaemia episodes with seizures have worse outcomes than hypoglycaemia episodes alone. At follow-up, many of those that had hypoglycaemia and seizures develop epilepsy of different types such as infantile spasms and partial seizures. Electroencephalographic recordings do not show specific patognomonic features that may result diagnostic (Alkalay, 2005).

Parieto-occipital diffusion restriction seen on MRI scans have been reported associated with neonatal hypoglycaemia and can result in long-term disability, epilepsy, and visual impairment (Finlan et al, 2006; Tam et al, 2008). The aetiology of this pattern of injury is unclear; however, transient hyperinsulinism may be an independent risk factor. Magnetic resonance brain imaging can help define the extent of brain injury and guide follow-up. In a 23 case follow-up, with severely low and persistent or recurrent glucose values, abnormal brain imaging findings were associated with profound hypoglycaemia and involved occipital lobes in 82% the cases. Half of these infants had visual impairment (Alkalay et al, 2005b).

In relation to this, a cohort of 45 neonates with diffusion-weighted MRI studies after hypoglycaemia was studied retrospectively to determine whether hypoglycaemic injury, as indicated by diffusion restriction in the occipital lobes, correlated with visual evoked potentials and long-term cortical visual dysfunction. They saw that diffusion-weighted imaging studies performed within 6 days after initial hypoglycaemia were sensitive in term (50% had restricted diffusion in occipital lobes) but not in preterm neonates (none had this alteration), as opposed to those performed after, and were associated with abnormal visual evoked potentials detected within 1 week after birth. Cortical visual impairment happened in a significant proportion of patients with recurrent hypoglycaemia and correlated significantly with low mesial occipital apparent diffusion coefficient values. They concluded that diffusion restriction, with low apparent diffusion coefficient values, in the mesial occipital poles, may indicate poor visual outcomes in acute settings after neonatal hypoglycaemia (Tam et al, 2008).

While occipital lobe injury patterns have been widely described, other brain injury patterns have also been identified when studying MRI scans performed on term neonates with symptomatic hypoglycaemia and compared to neurologically normal infants. White matter abnormalities occurred in 94% of the infants (43% of theses were severe lesions), with predominant posterior lobe alterations in 29% of the cases. Cortical abnormalities were identified in 51% of infants; 30% had white matter haemorrhage, 40% basal ganglia and or thalamic lesions, and 11% had an abnormal posterior limb of the internal capsule. Three infants had middle cerebral artery territory infarctions. It was noted that early MRI findings predicted neurodevelopmental outcomes better than the severity or duration of hypoglycaemia: 65% of these infants had impaired neurologic development at 18 months, which were related to the severity of white matter injury and involvement of the posterior limb of the internal capsule (Burns et al, 2008).

10. Prevention

Despite controversy and gaps in knowledge as to what level of hypoglycaemia and for how long, brain injury occurs, it is clear that hypoglycaemia can and must be prevented. In the majority of healthy newborn infants, if hypoglycaemia occurs, it is merely a transient adaptation process. However, although the majority of term newborns without risk factors will adapt correctly, there is up to 10% of these infants that will have significant hypoglycaemia in the first 3-4 hours of life, and will probably be asymptomatic. Helping these infants adapt is best achieved when promoting early skin to skin contact as soon as the baby is born (this promotes mother-child bonding, more effective breast feeding and better temperature control) and early and frequent breast feeding. On the other hand, infants with risk for hypoglycaemia are more vulnerable and may not adapt as easily as a healthy newborn, despite applying these strategies. Preventing significant hypoglycaemia in this subset population implies controlling these infants at risk in the first hours of life and thereafter periodically depending on the infants' clinical status and glucose levels, and adapting treatment options to the babies' situation.

11. Conclusions

Hypoglycaemia in the neonatal period is a frequent problem. In the majority of cases, in healthy term newborns, it is merely a transient adaptation process from intra-uterine life to extra-uterine conditions. However, there are infants who for different reasons are at risk of more significant and persistent hypoglycaemia, that will have less capacity to adapt to extra-uterine life and that will require frequent monitoring and treatment when necessary.

The goal is to maintain normoglycaemia in order to assure an adequate energy substrate for all organs but most importantly for the brain in order to prevent brain injury. To achieve this, many cut-off values have been proposed, and perhaps the most accepted concept is that of defining specific "operational thresholds" for different groups of infants at risk, that is, the glucose value for a given infant where treatment is required, the point where we must intervene. There is consensus in the need of preventing hypoglycaemia, which means looking out for it in infants at risk, and promptly treating it if present (from more frequent feeding to parenteral glucose infusion to glucagon if necessary).

Hypoglycaemic induced brain damage occurs when hypoglycaemia is severely low in a persistent or recurrent manner, and is more likely when acute neurological symptoms such as seizures are present. Occipital lobe affectation has been widely described, but recent research opens the scope of brain injury to white matter and to vascular lesions as well.

In the setting of persistent hypoglycaemia, persistent hyperinsulinemic hypoglycaemia, inborn errors of metabolism and endocrine disorders must be ruled out. Specifically, when considering persistent hyperinsulinemic hypoglycaemia, innovations in diagnosis at a molecular and radiological level have been particularly important in terms of differentiating focal from diffuse forms, which, if unresponsive to medical treatment may be candidates for curative partial pancreatectomy.

12. References

Achoki, R., Opiyo, N., English, M. (2010). Mini-revie : Management of hypoglycaemia in children 0-59 months. Journal Tropical Pediatrics, Vol. 56, No.4 (August 2010), pp. 227-34. doi:10.1093/tropej/fmp109. Available on PMC October 2010.

Alkalay, AL., Sarnat, HB., Flores-Sarant, L. et al.(2005a). Neurologic aspects of neonatal hypoglycemia. IMAJ Vol.7 (March 2005) pp:188-191

Alkalay, AL., Flores-Sarnat, L. Sarnat, HB et al. (2005b).Brain imaging findings in neonatal hypoglycemia : case report and review of 23 cases. Clinical Pediatrics (Philadelphia) Vol.44, No.9 (November-December 2005) pp: 783-90.

Arnoux, JB., De Lonlay, P., Hussain, K., et al. (2010). Congenital hyperinsulinism. Eraly Human Delivery. Vol.86, No.5 (June 2010) pp: 287-94

Beardsall, K. (2010). Measurement of glucose levels in the newborn. Early Human Delivery, Vol.86, No.5 (June 2010). pp: 263-7

Burns, CM., Rutherford, MA., Boardman, JP. (2008). Patterns of cerebral injury and neurodevelopmental outcomes after symptomatic neonatal hypoglycaemia. Pediatrics Vol.122 pp: 65-74

Chan, SW. (2011; last updated February 2011). Neonatal hypoglycaemia, in: *Up to Date reviews.* Available at: www.uptodate.com/contents/neonatal-hypoglycemia

Cornblath, M. & Hawdon, JM. (2000). Controversies regarding definition of neonatal hypoglycaemia: suggested operational thresholds. Pediatrics Vol.105, No.5 pp: 1141-5

Diderholm, B. (2009). Perinatal energy metabolism with reference to IUGR & SGA: Studies in pregnant women & newborn infants. Indian Journal Medical Research, Vol.130 (Novembre 2009) pp: 612-17

Desphande, S., Ward Plat, M. (2005). The investigation and management of neonatal hypoglycaemia. Seminars in Fetal and Neonatal Medicine, Vol.10, No.4 (August 2005) pp: 351-61.

Fernández Lorenzo, JR., Pico Couce, M., Fraga Bermúdez, JM. (2011). Hipoglucemia neonatal, in *Protocolos Diagnóstico-terapéuticos de neonatología de la SEN-AEP*, Ergon, ISBN 978-84-8473-908-1, Madrid, Spain.

Filan, PM., Inder, TE., Cameron, FK. et al. (2006). Pediatrics Vol.148, No.4. (April 2006) pp: 552-4

Fugelseth, D. (2001). Neonatal hypglycemia. Dsskr Nor Laegeforen Vol.121, No.14 (May 2001) pp: 1713-6

Garg, M. & Devaskar, SU. (2006). Glucose metabolsim in the late preterm infant. Clinical Perinatology Vol.33, No.4 (December 2006) pp: 853-70

Giurgea, I., Ribeiro, MJ., Boddaert, N., et al. (2005). Congenital hyperinsulinism in newborn and infant. Archives de Pediatrie Vol.12, No.11 (November 2005) pp:1628-35

Gustaffson, J. (2009). Neonatal energy substrate production. Indian Journal Medical Research, Vol.130 (November 2009) pp: 618-23

Hay Jr, WW., Raju, TN., Higgins, RD., Kalhan, SC., Devaskar, SU. (2009). Knowledge gaps and research needs for understanding and treating neonatal hypoglycaemia: workshop report from Eunice Kennedy Shriver National Institute of Child Health and HUmand Development. Journal Pediatrics, Vol.155, No.5 (Novembre 2009) pp: 612-7.

Hussain, K., Blankenstein, O., De Lonlay, P., Christesen, T. (2007). Hyperinsulinaemic hypoglycaemia : biochemical basis and the importance of maintaining normoglycaemia during management. Archives Disease Childhood Vol.92, pp: 567-8- doi: 10.1136/adc.2007.116327

(Kalhan, S. & Peter-Wohl, S. (2000). Hypoglycemia: what is it for the neonate? American Journal Perinatology Vol.17, No.1 pp: 11-8

Kapoor, RR., James, C., Hussain, K. (2009a) Advances in the diagnosis and management of hyperinsulinemic hypoglycemia. Natural Clinical Practice Endocrinology Metabolism Vol.5, No.2 (February 2009) pp: 101-12

Kapoor, RR., Flanagan, SE., James, C. et al. (2009b). Hyperinsulinaemic hypoglycaemia. Archives Disease Childhood Vol.94, No.6 (June 2009) pp: 450-7

Mitanchez, D. (2007). Glucose regulation in preterm newborn infants. Hormone Research Vol.68, (June 2007) pp: 265-71. doi: 10.1159/000104174

Mitanchez, D. (2008). Ontogenesis of glucose regulation in neonate and consequences in neonatal management. Archives de Pediatrie Vol.15, No.1 (January 2008) pp: 64-74.

Simmons, RA. (2007). Glucose metabolism in the newborn infant, in *Workbook in Practical Neonatology,* Richard A. Polin & Mervin C. Yoder, pp. 45-52, Saunders Elsevier, ISBN 978-1-4160-2637-2, Unites States of America.

Rozance, PJ. &Hay Jr, WW. (2006). Hypoglycemia in newborn infants: features associated with adverse outcomes. Biology Neonate. Vol.92, No.2 pp: 74-8

Rozane, PJ % Hay Jr, WW. (2010). Describing hypoglycemia- Definition or operational threshold? Early Human Delivery, Vol.86, No.5 (May 2010) pp: 275-80.

Straussman, S., Levitsky, LL. (2010). Neonatal hypoglycaemia. Current Opinion Endocrinology Diabetes Obseity Vol.17, No.1 (February 2010) pp: 20-4.

Tam, EWY., Widjaja, E., Blase, SI. Et al. (2008). Occipital lobe injury and cortical visual outcomes after neonatal hypoglycaemia. Pediatrics Vol.122 pp: 507-12

Vannucci, RC. & Vannucci, SJ. (2001). Hypoglycemic brain injury. Seminars in Neonatology Vol.6, No.2 (April 2001) pp: 147-55

Ward Platt, M., Desphande, S. (2005). Metabolic adaptation at birth. Seminars in Fetal and Neonatal Medicine Vol.10, No.4 (August 2005) pp: 341-50

Wayenberg, JL. & Pardou, A. (2008). Moderate hypoglycaemia in preterm infant: is it relevant? H Pediatrie Vol.15, No.2 pp: 153-6

Wight, NE. (2006). Hypoglycemia in breastfed neonates. Breastfeed Medicine Vol.1, No.4 (winter 2006) pp: 253-62

Wilker, RE. (2004). Hipoglucemia e hiperglucemia, in *Manual de Cuidados Neonatalesr,* John P. Cloherty & Ann R. Stark, pp. 615-623, Masson, ISBN 84-458-0740-4, Barcelona, Spain.

Williams, AF. (2005). Neonatal Hypoglycaemia: clinical and legal aspects. Seminars in Fetal and Neonatal Medicine Vol.10, o.4 (August 2005) pp: 363-48

6

Glucose Infusions into Peripheral Veins in Neonates with Hypoglycemia

Outti Tammela and Tarja Vanhatalo
Pediatric Research Centre, University of Tampere
Finland

1. Introduction

Intravenous glucose infusions into peripheral veins are often needed, in addition to oral feedings, to elevate blood glucose levels in the management of neonatal hypoglycemia. Central venous catheters are rarely inserted, when the duration of such treatment is less than a few days. More than half of peripheral venous cannulations extravasate by 36 h, or even faster, if medication is administered concomitantly (Möller et al., 1996, Hecker et al., 1991). Complications, including local swelling and in the worst cases damage to tissue may occur. Intravenous solutions containing 10 or 15 percent glucose are most commonly used in hypoglycemic infants. A glucose concentration of 15% has generally been regarded as the highest acceptable for use in solutions infused into peripheral veins in neonates. (Kien, 1993). However, 10% and even 15% glucose infusions increase fluid load especially in patients, who need high glucose intakes to reach sufficient energy intake or to maintain normal plasma glucose levels. Although large fluid volumes of short duration are well tolerated in neonates (Leake, et al, 1976), the effect of continuous rapid infusions on the fluid clearance have not been determined. First voiding might be delayed due to elevated Arginine vasopressin levels in newborn infants delivered vaginally after a prolonged and stressful labor (Vuohelainen T et al., 2007 and 2008). A poor fluid tolerance during the first days of life can be anticipated and cautious fluid administration might be indicated especially in such infants.

Earlier studies suggest that the development of phlebitis does not depend so much on the osmolarity of the solution as other factors causing phlebitis, for example material of the catheter (Madan et al., 1992). Factors affecting the development of infusion phlebitis include vein characteristics, size and material of the catheter, duration of infusion and the osmolarity and pH of the infusion solution. Experimental infusions of 10% glucose with electrolytes (pH 4.93, osmolarity 727 mOsm/kg) into rabbit ear veins cause phlebitis by reason of its acidity and an infusion of amino acids (pH 6.29, osmolarity 929 mOsm/kg) by reason of its high osmolarity. On the other hand, admixture of these solutions causes only minor phlebitic changes and the fluid components eliminate each others' damaging effects on the tissue (Kuwahara et al., 1998a). In the same animal model, the tolerance of peripheral venous endothelial cells was for 8 h in 820 mOsm/kg, 12 h in 690 mOsm/kg and 24 h in 550 mOsm/kg solutions, respectively, suggesting that a planned volume of solutions with high osmolarity should be infused rapidly rather than slowly to avoid the development of phlebitis (Kuwahara et al. 1998b). In the management of hypoglycemia, however, only continuous

infusions can be used. In such occasions the effect of the infusion rate on the risk of phlebitis seems not have been established. Earlier surveys suggest that high infusion flow rates might even markedly increase the risk of infusion failure (Hecker 1989, Hecker, et al 1991).
The occurrence of phlebitis has been evaluated in adults in a comparison of peripheral infusions of nutrient solutions with and without 20% fat emulsion (Daly et al., 1985). Adding fat to the fluids did not protect the veins from the development of phlebitis. Infiltration was more dependent on the catheters than on the osmolarity of solutions. In keeping with this, peripheral intravenous nutrition caused phlebitis in all patients using Teflon cannulas, but in only 7% using silicone catheters. The risk of phlebitis was very low even when nutrition solutions of an osmolarity of 1250 mOsm/kg were administered via the latter catheters (Madan et al., 1992).
Glucose solutions are acid and hyperosmolar, the 15% solution pH ranging between 3.5–5.5 and osmolarity 832.5 mOsm/kg and the 20% solution 4.0 and 1110 mOsm/kg. In spite of this, the latter solution might be a better choice in the management of hypoglycemia, because the fluid administration rate of the 20% solution to reach the same glucose intake is 25% lower compared to 15% glucose solution. Thus, risk of excessive fluid load can be decreased by using 20% glucose instead of 15% glucose infusion. As far as we know no earlier studies comparing the infusions of 15 % and 20% glucose into peripheral veins of newborn infants have been done.
The purpose of our study was to evaluate, whether peripheral intravenous 20% glucose solutions are as well tolerated as 15% glucose solutions in the management of neonatal hypoglycemia.

2. Patients and methods

The study was undertaken in the neonatal unit of Tampere University Hospital (Vanhatalo and Tammela, 2010). Newborn infants with hypoglycemia for which initiation of intravenous glucose infusion was prescribed at the discretion of the attending physician, were included in the study if they fulfilled the following criteria: (1) birth weight of 2000 g or more, (2) no significant malformations diagnosed, (3) intensive care not needed, (4) written informed consent obtained from the parents. Infants in intensive care were excluded in order to minimize confounding factors, including need of vasoactive infusions and/or multiple intravenous medications.
Hypoglycemia was defined as a plasma glucose level below 2.6 mmol/L and hyperglycemia as above 7.7 mmol/L. All infants received either their own mother's or banked pooled breast milk. On-demand breast and/or bottle feeding was preferred. Breast-fed infants were weighed before and after feedings, in order to measure the ingested milk volume. The minimum cumulative amount of breast milk was 80 mL, divided by 8-10 feedings, in the first day of life. The cumulative milk volume was daily increased by 80 mL, up to 170 mL/kg/day. Increasing the daily number of oral feedings was the first treatment for hypoglycemia. Gavage feeding was used in babies, who were sucking poorly. Intravenous glucose infusion was started at the discretion of the attending physician in cases with symptomatic hypoglycemia, recurrent blood glucose levels below 2.6 mmol/L, in spite of increased oral or tube feedings, and in hypoglycemic infants, who tolerated poorly enteral feedings. The infants were randomized to receive either 20% (group 20%, 60 infants) or 15% (group 15%, 61 infants) peripheral intravenous glucose infusions at an initiation glucose intake rate of 8 mg/kg/min, i.e. 2.4 mL/kg/h in the group 20% and 3.2 mL/kg/h in the 15% group.

The group allocation of each patient was written in a sealed envelope, which was opened after the written consent was received from the parents. Because infusion rates were dependent on the glucose concentration the group allocation was not possible to be blinded.
The infants' plasma glucose levels were measured every 4 h and the infusion rate reduced after each measurement by 0.5 mL/kg/h at blood glucose levels between 3.5-4 mmol/L and by 1 mL/kg/h at blood glucose levels above 4 mmol/L. The infusion was stopped when the plasma glucose level was 3.5 mmol/L or higher at an infusion rate of 2 mL/h. Plasma glucose surveillance was continued, until levels had remained normal (more than 2.9 mmoL/L) for 24 h after discontinuation of the glucose infusion. When the cannulation site had to be changed, local signs of phlebitis at the previous site were scored from 0 to 3 using a modified Maddox scale (Maddox and Rush, 1977), by the attending physician. Cumulative severity, i.e. the sum of scores for phlebitis, was calculated during the infusion period. Number of cannulation site changes, duration of intravenous infusions and daily weights of the infants were recorded. Weight changes were calculated as percentages of birth weight. Preterm infants were born at less than 37 weeks' gestational ages. Infants with birth weight less than 2 SD from the mean for gestational age were defined as small for gestational age (SGA).

0 No pain around the tip of the catheter, no color, no redness, no hardening, vein not hard when palpated.
1+ Pain around the tip of the catheter and redness
2+ Pain around the tip of the catheter, redness and swelling
3+ Pain around the tip of the catheter, redness, swelling and hardening

Table 1. Modified Maddox score scale (Maddox and Rush, 1977): observation criteria for phlebitis.

2.1 Statistical analysis

Irritation in the site of infusion, number of cannula site changes and weight gain were chosen as primary end points. The sample size was calculated on the assumption that either glucose solution might reduce the mean number of cannula site changes from 1.5 to 1.0. With 80% power and statistical significance level below 0.05 the sample size would be 57 in each group. The dropout rate was estimated to be about 5%, and thus the goal was to recruit 60 infants for both groups.
t-test, Mann-Whitney *U*-test and analysis of variance for repeated measures were used in the statistical analysis, as appropriate. P-value less than 0.05 was regarded as statistically significant.
The ethical committee of the hospital had approved the study.

3. Results

During the study period, hypoglycemia was diagnosed in 465 neonates. Of these, 108 did not fulfill the inclusion criteria; 357 were eligible. The parents refused consent in 12 of these cases and in 224 cases the attending physician had no possibility to request consent because of lack of time, or lack of possibility to contact the mother. Sixty infants were allocated to the group 20% and 61 to the group 15%. (Figure 1)

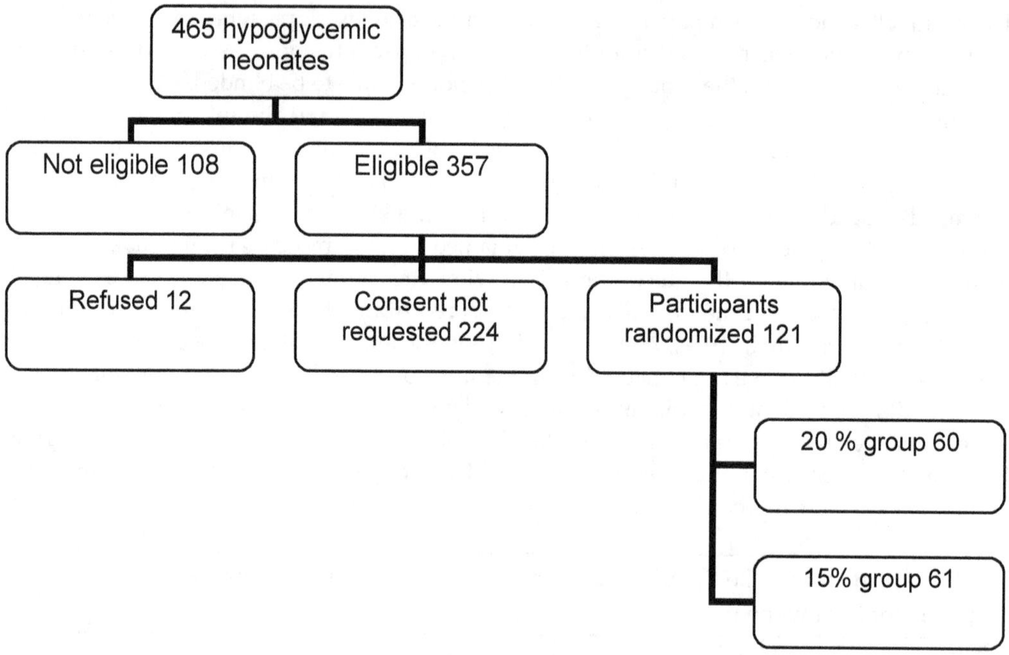

Fig. 1. Allocation of the study groups

The infants in the 20% and 15% groups were born at similar (mean (SD)) weeks' gestation (group 20% 39 (1.5) weeks vs. group 15% 39 (1.3) weeks) and birth weights (3605 (593) g vs. 3486 (626) g, respectively). Female/male ratios did not differ (23/38 vs. 24/36).
Similar percentages of infants in both groups had been delivered via caesarean section, were SGA or had birth weights >4500 g (Table 2). Few cases in either group were born from twin pregnancies and asphyxia was rare. Prematurity, need for phototherapy and antibiotic

	20% Glucose group	**15% Glucose group**
	N (%)	**N (%)**
Cesarean section	7 (12)	6 (11)
Small for gestational age (SGA)	0 (0)	2 (5)
Birth weight > 4500 g	2 (3)	3 (5)
Female/male	24/36	23/38
Twins	3 (5)	2 (3)
Premature	8 (13)	4 (7)
Five minute Apgar score < 7	2 (3)	4 (7)
Phototherapy	20 (33)	14 (23)
Intravenous antibiotics	12 (20)	6 (11)

The differences between the groups were not statistically significant

Table 2. Clinical characteristics of the infants in the study groups

treatment due to suspected or confirmed infection was more common in the group 20%, but the differences did not reach statistical significance. About half of the cases in both groups were infants of diabetic mothers (mean 30 (SD 49) % vs. 30 (SD 50) %). In the group 20%, 25 mothers and in the group 15%, 21 mothers had gestational diabetes, five versus nine mothers had type 1diabetes and seven versus 12 mothers were on insulin medication in the 20 and 15% groups, respectively, NS. Three mothers had pre-eclampsia in the group 20% and five in the group 15%. Ten mothers had hypertension in the group 20% and six in the group 15%. Ten mothers had signs of chorioamnionitis at delivery in the group 20% and six in the group 15%, respectively.

The concentrations of electrolytes in the glucose solutions, adjusted according to the plasma sodium and potassium levels, were similar in the two groups: the mean (SD) sodium concentrations being 38 (15) mmol/L versus 39 (12) mmol/L and potassium concentrations 12 mmol/L versus 13 mmol/L, respectively. Seven (12%) infants in the group 20% and 11 (18%) in the group 15% also received antibiotic treatment, the mean durations of antibiotic treatment being 6.0 (0.6) versus 5.2 (1.3) days, NS.

The mean (SD) duration of cannulation was in the group 20% 4.2 (1.4) days and in the group 15% 3.9 (1.3) days, NS. The number of cannulation site changes were median 1 (range 0–5) in the group 20% and 1 (range 0–6) in the group 15%, respectively, NS. In the 20% group 35 infants (59%) and in the 15% group 36 (60%) had some signs of phlebitis, NS. The cumulative severity score for phlebitis was low in both groups, in the 20% glucose group a median of 1 (range 0–7) and in the 15% group 1 (range 0–8), NS.

When the infants, who received antibiotics, were omitted, in infants receiving only intravenous glucose infusions, the mean (SD) duration of cannulation was in the group 20% 4.0 (1.3) days and in the group 15% 4.0 (1.3) days, NS. The number of cannulation site changes were median 1 (range 0–6), and 1 (range 0–5), respectively, NS. In the 20% group 31 (63%) and in the 15% group 33 infants (61%) had some signs of phlebitis, NS. The cumulative severity score for phlebitis was in the 20% group median 1 (range 0–8) and in the 15% glucose group 1.5 (range 0–8), NS.

Average plasma glucose levels were similar in both groups in the 20% group 4.6 (0.41) and in the 15% group 4.5 (0.37) mmol/L. High plasma glucose levels occurred in nine cases in the 20% glucose group and in 11 in the 15% group, and low levels in 37 versus 43 infants in the 20% and 15% groups, respectively, NS.

Weight as a function of infusion time and relative weight changes in the two groups were similar (Figure 2), NS.

4. Discussion

A recruitment bias is possible in this cohort in that the attending physician was not able to contact some mothers to obtain informed consent. A significant number of eligible infants were thus left out. This circumstance can be explained by the fact that a substantial proportion of hypoglycemia cases are admitted outside office hours, during which time the paediatricians on call are often too busy, and during the night reluctant to disturb the parents' sleep in order to recruit their baby for the study. It is also not possible to postpone the start of intravenous glucose infusion for long in hypoglycemic patients.

Maternal diabetes mellitus is one of the most important risk factors for neonatal hypoglycemia, and its severity might affect the need and duration of intravenous glucose infusion of the infants. Both small and large birth weight for gestational age might also be

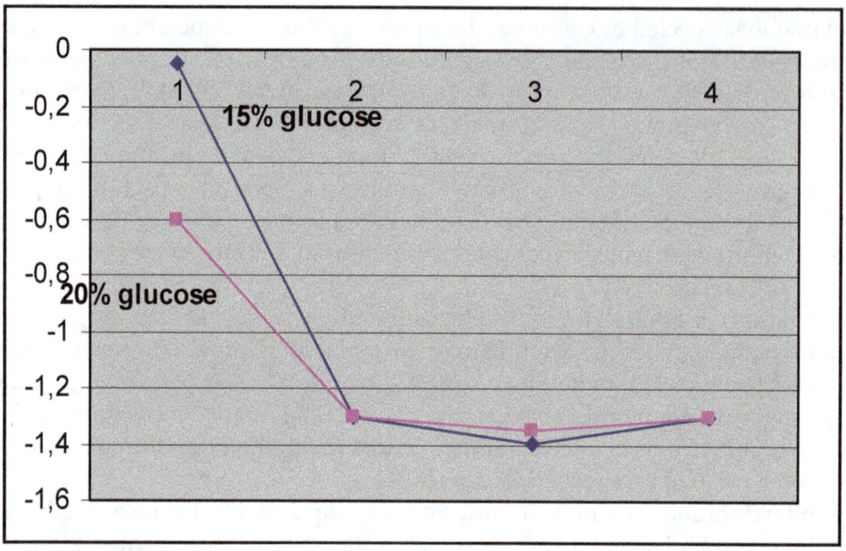

Fig. 2. Relative change in weight (% from birth weight) during intravenous glucose infusion. Circles indicate the 15% glucose and squares the 20% glucose group. X axis: weight changes. Y axis: time (days).

associated with a prolonged need of intravenous glucose infusion. The groups were, however, quite well matched for the percentages of mothers having gestational diabetes, type 1diabetes, for receiving insulin medication, and percentages of either SGA or LGA infants. Breast milk feeding is a cornerstone in the prevention and management of neonatal hypoglycemia, and weaning from intravenous glucose infusion is not possible without a successful feeding. The same feeding protocol was used in both groups.

Concomitant use of intravenous antibiotics during intravenous glucose infusion increases obviously the risk of phlebitis, and is therefore a confounding factor in the comparison between 15% and 20% glucose groups. The percentage of infants receiving antibiotics was somewhat, although not significantly higher in the 20% group. The higher osmolarity of the 20% glucose solution was, however, not associated with an increased rate or severity of phlebitis in our infants. In addition, omitting the antibiotic-treated cases did not change the result. The electrolyte concentrations in the 15 % and 20 % glucose infusion fluids were similar. As intravenous glucose was administered at the same rate (mg/kg/min) in both study groups, the 15% glucose group received fluids at a 33% higher rate than the 20% glucose group. The differences in fluid infusion rates might even have balanced the local effect of different glucose concentrations on the vessel wall at the infusion site.

The clinical classification of phlebitis also involves risk of bias, as observation and classification is subjective. The observers rating the severity of the phlebitis were not aware of the glucose concentration used in each case. Accidental detachment of intravenous lines occurs only rarely and the most common reason for a cannulation site change is local irritation and swelling at the infusion site. The number of cannulation site changes would thus seem to be a fairly objective measure of extravasation of fluids. According to earlier work, extravasation of peripheral fluid infusions occurs by 36 h in more than half of the patients (Möller, et al., 1996, Hecker et al.,1991). In our patients the mean duration of cannulation was about four days in both groups, suggesting that the median number of

cannulation changes in the cases on both groups is in accordance with the previous data. Thus, the duration of cannulation, number of cannulation changes and phlebitis severity scores were similar in both groups. One can assume, that the safety of peripheral 20 or 15% glucose intravenous infusions is similar also in neonates, who need intravenous glucose infusions for other reasons than hypoglycemia, including short-term parenteral nutrition.
The occurrence of phlebitis has been evaluated in adults in a comparison of peripheral infusions of nutrient solutions with and without 20% fat emulsion (Daly JM et al., 1985). Adding fat to the fluids did not protect the veins from the development of phlebitis. Infiltration was more dependent on the catheters than on the osmolarity of solutions. In keeping with this, peripheral intravenous nutrition caused phlebitis in all patients using Teflon cannulas, but in only 7% using silicone catheters. The risk of phlebitis was very low even when nutrition solutions of an osmolarity of 1250 mOsm/kg were administered via the latter catheters (Madan M et al., 1992). In our study, the same peripheral catheters were used in both groups and therefore the role of catheter type in the development of phlebitis cannot be established here.
Although infants in the 20% glucose group received 33% less fluids than those in the 15% group, no differences in weight changes were seen. Our infants were all quite healthy, having no or mild neonatal problems in addition to hypoglycemia and would thus seem to tolerate excess amounts of fluids well. Our study was not powered to establish, whether less fluid intake would be beneficial by decreasing risk of respiratory problems and need of oxygen supplementation in the 20% glucose group compared to the 15% glucose group. In patients who do not tolerate fluids normally, as in cases of birth asphyxia, renal failure, bronchopulmonary dysplasia or inappropriate antidiuretic hormone excretion, reduction of fluid intake by using 20% instead of 15% glucose might have beneficial effect on the outcome of the patient.

5. Conclusion

Intravenous 20% glucose solutions can be infused into peripheral veins as safely as 15% glucose solutions. The risks of excess fluid intake, in addition to oral feeding, need to be established in further studies in infants with neonatal hypoglycemia.

6. References

Daly JM, Masser RN, Hansen L, Canham JE. Peripheral vein infusion of dextrose/amino acid solutions ± 20% fat emulsion. *J Parent Ent Nutr* 1985; **9**: 296. ecker JF (1989) Failure of intravenous infusions from extravasation and phlebitis. *Anaesth Intensive care* Vol 17, No. 4 November 1989), pp 433-449, ISSN 0310-057X

Hecker JF, Duffy BJ, Fong T& Wyer M (1991) Failure of intravenous infusion in neonates. *J Paediatr Child Health* Vol. 27. No. 4. (June 1991), pp 175-179, ISSN 1034-4810

Kien CL. Carbohydrates. In: Tsang RC, Lucas A, UayR, ZlotkinS, editors. *Nutritional needs of the preterm infant: nutritional.* New York : Caduceus Medical Publishers Inc, 1993: 47–63.

Leake RD, Zakauddin S, Trygstad CW, Fu P, Oh W (1976) The effects of large volume intravenous fluid infusion on neonatal renal function. J Pediatr Vol 89, No. 6 (June 1976), pp 968-972, ISSN 0022-3476

Kuwahara T, Asanami S, Tamura T, Kaneda S. Effects of pH and osmolality on phlebitic potential of infusion solutions for peripheral parenteral nutrition. *J Toxicol Sci* 1998; 23: 77–85, ISSN 0388-1350

Kuwahara T, Asanami S, Kubo S. Experimental infusion phlebitis: tolerance osmolality of peripheral venous endothelial cells. *Nutrition* 1998; 14: 496–501, ISSN 0899-9007

Madan M, Alexander DJ, McMahon MJ. Influence of catheter type on occurrence of thrombophlebitis during peripheral intravenous nutrition. *Lancet* 1992; 339: 101–3, ISSN 0140-6736

Maddox RR, Rush DR. Double-blind study to investigate methods to prevent cephalotin-induced phlebitis. *Am J Hosp Pharm* 1977; 34: 29–34, ISSN 0002-9289

Möller JC, Reiss I, Schaible Th. Vascular access in neonates and infants - indications, routes, techniques and devices, complications. *Intensive Care World* 1995; 12: 48–53.

Vanhatalo T, Tammela O. Glucose infusions into peripheral veins in the management of neonatal hypoglycemia--20% instead of 15%?. *Acta Pædiatr* 2010;99:350-353, ISSN 0803-5253

Vuohelainen T, Ojala R, Virtanen A, Laatta J, Mörsky P, Uotila J and Tammela O (2002). Predictors of AVP and TSH levels and the timing of first voiding in the newborn. *Pediatr Res* 2007, Vol 62, No 1 (Jul 2007), pp. 106-110, ISSN 0031-3998

Vuohelainen T, Ojala R, Virtanen A, Holm P and Tammela O (2001). Predictors of delayed first voiding in newborn. *Acta Paediatr* 2008, Vol 97, No 7 (July 2008), pp. 904-908, ISSN 0803-5253

7

An Update on Neonatal Hypoglycemia

Praveen Kumar and Shiv Sajan Saini
Neonatal Unit, Department of Pediatrics,
Postgraduate Institute of Medical Education and Research, Chandigarh
INDIA

1. Introduction

Glucose is the predominant source of energy for the fetal and neonatal brain. During the process of adaptation from a continuous supply of glucose in-utero to an intermittent supply after birth, the neonate is prone to periods of low blood glucose. Transient mild decreases in blood glucose levels are a common feature of perinatal adaptation. This period is characterized by an up-regulation of hormonal and metabolic pathways of gluconeogenesis, hepatic glycogenolysis and ketogenesis. However, in some neonates, these may be delayed and hypoglycemia may get prolonged or severe. Persistent, recurrent or severe hypoglycemia may cause irreversible injury to the developing brain. Hence, the neonatologist needs to be proactive in suspecting, diagnosing and treating hypoglycemia in the newborn.

The normal range of blood glucose is different for each newborn and depends upon birth-weight, gestational age, body stores, feeding status, availability of energy sources as well as the presence or absence of disease. Population based meta-analyses have revealed that the blood glucose levels rise with increasing post natal age. Although, there are controversies surrounding the definition, a blood glucose <40 mg/dL is considered as the operational threshold to treat hypoglycemia in all neonates in first few days of life, irrespective of gestation. Hypoglycemia is the most common metabolic disorder in the neonatal intensive care unit. The reported incidence of hypoglycemia varies with the definition, population, glucose measurement technique and feeding schedule. Preterm infants and those with intrauterine growth retardation are at a high risk of developing hypoglycemia in the first week of life because of lack of sufficient glycogen and fat stores, which are normally accumulated in the third trimester. In some preterm infants, developmental delays in the postnatal up-regulation of enzymes of glucose homeostasis may persist even at the time of discharge from hospital. Large for gestational age infants and infants of diabetic mothers are the other important high risk groups because of relative hyperinsulinemia. A proportion of small for gestational age infants also have high insulin levels which contribute to hypoglycemia and can persist for few weeks to months. Recently, late preterm ($34^{0/7}$ to $36^{6/7}$weeks) infants have been identified as another important group prone to hypoglycemia. In addition, any sick newborn warrants screening for low blood glucose. Term healthy infants without any risk factors need not be monitored routinely. All asymptomatic, at-risk neonates should be screened at two hours after birth and surveillance should be continued 4-6 hourly thereafter, until feedings are well established and glucose values have normalized; which may take 48-72 hours. Monitoring before 2 hours may be required if mother has been starving or vomiting. The maximum risk for hypoglycemia is in first 24 hours but usually persists till 72 hours.

The prevention of hypoglycemic brain injury requires early detection in infants considered 'at risk' and appropriate timely intervention. Detection and treatment of hypoglycemia requires accurate, rapid and reliable measurement of blood glucose. This is usually done on the bedside by glucose reagent strips. If the values are low, a blood sample is sent to the laboratory for confirmation by glucose oxidase or glucose electrode method. The treatment should be given on the basis of screening test and not await laboratory results. Most of the point-of-care strip based glucometers are however unsuitable for neonates because they were primarily developed to measure higher blood glucose levels in diabetic patients. Their accuracy in low blood glucose ranges is not good. Current blood gas machines incorporate a glucose sensor which is more accurate but may require a larger blood volume. Treatment of hypoglycemia should be based upon 'operational thresholds' and clinical assessment. Symptomatic hypoglycemia with neurological signs requires more urgent treatment by intravenous route, as compared to the 'asymptomatic' baby, irrespective of blood glucose value. Supervised and measured volume milk feeding may be an initial treatment option for asymptomatic hypoglycemia in healthy infants. However, symptomatic hypoglycemia should always be treated with a continuous infusion of parenteral dextrose. Intravenous dextrose infusion should be started in babies with asymptomatic hypoglycemia if the blood glucose is <25 mg/dL, blood glucose remains below 40 mg/dL despite one attempt of feeding milk, enteral feeding is contraindicated or if the baby becomes symptomatic. If there is no contraindication to feeding, oral feeds of breast or formula milk should be continued along with and their proportion increased as the intravenous infusion is tapered. Oral feeding ensures a more stable glycemic control.

Symptomatic hypoglycemia, especially if manifesting as seizures, is associated with abnormal neurodevelopmental outcomes in 50% of infants. Moderate asymptomatic hypoglycemia persisting for 3 to 5 days is also associated with 30% to 40% incidence of neurodevelopmental sequelae. Neuroimaging in infants with severe hypoglycemia shows involvement of the occipital lobes in 82%. Occipital brain injury can cause visual impairment, epilepsy and long-term disability. Cortical visual deficits are seen in a significant proportion of infants with recurrent hypoglycemia and correlate significantly with low mesial occipital apparent diffusion coefficient values on diffusion weighted MRI. All infants with hypoglycemia should be followed up for neurodevelopmental sequelae.

Refractory or persistent hypoglycemia should be suspected and investigated if the glucose infusion requirement is >12 mg/kg/min or the hypoglycemia persists >5-7 days, respectively. Hyperinsulinemic hypoglycemia is the most important cause of severe and persistent hypoglycemia after initial few days. The risk for brain injury and subsequent neurodevelopment handicap is significantly greater with hyperinsulinemic hypoglycemia. Hyperinsulinemic hypoglycemia may persist for many weeks to months and then remit spontaneously, particularly in growth retarded and stressed neonates. In such infants, the hypoglycemia nearly always responds to medications like diazoxide. Several forms of congenital hyperinsulinism also present with hypoglycemia in neonates that does not remit. Depending on the type of genetic mutation, hypoglycemia in these infants with congenital hyperinsulinism may be controlled medically or may require surgery. The extent of surgery required in infants with ATP-dependent potassium channel mutations unresponsive to diazoxide is dependent upon whether the histological subtype is focal or diffuse. Advances

in molecular genetics, positron emission tomography scanning and minimally invasive surgery have completely changed the clinical approach to these infants.
Certain clinical practices can help prevent the occurrence of hypoglycemia. These include support and promotion of early exclusive breastfeeds within first hour of life in all healthy newborns. Delayed initiation of breast feeds is an important risk factor for hypoglycemia. Maintenance of thermoneutral environment in small infants helps prevent hypoglycemia and skin to skin contact with mother should be encouraged as a strategy for temperature maintenance. Oral dextrose solutions should not be used as a substitute for breast milk. Plain dextrose feeding can induce vomiting and will cause increased insulin secretion, decreased glucagon, delayed gluconeogenesis and rebound hypoglycemia. In infants receiving intravenous infusions, it should be ensured that there is no interruption in the glucose infusion by maintaining a good intravenous access and using a syringe infusion pump to deliver at a steady rate.
In this chapter, we discuss the controversies behind the definition of hypoglycemia, glucose metabolism in fetal and neonatal brain, biochemical derangements during hypoglycemia, clinical correlates and pathological manifestations of hypoglycemia, management issues and the rare entity of persistent hypoglycemia of infancy.

2. Definition

The literal meaning of hypoglycemia is low level of glucose in blood. The 'low level' is however difficult to define in neonates due to the several reasons. First, their nervous system does not have sufficient maturity and capacity to manifest the signs and symptoms of hypoglycemia in a consistent fashion, below the 'low level' of blood glucose. The 'critical limit' of blood glucose required for normal integrity of neonatal brain function is currently not fully understood. Secondly, the 'low blood glucose' levels often occur in association with other biological insults. In presence of these insults, the 'low blood glucose level' limits are likely to be higher as compared to isolated cases of hypoglycemia. These insults e.g. hypoxemia, ischemia, asphyxia, acidosis etc. might have a role in potentiating hypoglycemic brain injury in the vulnerable sick newborn (Volpe, 2008). Hence, the 'normal' range of blood glucose is different for each newborn and depends upon birth-weight, gestational age, body stores, feeding status, availability of energy sources as well as the presence or absence of disease.

2.1 Clinical definition

In early nineteenth century, clinical manifestations (lethargy, tremor, sweating, cyanosis, jitteriness, hypotonia, coma, and seizures) were recognized as the only responses to hypoglycemia. Working definition of hypoglycemia was the 'low blood glucose levels' at which the clinical manifestations were noticed (Hartmann et al., 1960; Brown & Wallis 1963; Cornblath et al., 2000). These clinical manifestations are however nonspecific and can occur with many other neonatal illnesses e.g. sepsis, hypothermia, hypoxic-ischemic brain injury etc. Certain signs like jitteriness can be present even in normal healthy neonates. Therefore clinically significant hypoglycemia is diagnosed if Whipple's triad (Whipple & Frantz 1935) is present. Whipple's triad is defined as: (a) the presence of characteristic clinical manifestations, (b) clinical manifestations occurring in presence of low plasma glucose concentrations, and (c) the clinical signs resolve within minutes to hours, after normalization of blood glucose. It is possible to make clinical diagnosis confidently when all three requirements are met.

However, there are several limitations with this clinical definition. The levels of blood glucose at which clinical manifestations appear may be different from the levels at which biochemical injury occurs leading to long term neurological sequelae. This clinical definition does not take into account clinically asymptomatic neonates who have 'low blood glucose' i.e. "asymptomatic hypoglycemia". Asymptomatic hypoglycemia can also cause hypoglycemic brain injury (Griffiths, 1968; Griffiths & Bryant, 1971; Lucas et al., 1988). The presence or absence of such signs cannot be used reliably to discriminate between normal and low blood glucose levels. Nevertheless presence of clinical signs of encephalopathy such as decreased level of consciousness or seizures should alert the physician for possibility of cerebral fuel deficiency.

2.2 Metabolic definition

Low blood glucose concentrations stimulate counter-regulatory hormonal response in order to increase the blood glucose. With the decrease in blood glucose levels, plasma insulin levels decrease and plasma glucagon levels increase (Sperling et al., 1974). There is increase in serum levels of cortisol, epinephrine, and growth hormone levels as well. The concentration of alternative brain fuels e.g. lactate and ketone bodies also increase in presence of low blood glucose (Persson et al., 1972; Adam et al., 1975; Vannucci et al., 1981). The concentration of blood glucose at which counter-regulatory hormonal response is elicited, may be utilized to define 'acceptable' lower limit of blood glucose. However, there is little information available for the thresholds levels of blood glucose in neonates for the counter-regulatory hormonal stress response, autonomic and neuroglycopenic signs, as well as impaired cognitive function; which have been described in adults (Mitrakou et al., 1991; Ward Platt & Deshpande, 2005). Additionally, preterm neonates are unable to mount a mature counter-regulatory response to low blood glucose levels, making this judgment unsuitable for this population (Hawdon et al., 1992).

2.3 Neurophysiological definition

With fall in blood glucose levels, there may be changes in neurophysiological functions, which can be recorded in form of evoked potentials. Few authors have attempted to measure neurophysiological changes in response to neuroglycopenia. Koh et al. described abnormalities of brain-stem auditory or somatosensory evoked potentials in some children having blood glucose less than 2.6 mmol/L (Koh et al., 1988). None of the children with blood glucose concentrations of ≥2.6 mmol/L showed changes in neurophysiological functions. The authors suggested that 2.6 mmol/L of blood glucose may be taken as a safe threshold in neonates and children. However, there were only five term neonates included in this study. The concentrations of alternative fuels were not measured consistently during this study. Moreover, researchers failed to reproduce distinct threshold to diagnose hypoglycemia on the basis of evoked potentials in both term and preterm babies (Pryds et al., 1988; Cowett et al., 1997).

Positron emission tomography has been utilized to study changes in cerebral blood flow during hypoglycemia among preterm newborn infants (Koh et al., 1988; Pryds et al., 1988). However, resolution of these abnormalities in response to glucose administration needs to be documented to attribute these abnormalities to significant hypoglycemia. Pryds et al. compared hypoglycemic infants (N=13, mean birth weight - 1,500 g) and normoglycemic controls (N=12, mean birth weight - 1,310 g) for the cerebral blood flow and plasma epinephrine and norepinephrine responses. Hypoglycemia was defined as a blood glucose less than 30 mg/dL. Cerebral blood flow and plasma epinephrine concentrations were increased among hypoglycemic infants. There was no difference in norepinephrine levels. Among hypoglycemic neonates, cerebral flow decreased by 11% after correction of blood glucose. The data suggests that counter-regulatory mechanisms are stimulated below blood glucose values of less than 30 to 45 mg/dL (Pryds et al., 1990).

2.4 Neurodevelopmental approach to define hypoglycemia

Clinical risk of hypoglycemia can be correlated with neurodevelopmental outcome. In a follow-up study of 661 infants weighing less than 1850 g at birth, Lucas et al identified a significantly strong association between the number of days (≥5d) on which blood glucose concentrations of <2.6 mmol/L(<47 mg/dL) were found and lower Bayley developmental scores at 18 months of age (Lucas et al., 1988). The major limitations of this study were non-standardized monitoring of blood glucose, and effect of unidentified confounders with the result that the 'safe' plasma glucose concentrations still cannot be reliably extrapolated. The low plasma glucose concentrations may have been a proxy for extreme illness because such protracted hypoglycemia lasting for 5 days is rare. At 8 years, however, this association was not sustained, and another study in a different large cohort has also failed to replicate this finding (Cornblath & Schwartz, 1999; Williams, 2005).

2.5 Statistical definition

Conventionally, hypoglycemia is defined by a value lying outside the 'normality distribution of the range of values obtained in a healthy population'. 'Low' is arbitrarily defined as a value, 2-standard deviations (SD), below the mean of the population. The major caveat is this approach is that the blood glucose concentrations in a cohort of normal population represent a continuum, and it is not possible to pick a single value that could represent a threshold of abnormality. Those 'minus 2-SD' cutoff value would vary with the gestational age, postnatal age, type of feeding and physiological state e.g. post or pre-feed (Srinivasan et al., 1986; Hawdon et al., 1992; de Rooy & Hawdon, 2002). Moreover, this 'statistical' abnormality cannot be taken as 'biological' abnormality. Technical issues, including discrepancy between values obtained from whole blood and plasma, and the low sensitivity of reagent strip for hypoglycemic range of blood glucose, are also deterrent for such an approach. This may partly explain the lack of consensus between physicians and standard texts in the field. A major criticism of the 'normal range' approach to deriving a treatment yardstick is that it does not consider the complexities of the metabolic milieu, the availability of alternative substrates and the clinical condition of the baby (Koh et al., 1988; Williams, 1997; Williams, 2005).

2.6 Operational thresh-holds

Cornblath et al have suggested a pragmatic way to give cut-off values of blood glucose on which the action should be taken (Cornblath et al., 2000). An "operational threshold " is not diagnostic of a disease, but an indication for action. These recommendations are conservative approximations of designating the lower level of normoglycemia that one can safely tolerate in specific infants, at specific ages and under established conditions. It is difficult to define significant hypoglycemia by a single cut-off value that can be applied universally. Rather, it is characterized by a value(s) that is unique to each individual and varies with both their state of physiologic maturity and the influence of pathology. It can be defined as the concentration of glucose in the blood or plasma at which the individual demonstrates a unique response to the abnormal milieu caused by the inadequate delivery of glucose to a target organ (for example, the brain).

The operational thresholds may not be applicable to breastfed infants as they have higher concentrations of ketone bodies than formula-fed infants despite having lower blood glucose concentrations (Hawdon et al., 1992; Swenne et al., 1994). The production of ketone bodies among breastfed infants is directly proportional to postnatal weight loss. These data suggest that the provision of alternate fuels constitutes a normal adaptive response to transiently low nutrient intake during the establishment of breastfeeding. These infants may well tolerate lower plasma glucose levels without any significant clinical manifestations or sequelae. However any symptomatic infant with clinical signs consistent with low blood glucose concentration should be treated if the blood glucose levels are <45 mg/dL (2.5 mmol/L). Operational thresh-holds are different among neonates, who are at risk of hypoglycemia as a result of alteration in maternal metabolism, intrinsic neonatal problems, or anticipated or perceived endocrine or metabolic disorders. If the plasma glucose concentration is less than 36 mg/dL (2.0 mmol/L), a close surveillance should be maintained, and intervention is recommended if plasma glucose remains below this level, if the level does not increase after a feed, or if abnormal clinical signs develop. At very low glucose concentrations (<20–25 mg/dL, 1.1–1.4 mmol/L), intravenous glucose infusion aimed at raising the plasma glucose levels above 45 mg/dL (2.5 mmol/L) is indicated. The higher therapeutic goal is chosen to include a significant margin of safety in the absence of any data evaluating the correlation between glucose levels in this range and long-term outcome in full-term infants. The operational thresh-hold suggested for the infants on parenteral nutrition is 45 mg/dL (Cornblath et al., 2000).

It is clear from the above discussion that it is very difficult to give a single value to define hypoglycemia. The approach for the diagnosis and treatment of hypoglycemia should take into account the gestational age as well as sickness level of the baby.

3. Fetal glucose metabolism and metabolic adaptation at birth

In the in-utero life, the fetus is dependent largely on maternal circulation for transplacental transfer of nutrients including glucose. However fetus is capable of endogenous glucose production during placental insufficiency and maternal starvation (Hay & Sparks, 1985). The fetal blood glucose concentrations are lower than but close to those of mother (Bozzetti et al., 1988). Glucose crosses the placenta by facilitated diffusion along a concentration gradient. Human liver contains glycogenic enzymes as early as 8 weeks of gestation, and glycogen deposition begins in early pregnancy. Hepatic glycogen content increases from only 3.4 mg/g at 8 weeks of age to 50 mg/g by term (Capkova & Jirasek, 1968; Williams, 2005). In humans, the enzymes for gluconeogenesis develop by 2 months of gestational age. However under normal physiological circumstances, the gluconeogenesis is not expressed in-utero (Kalhan et al., 1979). Only 40-50% of the maternal glucose taken up by the placenta is transferred to the fetus and rest is utilized by the placenta, which converts it to lactate. This lactate is released into the fetal and maternal circulation in a ratio of 1:3. Fetal lactate uptake is about half of the fetal glucose uptake and provides a major substrate for both oxidative and non-oxidative (such as glycogen synthesis) fetal metabolism. Glucose, however, remains the principal energy substrate for the human fetus under physiological conditions (Williams, 2005).

The blood glucose concentration in the umbilical venous blood is 80-90% of that in the maternal venous blood at the time of birth. Clamping of the umbilical cord causes rapid decrease in neonatal glucose concentration, reaching a nadir by 1 h of age and then increasing to stabilize by 3 h of age even in the absence of any exogenous nutritional intake (Fig. 1) (Srinivasan et al., 1986; Heck & Erenberg, 1987). The cascade of events in successful adaptation to extrauterine life includes metabolic changes such as hepatic glycogenolysis, lipolysis, fatty acid β-oxidation with generation of ketone bodies, and proteolysis that generates lactate and other substrates for gluconeogenesis.

These changes in glucose concentration are modified by a number of factors, including prior fetal glucose homeostasis influenced by antepartum and peripartum events, umbilical concentrations of glucose, plasma insulin concentrations, and the onset of neonatal glucose production from glycogenolysis and gluconeogenesis. There is considerable variability in glucose concentrations during this early postnatal period, both within individual neonates and among groups of neonates of different gestational ages and growth patterns. During this period, plasma insulin levels fall and plasma glucagon levels markedly rise from the baseline levels (Bloom & Johnston, 1972; Sperling et al., 1974). The stress of the birth process causes catecholamine surge. Growth hormone concentration also increases markedly after birth. However its physiological significance is not clear. The initial glucagon surge with low insulin/glucagon molar ratio is the key hormonal adaptation in the newborn infant (Ward Platt & Deshpande, 2005).

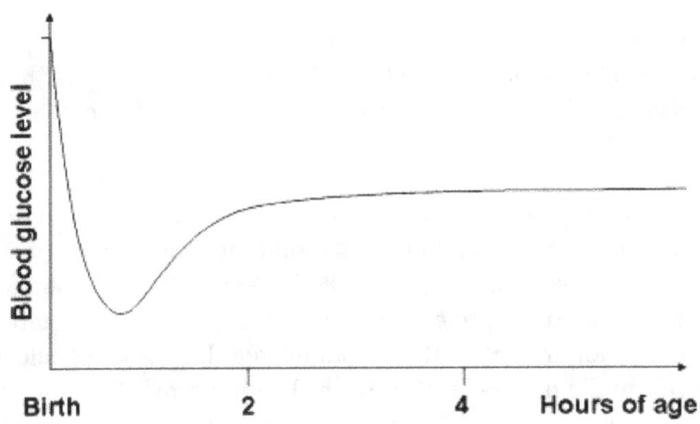

Fig. 1. Profile of blood glucose concentrations in the immediate postnatal period (Srinivasan et al., 1986)

Ketone bodies and lactate serve as alternative fuels with glucose-sparing effects, and are important in maintaining cerebral energy supply. Oxidative metabolism of glucose in fasting human newborns can only supply 70% of the estimated energy needs of the brain (Denne & Kalhan, 1986). Alternative energy substrates such as ketone bodies and lactate are required during fasting for energy production in brain. The capability of newborn brain to utilize ketone bodies is about 5-40 fold greater than that of infant or adult brain (Persson et al., 1972). Even in regularly fed newborn infants, ketogenesis and ketone body consumption provide around 12% of the cerebral oxygen consumption in neonates after a 6-h fast (Hawdon et al., 1992; Ward Platt & Deshpande, 2005). Lactate appears to be an important energy substrate for the infant in the immediate postnatal life. It is metabolized via oxidation by lactate dehydrogenase in the brain. Although the lactate pool is small (2.4 mM), the concentrations tend to be higher in the crucial first 2-3 postnatal hours (Kalhan et al., 2001).

In the post-natal life, blood glucose concentrations depend upon the feeding practices. Postnatal age and blood glucose concentrations are positively correlated, with the lowest values usually found on day-1 of life (Hawdon et al., 1992; Ward Platt & Deshpande, 2005). The rate of glucose production in the human neonate during the first few postnatal days is estimated to be 4-6 mg/kg/min. Approximately one-third of glucose is produced by glycogenolysis (Shelley & Neligan, 1966). Gluconeogenesis is important for continued glucose supply at this time. The activity of cytosolic phosphoenolpyruvate carboxykinase (PEPCK), which is responsible for gluconeogenesis, markedly increases after birth. Its secretion is stimulated by a fall in the plasma insulin/glucagon molar ratio. The concentrations of gluconeogenic precursors such as alanine and lactate are higher in term neonates as compared to older children or adults (Stanley et al., 1979; Hawdon et al., 1992). It may be due to slow postnatal maturation of PEPCK enzyme, or may be due to catabolic status of the neonate. Gluconeogenesis starts as early as 2 h after birth in the term human neonate (Kalhan et al., 1980). Long-chain fatty acids are required for the postnatal induction of enzymes of mitochondrial fatty acid β-oxidation (Pegorier et al., 1998). Owing to the limited capacity for hepatic ketogenesis in the immediate postnatal life, newborn infants have low plasma ketone body concentrations despite adequate levels of precursor free fatty acids (FFAs) in the first 8 h after birth (Stanley et al., 1979). From 12 h of age onwards, healthy term infants have high ketone body turnover rates (12-22 mmoL/kg/min) (Hawdon et al., 1992). The vigorous ketogenesis appears to be an integral part of extrauterine metabolic adaptation in the term human neonates.

Among preterm neonates, blood glucose levels have a greater fall after birth as compared to term infants. Circulating levels of gluconeogenic substrates are higher in preterm infants (Hawdon et al., 1992). However, the activity of microsomal glucose-6-phosphatase (the final enzyme of glycogenolysis and gluconeogenesis) in preterm infants is extremely low as compared to term infants (Hume & Burchell, 1993). In contrast to these findings, Sunehag et al. showed that preterm infants (25-26 weeks gestation) can have glucose production rates similar to the term neonates (Sunehag et al., 1993; Ward Platt & Deshpande, 2005). Similar observations were reported in preterm infants of 26-31 weeks gestational age. Preterm infants, however, cannot mount mature counter-regulatory ketogenic responses to low blood glucose levels in the first week after birth. The preterm infants demonstrate a positive relationship between blood ketone body concentrations and the volume of enteral feed (Hawdon et al., 1992). This immaturity of counter-regulatory ketogenesis is shown to persist during first 8 postnatal weeks. It may persist even till 2-6 months of postmenstrual age. Preterm neonates have a higher basal insulin secretion (plasma immunoreactive insulin concentrations at low blood glucose levels) as compared to term infants or children. The basal insulin concentrations have been shown to decrease with increasing maturity, however, they remained persistently high in the longitudinal evaluation of metabolic counter-regulation in preterm infants (Ward Platt & Deshpande, 2005).

4. Glucose metabolism and brain

Glucose and oxygen are the principle substances required for energy production in brain. To understand the injury caused by hypoglycemia it is essential to understand the metabolism of glucose in human brain.

4.1 Glucose uptake

Glucose supply to the brain is regulated by the plasma glucose concentration and mediated through a process of facilitated diffusion utilizing glucose transporter 1 (GLUT1) and glucose transporter 3 (GLUT3) proteins. This transport is not energy dependent. The levels of these proteins are relatively low in immature neonates and are a limiting step for glucose transfer and utilization (Koh et al. 1988; Cornblath et al., 2000; Volpe, 2008). GLUT1 is expressed in the blood-brain barrier endothelial cells, astrocytes, oligodendrocytes and choroid plexus while GLUT3 is expressed primarily in neurons and their synaptic membranes (Mantych et al., 1993; Kalhan et al., 2001). The brain glucose transporter is concentrated in capillaries and the concentration increases with maturity. The limiting factor for the passage of glucose to the brain tissue is the concentration of glucose transporters rather than the affinity of the receptors. The number of available endothelial receptors in human premature neonates is one third to half as compared to the adult brain (Powers et al., 1998; Volpe, 2008).

4.2 Glucose utilization in brain

Glucose is acted upon by hexokinase to form glucose-6-phosphate. It may be utilized via glycolytic pathway to produce energy (ATP), Hexose mono-phosphate (HMP) shunt to produce reducing equivalents or conversion to glycogen. Glycogen thus formed is stored in astrocytes and is used for energy production later on during periods of low blood glucose levels. Reducing equivalents from HMP shunt are required for lipid synthesis and nucleic acid synthesis. Glucose utilization is highest in brainstem gray matter structures, declining in a caudal to rostral manner, to the cerebral cortex. Cerebral glucose utilization in the human studies was found to be highest in the sensorimotor cerebral cortex, thalamus, mid-brain-brainstem, and the cerebellar vermis. By 3 months of age, glucose metabolic activity in the human infants had increased in the parietal, temporal, and occipital cortices and in the basal ganglia. Subsequently it increased in frontal and various association regions of cerebral cortex by 8 months. Little further change was observed between 8 and 18 months of postnatal age (Vannucci & Vannucci, 2000). Glucose acts as a primary metabolic fuel in the mature and immature brain. The studies in the newborn dogs indicate that glucose consumption accounts for 95% of the cerebral energy supply (Volpe, 2008). If the glucose supply to the brain is limited, alternative substances such as lactate and ketone bodies can be utilized to protect the brain functions and structure. Ketone bodies can be taken up by carrier mediated transport system, converted to acetyl CoA and metabolized to produce energy. Ketone bodies account for approximately 12% of total cerebral oxygen consumption after 6-hr fasting in newborns. However, availability of ketone bodies in such circumstances depends on the liver's capacity to deliver them in blood. The role of exogenous ketone bodies as a source of energy in settings of hypoglycemia is yet to be explored (Plecko et al., 2002). Lactate uptake from the blood also increases during periods of low blood glucose levels and it gets oxidized to pyruate by lactate dehydrogenase. The activity of lactate dehydrogenase in perinatal animal models is higher than adults (Lehrer et al., 1970; Wilson, 1972; Nehlig & Pereira de Vasconcelos, 1993). The association of increased lactate utilization and relative sparing of neonatal brain is strong but the exact role is yet to be explored. It is argued that the lactate utilization in perinatal animal could be an adaptive response to increased lactate levels in blood in perinatal period to avoid lactic acidemia (Volpe, 2008).

5. Biochemical alterations during hypoglycemia

In the event of low blood glucose, certain biochemical changes occur in the neonatal brain. With continuing hypoglycemia, changes secondary to hypoxia, ischemia and seizures may add to the insult. These combined effects are of major concern as it increases the chances of brain injury even if individual insults are not of sufficient magnitude to cause injury by themselves (Volpe, 2008).

5.1 Initial changes

The initial response to the low blood glucose levels is an increase in cerebral blood flow so as to increase glucose supply to brain. This effect has been shown in adult models (Siesjo, 1988), neonatal animal models (Anwar & Vannucci, 1988; Mujsce et al., 1989), and human infants (Pryds et al., 1988, 1990; Pryds, 1991; Skov & Pryds, 1992). In human infants, a sharp increase in cerebral blood flow has been observed below a blood glucose of 30 mg/dL (Pryds et al., 1990). Initial biochemical changes include metabolic attempts to preserve cerebral energy status by utilizing alternatives to glucose. Glycogenolysis starts to provide glucose to brain tissue. Researchers have noticed that initially there is not much change in cerebral oxygen consumption. This discrepancy between falling blood glucose levels and relatively preserved oxygen utilization in initial phases of hypoglycemia implies that alternative substrates like lactate and ketone bodies might be sufficient to meet cerebral energy needs (Norberg & Siesio, 1976; Ghajar et al., 1982). Amino acids may be other alternative substrates as a sharp decrease in brain concentrations of most amino acids occurs along with increase in brain ammonia levels (Volpe, 2008).

There is dissociation between cerebral energy metabolism and brain functions during hypoglycemia. The changes in level of consciousness (from alert state to depressed state) and from normal EEG to slowing can occur with relatively little change in levels of ATP in various regions of brain (Siesjo, 1988; Vannucci et al., 1981; Vannucci & Vannucci, 2000; Volpe, 2008). This phenomenon can be attributed partially to metabolic changes happening during early periods of hypoglycemia. The concentration of ammonia goes up as the levels of amino acids decrease so as to preserve ATP production. The level of ammonia production is considered sufficient to produce stupor in adult hypoglycemic animals. Mature rats, who were made hypoglycemic, displayed impaired acetylcholine synthesis in early phase of hypoglycemia (Gibson & Blass, 1976; Ghajar et al., 1982). Only modest hypoglycemia was able to decrease acetylcholine levels by 20-45%. Moreover there was 40-60% decrease in synthesis of this neurotransmitter in cortex and striatum (Ghajar et al., 1982). The likely mechanism for the dissociation between cerebral energy metabolism and brain functions during hypoglycemia, is decrease in acetyl-coA concentration secondary to low blood glucose and hence glycolysis (Volpe, 2008). However in newborn animal models, hypoglycemia severe enough to deplete glucose from brain is accompanied by some preservation of glycolytic intermediates such as pyruate and lactate; and almost complete preservation of ATP levels. Newborn animal models showed resistance to neurological deterioration even at plasma glucose levels of 15 mg/dL when maintained for a period of 2 hours (Vannucci & Vannucci, 1978). In newborn dog, the EEG slowing was observed only below 20 mg/dL (Vannucci et al., 1981). There are various reasons for the relative resistance of newborn brain towards neuronal injury to hypoglycemia. These include lower cerebral energy requirements, marked increase in cerebral blood flow in early phases of hypoglycemia, increased capacity of neonatal brain to utilize lactate as an alternative brain fuel and relatively less effect on cardiovascular system as compared to adults due to abundant endogenous carbohydrate stores (Volpe, 2008).

5.2 Later changes

If hypoglycemia continues, generation of fatty acids increases due to phospholipid degradation, to provide additional source of energy. However, this energy source is not sufficient to provide for the deficit of high energy phosphate compounds and prevent clinical and EEG deterioration (Ghajar et al., 1982; Siesjo, 1988). In advanced phases of hypoglycemia, there are changes in intracellular Ca^{++} and extracellular K^+ concentration (Agardh et al., 1981; Wieloch et al., 1984; Siesjo, 1988). The neuron loses its ability to maintain normal ionic gradients. The failure of energy dependent Na^+/K^+ ATPase is the likely reason responsible for these changes. With energy failure, Na^+ accumulates intracellularly and K^+ accumulates in extracellular space leading to sustained membrane depolarization. Increase in intracellular Na+ would lead to activation of Na^+/Ca^{2+} exchange system and intracellular accumulation of Ca^{2+} ions. There is also failure of energy dependent Ca^{2+} transport across the cell membrane, which again leads to intracellular accumulation of Ca^{2+} ions. The increased concentration of cytosolic Ca^{2+} ions leads to phospholipase activation and cellular injury. This explanation is supported by the observed corresponding decline in phospholipid concentration and increase in fatty acid levels with increase in intracellular Ca^{2+}. Additionally, the increase in cytosolic calcium concentration causes increase in release of excitatory amino acids (e.g. aspartate and glutamate) from synaptic nerve endings and reduced uptake secondary to failure of glutamate transport. Antagonists of N-Methyl-D-Aspartate type of glutamate receptors have been shown to attenuate neuronal injury in cultured neurons and in vivo models (Wieloch, 1985; Volpe, 2008). The excess cytosolic Ca^{2+} also leads to increase in reactive oxygen and nitrogen species. These free radical species result in DNA damage and as a consequence DNA repair enzyme, poly (ADP-ribose) polymerase-1 (PARP). Excessive activation of PARP, leads to apoptosis. PARP inhibitors have been shown to protect neurons from hypoglycemic injury in in- vivo and in-vitro models (Suh et al., 2003; Volpe, 2008).

6. Pathological changes in hypoglycemic brain injury

It is difficult to define exact neuropathology in newborns suffering from hypoglycemia as it almost always coexists with other morbidities. However the literature suggests that the topography of the hypoglycemic brain injury is peculiar and is different from that of hypoxic ischemic brain injury. Adolescent monkeys when exposed to blood glucose of <20 mg/dL for more than 2 hours showed neuronal injury predominantly in the regions of parieto-occipital cortex. Less commonly involved regions were hippocampus, caudate nucleus, and putamen. The injury was most severe in regions contiguous to cerebrospinal fluid such as superficial cerebral cortical layers (Agardh et al., 1980; Auer et al., 1984, 1985; Kalimo et al., 1985; Siesjo, 1988). Similar topographical distribution of neuropathology was observed in premature infants using autopsy studies, computed tomography, magnetic resonance imaging and single photon emission computed tomography blood flow scans (Anderson et al., 1967; Spar et al., 1994; Chiu et al., 1998; Volpe, 2008). The hypoglycemic brain injury primarily involves neurons but glia are also affected (Anderson et al., 1967). Studies of oligodendrocyte precursor cells and cerebellar slice cultures showed that hypoglycemia induces apoptotic cell death and inhibits differentiation and myelination (Yan & Rivkees 2006). Additionally hypoglycemia alone if not severe enough to cause neuronal injury, may contribute to the injury caused by other insults. The sequelae of hypoglycemic brain injury include microcephaly, widened sulci and atrophic gyri, diminished cerebral white matter and dilated lateral ventricles. The pathological effects of marginal hypoglycemia with or without other concomitant insults are not known.

7. Clinical profile

Hypoglycemia is a concomitant finding in variety of neonatal disorders. The incidence of hypoglycemia depends upon the proportion of term and preterm in a given population, type of milk feeding, the pattern of feeding, screening timings and methods, temperature, sickness level and definition used for the diagnosis of hypoglycemia. In a large series of 661 preterm neonates with birth weight <1850 g, 10% had at least one value of blood glucose <0.6mmol/L (<10mg/dL approximately), 28% had at least one value <1.6mmol/L (<30mg/dL approximately), and 66% had at least one value of blood glucose <2.6 mmol/L (<45mg/dL approximately) (Lucas, Morley et al. 1988). Among breastfed healthy term neonates, approximately 17% of the neonates had plasma glucose value of <2.16mmol/L (<40 mg/dL) at 3 hours of postnatal life. Ten percent of neonates had similar values at 72 hours of life (Diwakar & Sasidhar, 2002).

The clinical manifestations of hypoglycemia are largely related to central nervous system. Common clinical signs include jitteriness, irritability, varying degree of altered consciousness, seizures, tachypnea, apnea and hypotonia. It is important to realize that there might be no symptoms in presence of biochemical evidence of hypoglycemia (Asymptomatic hypoglycemia)(Volpe, 2008). Neonates with 'symptomatic hypoglycemia' can be classified into four categories according to the clinical setting of hypoglycemia, time of presentation, and severity of presentation (Volpe, 2008):

7.1 Early transitional adaptive hypoglycemia

It occurs in first 6-12 hours of life, after sudden withdrawl of maternal nutrient supply due to cord clamping. This manifests in neonates, who fail to mount adequate metabolic adaptive response in the face of falling blood glucose levels, in immediate postnatal life. If the mother receives excess glucose in intravenous fluids during intrapartum period, the glycolytic and gluconeogenic responses of the neonate are blunted and insulin secretion increases in immediate postnatal period. Large for gestational age infants born to diabetic (IDM) or non-diabetic mothers, neonates who experience hypothermia or asphyxia are at risk for very early hypoglycemia. This type of hypoglycemia lasts for brief duration, is mild in severity and responds rapidly to treatment. The prognosis depends largely on the underlying cause.

7.2 Secondary associated hypoglycemia

This can occur as an associated finding with a variety of illnesses. It is often seen in appropriate for gestational age (AGA) term and preterm neonates, and is associated with illnesses particularly involving central nervous system e.g. birth asphyxia, intracranial hemorrhage, congenital anomalies and systemic disorders. The association with brain disorders is of particular interest as these may have adverse impact on regulation of hepatic glucose production. This variety of hypoglycemia is also characterized by short duration, mild severity and rapid response to treatment (Volpe, 2008).

7.3 Classic transient neonatal hypoglycemia

This group encompasses predominantly small for gestation (SGA) term infants, who may also have polycythemia concomitantly. The onset of hypoglycemia is in later part of first day. Hypoglycemia is usually moderate to severe, duration can be prolonged and often high glucose infusion rates are required to maintain euglycemia.

7.4 Severe recurrent hypoglycemia

Recurrent and persistent hypoglycemia is the hallmark of this variety. This type occurs in term AGA neonates who have either hyperinsulinism or endocrinopathies or hereditary metabolic defects. The hypoglycemia is variable in onset according to the underlying cause, usually severe, difficult to treat, prolonged and invariably symptomatic. The prognosis depends on the timely detection of the disorder, institution of specific therapy, and the ability to maintain normal blood glucose levels.

8. Monitoring of blood glucose

8.1 Who should be monitored?

All preterm and SGA neonates merit blood glucose screening as they have decreased body stores of glycogen and they often harbor co-morbidities putting them at risk for hypoglycemia. The large for gestation age infants and IDM neonates usually have excess insulin secretion in the immediate neonatal period putting them at risk of hypoglycemia. All 'unwell' neonates should also be routinely monitored for hypoglycemia. (Deshpande & Ward Platt 2005). The indications of monitoring blood glucose in neonatal age group are shown in Figure 2.

Due to maternal indications

- Maternal drug ingestion eg β-blockers, oral hypoglycemics, β-sympathomimetics
- Insulin dependent diabetic mothers
- Gestational diabetic mothers
- Massively obese mothers
- Mothers given large amounts of parenteral glucose during labor and delivery
- Mothers given parenteral glucose too rapidly prior to delivery

Neonatal indications

- Prematurity
- Small or large for gestational age
- Hypothermia
- 'Sick looking' or 'unwell' neonate
- Sepsis
- Hypoxia ischemia
- Polycythemia
- Congenital heart diseases
- Total parenteral nutrition
- Blood exchange transfusion
- Suspected inborn errors of metabolism

Fig. 2. Indications of monitoring blood glucose

8.2 What should be the monitoring schedule?

The neonates in whom there is increased consumption of glucose because of increased insulin levels become symptomatic very early in postnatal life. It is also evident that the levels of alternative 'brain fuels' would also be less due to presence of anabolic hormone insulin. Hence IDM and severely intrauterine growth retarded neonates can become symptomatic very early in life and merit screening right from cord blood. Some severely IUGR infants may develop hypoglycemia in-utero (Soothill et al., 1987; Economides &

Nicolaides, 1989) and would not be expected to achieve normal metabolic adaptation soon after birth. These neonates merit cord blood glucose estimation and routine screening in the postnatal life at least for initial 48 hours. The neonates with low body glycogen stores like preterm and IUGR neonates should get first screening within 1 hour of life. All neonates who are symptomatic should get blood glucose levels checked immediately. Many textbooks and guidelines recommend blood glucose monitoring at pre-fixed time periods after birth, such as at 1 h, 2 h, 3h,6h and then 6 hourly till 48-72 hours by when feeding is likely to be established. Blood glucose estimation should be done immediately before a feed, as the purpose of screening is to identify the minimum blood glucose level (Lucas et al., 1981).

8.3 How should blood glucose be measured?

An ideal diagnostic method should be precise, rapid, inexpensive, available at bedside, and should require small blood volume. At beside, the blood glucose measurements are done by point of care glucose meters. They measure blood glucose within few seconds and require small sample volumes (as small as 0.3 µL). For treatment decisions, the clinical practices are dependent on point of care measurements rather than laboratory estimations. The small volume of blood required by such approach has been shown to reduce the need for blood transfusions (Madan et al., 2005). Apart from the devices used, the estimation of blood glucose levels can also be affected by the properties of sample used for analysis.

8.3.1 Devices for screening of blood glucose

Since the introduction of reagent strip blood glucose tests in the 1970s for blood glucose screening in newborn infants, the world has witnessed dramatic developments in point of care devices for blood glucose measurements. Dextrostix was the first dry reagent, which was interpreted with change in color and hence was dependent on subjective interpretation. Then came the era of photometric devices (reflectance meters). In this method, the blood was required to be placed on the strips for specific time periods, wiped and then inserted into a meter . Sources of error in glucose estimation while using these methods are possible contamination by alcohol skin-cleansers, not covering the whole surface of the test-pad with blood, and failure to time the reaction accurately before wiping the strip. The paper-strip methods tend to underestimate the neonatal blood glucose values even when these precautions are adopted. The common glucose strips used in neonatal practice were Dextrostix (Ames Co., Slough, England) (Chantler et al., 1967; Wilkins & Kalra 1982; Williams, 1997), BM-test-Glycemie (Boehringer Mannheim, Mannheim, Germany) (Wilkins & Kalra, 1982; Reynolds & Davies, 1993), and Chemstrip bG (Boehringer Mannheim, Mannheim, Germany) (Kaplan et al., 1989; Holtrop et al., 1990). Recently, point of care testing is being done by glucose meters, which utilize enzyme reactions (glucose oxidase or glucose dehydrogenase) to generate electric signals, which are measured by a meter. The size of the current is proportional to the amount of glucose in the blood sample leading to increased accuracy (Beardsall, 2010).

However it is important to know that these methods were primarily designed for diabetic patients and not for the glucose screening of newborns. The sensitivity of these methods is likely to be highest at blood glucose levels in diabetic range and may drop at extreme values. In intensive care units, a number of potential inaccuracies may arise because of presence of metabolic acidosis (Tang et al., 2000), hypoxia (Tang et al., 2001), hypoperfusion

(Atkin et al., 1991) or edema (Critchell et al., 2007). If the devise uses glucose oxidase method, it may give abnormally low glucose values at high blood oxygen levels (Tang et al., 2001). High hematocrit levels in preterm and IUGR neonates might display falsely low glucose levels with these methods and this effect is most marked at low blood glucose levels (Kaplan et al., 1989; Tang et al., 2000). High bilirubin levels can also interfere with some analyzers (Jain et al., 1996). The data of their use in neonatal age group is limited. In a study comparing five glucometers namely Reflolux S (Boehringer), Advantage and Glucotrend (Roche); Elite XL (Bayer) and Precision (Abbott) with plasma glucose measured in the laboratory (Aeroset; Abbott); none of the five glucometers was satisfactory as the sole measuring device. For detection of glucose concentrations <2.6 mmol/L, the Precision glucometer had the highest sensitivity (96.4%) and negative predictive value (90%). For lower glucose concentrations (<2.0 mmol/L), the Glucotrend glucometer performed even better (sensitivity 92.3%, negative predictive value 96.3%) (Ho et al., 2004). A recent retrospective study compared three meters (Elite™ XL, Ascensia™ Contour™ and ABL 735) with laboratory hexokinase reference method. All three POCT systems tended to overestimate glucose values. The Elite XL appeared to be more appropriate than Contour to detect hypoglycemia, however with a low specificity. Contour additionally showed an important inaccuracy with increasing hematocrit. The sensitivity to detect hypoglycemia with a cutoff value <2.5 mmol/L was 86% and 43% for Elite XL and Contour respectively (Beardsall, 2010).

With modern blood gas and electrolyte analyzers, it is possible to directly measure blood glucose levels by electrochemical biosensors. The comparative data for glucose biosensor technology versus traditional methods of blood glucose estimation in the neonatal age group is sparse. In a recent study, an amperometric electrode with glucose oxidase membrane incorporated in a multi-analyte analyzer was compared with hexokinase/glucose-6-phosphate dehydrogenase method. It showed a sensitivity and specificity of 55% and 100% respectively below a cutoff of <2.5mmol/L and 89% and 95% respectively below a cutoff of <3.0mmol/L of laboratory reference value (Beardsall 2010). Another study compared blood glucose measurements obtained by point-of-care testing using an AVL Omni 9 blood gas analyzer with those obtained in the central laboratory using a DADE Dimension RXL analyzer. There was a good correlation (r = 0.92) between the two for glucose values <3 mmol/L. The limits of agreement for the AVL Omni 9 when compared with the DADE Dimension RXL analyser were -0.1 +/- 0.5 mmol/L. (Newman et al., 2002). Laboratory analyses are done by a number of different enzymes which measure glucose e.g. glucose oxidase, hexokinase or glucose dehydrogenase. Glucose measured by these methods is the most practical method for measurement of glucose levels. The plasma glucose levels measured by these enzymes are less affected by interference by metabolites and are not affected by hematocrit (Beardsall, 2010).

8.3.2 Continuous glucose monitoring

Continuous glucose monitoring is possible by placement of subcutaneous glucose monitoring sensors. This glucose oxidase based platinum sensor catalyzes interstitial glucose and an electrical current is produced every 10 seconds. This current is recorded by a monitor and displayed as real time trend. The glucose value is averaged for past 5 min and thus profile of glucose trend is generated. This displays trend of tissue glucose levels over time, like continuous saturation monitors. The glucose levels in newborns can fluctuate

widely especially those requiring intensive care. This means that by periodic spot monitoring we may miss undetected periods of hypoglycemia as well as hyperglycemia (Beardsall et al., 2005). Their use in management of adults and children with diabetes has led to stringent control over blood glucose levels, with reduction in episodes of hyperglycemia and hypoglycemia. Commercial devices are available such as CGMS Gold or Guardian (Medtronic Watford UK) or Free Style Navigator (Abbott Maidenhead, Berks, UK). The initial devices could not display real time trends limiting their clinical potential. However it is possible with more recent models, which have been successfully used to monitor post-cardiac surgery pediatric patients. During the management of infants with neonatal diabetes, these can be linked to subcutaneous insulin pumps (Corstjens et al., 2006). Their clinical application can be extended to the management of preterm and sick neonates who are at risk of hypoglycemia and hyperglycemia. However the benefits and risks need to be fully evaluated before their introduction into clinical care. Microdialysis is another method of continuous glucose monitoring. A semi-permeable dialysis fiber or double lumen catheter with micro-holes is placed in subcutaneous tissue. Isotonic glucose free fluid passes through the device collecting dialysate of interstitial fluid. Thus the dialysate contains glucose equal in concentration to that of interstitial fluid. Commercial devices are available such as the CMA Microdialyses catheter (Solna Sweden), which can be used in neonates. However these devices are expensive, invasive, need calibration, and there is a significant lag time in collection and measurement. Although they have been used as research tool, their routine clinical use is limited (Baumeister et al., 2001). In a recent study comparing Continuous Glucose Monitor Sensor (CGMS system gold, Medtronic, MiniMed, Northridge, California) with glucose oxidase method in blood gas analyzer (Radiometer, ABL800Flex, Copenhagen, Denmark), 81% of total 265 episodes of low interstitial glucose concentrations were not detected with blood glucose measurement (Harris et al., 2010). The non-invasive devices utilizing optical sensors (spectrophotometry) or transdermal devices using reverse iontophoresis are being evaluated for possible clinical utilization. They are in early phase of development and their clinical potential is yet to be evaluated in neonates (Beardsall, 2010).
Thus, at present, there is no reliable and accurate point-of-care method for blood glucose estimation in the low ranges of blood glucose encountered in newborn infants. Laboratory systems that provide timely results may be the preferred option; these facilities require certification by the institutional clinical pathology services and other accrediting agencies, as well as initial and ongoing assessment and maintenance of instrument function, technical training of the users, and data quality monitoring. Thus far, there are no satisfactory methods for noninvasive monitoring of glucose or alternate substrates. Such monitoring devices, however, would have a major impact on clinical decision making. Continuous glucose monitoring with subcutaneous perfusion devices has been used to a limited extent.

8.3.3 Properties of the sample and sources of error

Arterial blood has a slightly higher glucose concentration than venous, while the capillary blood has intermediate values. This difference is usually not clinically significant. The difference of blood glucose levels between arterial and venous blood depends upon tissue glucose demands and is greatest in anaerobic conditions. In presence of peripheral circulatory failure, capillary sampling is unreliable as the blood flow is reduced. The blood sample must be a free-flowing sample and squeezing the tissues to get blood causes hemolysis. The glucose estimations performed with 'squeezed' sample are not true values and deproteinization is required to get true values. Contamination by the alcohol antiseptic solutions during skin preparations might give erroneously high values (Grazaitis & Sexson 1980; Togari et al., 1987). The sample should be analyzed immediately or it should be deproteinized (e.g. using perchloric acid) and chilled to avoid glycolysis. Sodium fluoride added to blood inhibits glycolysis and gives freedom to process sample after some time. But the fluoride is not able to completely prevent glycolysis, thus getting falsely low blood glucose values in samples sent to a distant laboratory (Elimam et al., 1997). Commercially available sodium-fluoride coated tubes do not always ensure a fluoride concentration sufficient to inhibit glycolysis (Joosten et al., 1991). Chan et al. observed that glucose levels in blood fall about 0.3–0.34 mmol/L over the first hour, in samples collected into either heparin or sodium fluoride containing tubes (Chan et al., 1989). High hematocrit values may be associated with falsely low blood glucose estimation. Red blood corpuscles contain less proportion of water than an equivalent volume of plasma. Thus in equal volume of blood and plasma, the glucose concentration is expected to be higher in plasma, on average by about 18% (Aynsley-Green, 1991). Furthermore, the diffusion of plasma into the testpad of the strip is impeded due to higher sample viscosity. This problem can be tackled by estimating plasma glucose after getting plasma from a heparinized microhaematocrit tube (Kaplan, Blondheim et al. 1989). Presence of hemolysis also gives falsely low values. The presence of hemoglobin or release of reduced glutathione competes with the chromogen for hydrogen peroxide released in the assay. Deproteinization of the sample reduces the interference with blood glucose estimations by hemolysates, uric acid, and bilirubin (Williams, 1997).

9. Prevention

The earliest and common cause of low blood glucose levels is delay in the normal metabolic adaptation after birth. Hence oral feeds within half hour of life should be promoted in healthy appropriately grown term infants. In preterm infants of <32 weeks gestation or those with asphyxia or respiratory distress or any illness interfering with enteral nutrition, intravenous dextrose infusions should be started. Glucose delivery through intravenous infusions should match the amount of glucose production by endogenous hepatic output. For most well-grown preterm infants, it is approximately 6 mg /kg/ min (around 90 mL 10% dextrose/kg per day (Sunehag et al., 1993). The occurrence of hypoglycemia should be unusual with such fluid regimens, in these preterm infants, (Hawdon et al., 1992) and enteral feeds can be gradually increased along with. Near-term infants of 33-36 weeks gestational age require careful nursing as they may not be able to establish good feeding due to physiological handicaps and increased demands. Supplementary feeds may be required if breastfeeding is not fully established. If possible first option should be expressed breast milk, and formula milk can be used if breast milk is unavailable or inadequate. In neonates who remain hypoglycemic despite an adequate enteral intake, or for those unable to tolerate milk, an intravenous dextrose infusion is necessary. Some IUGR infants require glucose intake in excess of 10 mg/kg/min. Hyperinsulinism may be the likely mechanism of such high glucose requirements (Collins et al., 1990) and these babies may have insulin values above those seen in healthy term babies (Hawdon et al., 1993a, 1993b). They may be described as 'functionally' hyperinsulinemic as they also demonstrate increased insulin sensitivity (Bazaes et al., 2003).

10. Treatment of neonatal hypoglycemia

A 'symptomatic' neonate should be treated with intravenous dextrose and this should be instituted as early as possible if the blood glucose concentrations are below 45-50 mg/dL (Volpe, 2008). Glucose 'minibolus' (200 mg glucose/kg, 2 mL/kg of 10% dextrose) is effective in rapidly correcting neonatal hypoglycemia. A minibolus should be given when blood glucose concentration needs to be raised quickly, such as in a symptomatic neonate with neurological signs in association with a low blood glucose concentration. A minibolus should always be followed by intravenous glucose infusion. The glucose infusion should be started at an infusion rate of 6-8 mg/kg per min (Lilien et al., 1980). The glucose infusion rate (GIR) should then be titrated with repeated blood glucose estimations. Blood glucose should be frequently monitored until it stabilizes. After commencing intravenous infusion, blood glucose should be repeated with in half an hour. The glucose infusion rate should be hiked by 2 mg/kg per min if the repeat screen is also in 'hypoglycemic' range. Once blood glucose levels are stabilized, preprandial blood glucose may be monitored at 4 to 8 hour intervals (Cornblath & Ichord, 2000). Boluses of hypertonic glucose solution should be avoided as they can precipitate rebound hypoglycemia. Baby should be offered enteral feeds if clinically there is no contraindication. Amino-acids like alanine promote gluconeogenesis and help to maintain blood glucose levels. Breast milk in particular promotes ketogenesis (de Rooy & Hawdon, 2002). After 12-24 hours of intravenous glucose infusion, addition of sodium 1 to 2 mEq/kg/day is indicated to prevent iatrogenic hyponatremia. After 24-48 hours, 1 to 2 mEq/kg/day of potassium should be added to the parenteral fluids (Cornblath & Ichord, 2000). If baby remains symptomatic or if plasma glucose concentrations cannot be maintained over 45 mg/dL (2.6 mmol/L), even at glucose infusion rate of 12 mg/kg/min, hydrocortisone (5 mg/kg intravenously every 12 hours) should be added to the regimen (Volpe, 2008). If the concentration of glucose infusion exceeds 12.5% to 15% through peripheral vein, a PICC (peripherally inserted central catheter) line should be placed, as concentrated solutions can cause injury to peripheral veins. If the rate of glucose infusion exceeds 10-12 mg/kg/min or the hypoglycemia is present after 5 to 7 days, the infant may have refractory or persistent hypoglycemia (Cornblath & Ichord, 2000).

Once the blood glucose levels are maintained in euglycemic range of 70-100mg/dL, the glucose infusion should be tapered by 2mg/kg/min every 6 to 12 hourly. The gradual reductions in the rate of intravenous glucose infusion should be attempted as they avoid wide swings in blood glucose concentrations. The glucose infusion rate should be reduced while increasing oral intake (Williams, 1997) and glucose levels should be closely monitored to keep them >50mg/dL (Volpe, 2008). Intramuscular glucagon (see below) may act as a temporary measure to raise blood glucose, if there is difficulty in placing intravenous line quickly. Glucagon promotes early neonatal glycogenolysis from liver and also stimulates gluconeogenesis and ketogenesis (Milner & Wright, 1967). An intramuscular bolus dose of 200 µg/kg increases the blood glucose level (Hawdon et al., 1993c). It has been used successfully to treat hypoglycemia in infants of diabetic mothers (Wu et al., 1975) and growth-restricted infants (Carter et al., 1988). Side-effects of glucagon include vomiting, diarrhea, and hypokalemia; at high doses it may stimulate insulin release. Controlled studies of the relative efficacy of glucagon and the more conventional alternative of glucose infusion at concentrations >6mg/kg per min are needed (Williams, 1997). An algorithm for the management of a neonate with hypoglycemia is presented in Figure 3 (Narayan & Wazir, et al. 2010).

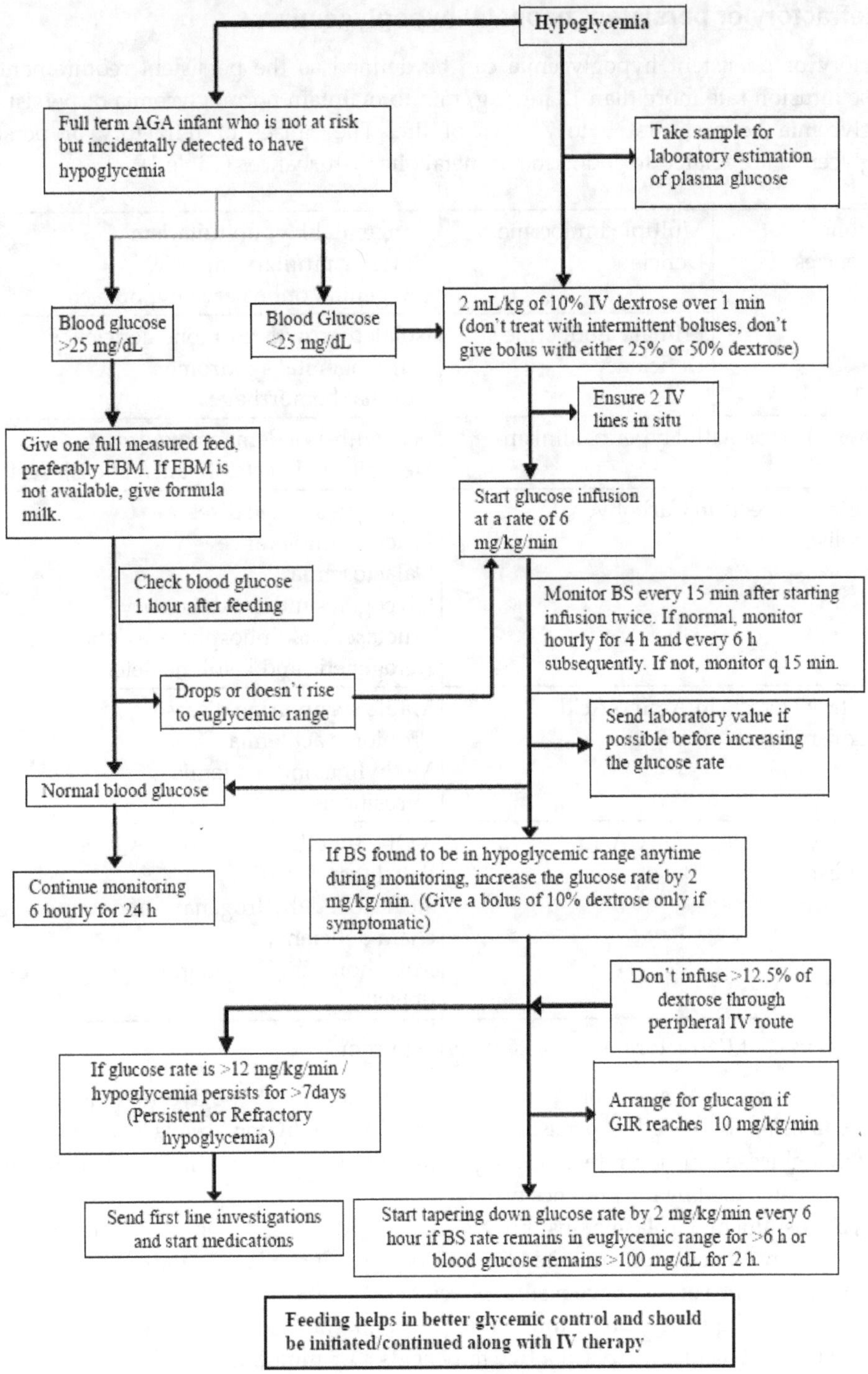

GIR: Glucose Infusion Rate BS:Blood Sugar(Glucose)

Fig. 3. Management algorithm for neonatal hypoglycemia

11. Refractory or persistent neonatal hypoglycemia

Refractory or persistent hypoglycemia can be defined as the persistent requirement of a glucose infusion rate more than 12 mg/kg/min to maintain normoglycemia or persisting or hypoglycemia beyond first 5 to 7 days of life. The causes of refractory or persistent hypoglycemia are related to endocrine or metabolic disturbances (Table 1)

Hormone Deficiencies	Multiple Endocrine Deficiency	Congenital Hypopituitarism Anterior pituitary "aplasia" Congenital optic nerve hypoplasia
	Primary Endocrine Deficiency	Isolated growth hormone deficiency Adrenogenital syndrome Adrenal hemorrhage
Hormone Excess with Hyperinsulinism		Beckwith-Wiedemann syndrome Hereditary defects of pancreatic islet cells
Hereditary Defects in Carbohydrate Metabolism		Glycogen storage disease Fructose intolerance Galactosemia Glycogen synthase deficiency Fructose, 1-6 diphosphatase deficiency Ketogenetic and ketolytic defects
Hereditary Defects in Amino Acid Metabolism		Maple syrup urine disease Propionic acidemia Methylmalonic acidemia Tyrosinosis
Hereditary Defects in Fatty Acid Metabolism		3-OH-3-methyl glutaryl CoA lyase deficiency Acyl CoA dehydrogenase--medium, long chain deficiency Mitochondrial/3-oxidation & degradation defects

Table 1. Causes of Refractory or Persistent Hypoglycemia

The most common cause of persistent or refractory hypoglycemia is congenital hyperinsulinism, also called as persistent hyperinsulinemic hypoglycemia of infancy (PHHI). Although a glucose infusion rate exceeding 12 mg/kg per min suggests hyperinsulinism, the diagnosis is confirmed by the presence of-

1. Hyperinsulinemia (plasma insulin >2 μU/mL, depending on sensitivity of insulin assay), in presence of documented laboratory hypoglycemia (<50 mg/dL)
2. and/or evidence of excessive insulin effect
   a. Increased glucose consumption rate (>8 mg/kg/min)
   b. Hypofattyacidemia (plasma free fatty acids <1.5 mmol/L)
   c. Hypoketonemia (plasma β-hydroxybutyrate <2.0 mmol/L)
   d. Glycemic response to 1 mg IV glucagon 50 μg/kg (max 1mg) (increase in glucose >30 mg/dL)

Insulin level should be obtained only during presence of hypoglycemia. Simultaneous measurement of blood glucose level may be done to find out the insulin-glucose ratio. Elevated insulin-glucose ratios are found in hyperinsulinemic states (normal - up to 0.2; elevated - >0.4). A 'normal' level of insulin is abnormal if it occurs in the face of hypoglycemia, especially in the context of high glucose requirement to maintain normoglycemia.

PHHI results from an inappropriate insulin secretion by the β-cells of pancreatic islets of Langerhans (Arnoux et al., 2010). Insulin decreases plasma glucose concentration by inhibiting glucose release from the liver (by glycogenolysis and gluconeogenesis), and by increasing glucose uptake in muscle and adipose tissues. It also inhibits lipolysis and hence production of fatty acids and ketone bodies is markedly reduced. Hence, the brain is unable to get alternative fuels in presence of hypoglycemia and thus is particularly vulnerable to hypoglycemic injury.

PHHI presents as severe hypoketotic hypoglycemia. There is a risk of neonatal seizures and brain damage if it is left untreated. Hypoglycemia occurs early within 72 h after birth and half of the patients become symptomatic in the form of seizures. Majority of neonates are macrosomic. The affected neonates may present with abnormal movements as tremulousness, hypotonia, cyanosis, hypothermia or a life-threatening event. On external examination, they may have mild hepatomegaly. Sometimes typical facial features in form of high forehead, large and bulbous nose with short columella, smooth philtrum and thin upper lip can be appreciated. However, hyperinsulinism can be associated with syndromes such as Beckwith–Wiedemann syndrome (BWS), Perlman syndrome, Kabuki syndrome, Sotos syndrome, congenital disorders of glycosylation type Ia or Ib (CDG) (de Lonlay et al., 1999), or Usher syndrome type Ic. Hypoglycemia may be detected in such neonates by routine measurement of blood glucose. The hypoglycemia is severe and rates of intravenous glucose administration to maintain euglycemia are usually in excess of 12 mg/kg per min. Subcutaneous or intramuscular administration of glucagon can be used to raise blood glucose concentrations transiently.

Hyperinsulinemia in the neonatal age group may also be seen for transient periods in conditions like acute fetal distress, small weight for gestational age and gestational diabetes. The severity is usually mild in such cases. These neonates respond to diazoxide, and hyperinsulinemia resolves spontaneously within several days or weeks. All neonates with hyperinsulinemia should be screened for hyperammonemia to diagnose hyperinsulinemia hyperammonia (HI/HA) syndrome (GLUD1 gene), urine organic acids to diagnose short chain hydroxyacyl-CoA dehydrogenase (SCHAD) deficiency (HADH gene) and plasma acylcarnitines chromatographies, for CDG syndromes, as these 3 diseases may present in the neonatal period as apparently isolated hyperinsulinism (Arnoux et al., 2010). Other genes which can be suspected are SLC16A1 gene (Otonkoski et al., 2003) and HNF4A gene when the newborn is macrosomic with a family history of maturity onset diabetes of young (Pearson et al., 2007). Finally, familial forms or consanguinity and syndromic forms have to be checked as these are associated with diffuse HI (Arnoux et al., 2010).

The treatment of such a condition should be aggressive as the glucose levels are very low and there is deficiency of alternative brain fuels in hyperinsulinemic neonates. Majority of these neonates are already on intravenous glucose administration when the diagnosis of hyperinsulinemia is established. Medical management consists of drugs such as Diazoxide,

Nifedipine and Octreotide. Diazoxide blocks insulin secretion by activating (opening) the SUR1 receptors. Transient and persistent hyperinsulinemia (involving genes other than those encoding SUR1 and Kir6.2) respond to diazoxide. However, most of neonatal and isolated persistent HI is resistant to diazoxide. Diazoxide is tolerated well by neonates except in premature neonates because of sodium and fluid retention, which may lead to edema, pulmonary hypertension or heart failure. The most frequent adverse effect of prolonged use is hypertrichosis. Hematological side effects are very rare in routine doses. Diazoxide unresponsiveness is defined by the occurrence of 2 episodes of hypoglycemia [<54 mg/dL (<3 mmol/L)] in 24-hour period. In such cases, Octreotide must be tried before considering surgery (Thornton et al., 1993). Doses vary from 10 to 50 µg/kg/day intravenously, administered continuously or subcutaneously every 6 or 8 h. Higher doses may worsen hypoglycemia by suppressing both glucagon and growth hormone. Some patients may have vomiting and/or diarrhea and abdominal distension after starting therapy, which spontaneously resolves within 7–10 days. Gallbladder sludge or stones may appear during therapy. The dose of octreotide should be progressively increased according to the weight gain of the baby, to prevent recurrence of hypoglycemia. Other drugs such as calcium channels blockers (nifedipine, 0.5– 2 mg/kg/day in 2 oral doses) can be tried. Surgery is the other treatment option if medical management fails. Patients requiring surgical treatment must be assessed for histological form of HI (Shilyansky et al., 1997; Rahier et al., 1998). HI has two histological forms (focal form and diffuse form) and the choice of surgery is different for each form. The focal form is defined by focal adenomatous hyperplasia of islets β-cells within the pancreatic tissue and it requires partial and selective pancreatectomy (Goossens et al., 1989; Arnoux et al., 2010). However all the β-cells of the pancreas are abnormal in diffuse form, so that a subtotal pancreatectomy may improve the patient's condition. Positron emission tomography (PET) utilizing 18F-fluoro-L-DOPA isotope localizes the focal lesion (Ribeiro et al., 2007; Barthlen et al., 2008) and differentiates between the two histological forms. Pancreatic catheterization with pancreatic venous sampling was previously used to distinguish the two forms but now it has been replaced by PET scan (Arnoux et al., 2010).

12. Summary

Neonatal hypoglycemia is a common metabolic disorder and the operational threshold values of blood glucose <40 mg/dL (plasma glucose< 45 mg/dL) should be used to guide management. All "at risk" neonates and sick infants should be monitored for blood glucose levels. Term healthy AGA infants without any risk factors need not be monitored routinely. Screening for hypoglycemia can be done by point of care devices but confirmation requires laboratory estimation of blood glucose levels. Treatment however should not be delayed while awaiting laboratory confirmation. Asymptomatic hypoglycemia can be managed with a trial of measured oral feed if blood glucose is >25 mg/dL and there is no contraindication to feeding. Symptomatic hypoglycemia should be treated with a mini-bolus of 2 ml/kg 10% dextrose followed by continuous infusion of 6-8 mg/kg/min of 10%dextrose. Refractory or persistent hypoglycemia should be suspected and investigated if the glucose infusion requirement is consistently more than 12 mg/kg/min or the hypoglycemia persists more than 5-7 days. Babies with hypoglycemia should be followed up for neurodevelopmental sequelae.

13. References

Adam, P. A., Raiha, N. Rahiala, E. L., Kekomaki, M. (1975). Oxidation of glucose and D-B-OH-butyrate by the early human fetal brain. *Acta Paediatr Scand* 64(1): 17-24.

Agardh, C. D., Chapman, A. G., Nilsson, B., Siesjo, B. K. (1981). Endogenous substrates utilized by rat brain in severe insulin-induced hypoglycemia. *J Neurochem* 36(2): 490-500.

Agardh, C. D., Kalimo, H., Olsson, Y., Siesjo, B. K. (1980). Hypoglycemic brain injury. I. Metabolic and light microscopic findings in rat cerebral cortex during profound insulin-induced hypoglycemia and in the recovery period following glucose administration. *Acta Neuropathol* 50(1): 31-41.

Anderson, J. M., Milner, R. D., Strich, S. J. (1967). Effects of neonatal hypoglycaemia on the nervous system: a pathological study. *J Neurol Neurosurg Psychiatry* 30(4): 295-310.

Anwar, M., Vannucci R. C. (1988). Autoradiographic determination of regional cerebral blood flow during hypoglycemia in newborn dogs. *Pediatr Res* 24(1): 41-45.

Arnoux, J. B., de Lonlay, P., Ribeiro, M. J., Hussain, K., Blankenstein, O., Mohnike, K. et al. (2010). Congenital hyperinsulinism." Early Hum Dev 86(5): 287-294.

Atkin, S. H., Dasmahapatra, A., Jaker, M. A., Chorost, M. I., Reddy, S. (1991). Fingerstick glucose determination in shock. *Ann Intern Med* 114(12): 1020-1024.

Auer, R. N., Kalimo, H., Olsson, Y., Siesjo, B. K. (1985). The temporal evolution of hypoglycemic brain damage. II. Light- and electron-microscopic findings in the hippocampal gyrus and subiculum of the rat. i 67(1-2): 25-36.

Auer, R. N., Wieloch, T., Olsson, Y., Siesjo, B. K. (1984). The distribution of hypoglycemic brain damage. *Acta Neuropathol* 64(3): 177-191.

Aynsley-Green, A. (1991). Glucose: a fuel for thought! *J Paediatr Child Health* 27(1): 21-30.

Barthlen, W., Blankenstein, O., Mau, H., Koch, M., Hohne, C., Mohnike, W., et al. (2008). Evaluation of [18F]fluoro-L-DOPA positron emission tomography-computed tomography for surgery in focal congenital hyperinsulinism. *J Clin Endocrinol Metab* 93(3): 869-875.

Baumeister, F. A., Rolinski, B., Busch, R., Emmrich, P. (2001). Glucose monitoring with long-term subcutaneous microdialysis in neonates. *Pediatrics* 108(5): 1187-1192.

Bazaes, R. A., Salazar, T. E., Pittaluga, E., Pena, V., Alegria, A., Iniguez, G., et al. (2003). Glucose and lipid metabolism in small for gestational age infants at 48 hours of age. *Pediatrics* 111(4 Pt 1): 804-809.

Beardsall, K. (2010). Measurement of glucose levels in the newborn. *Early Hum Dev* 86(5): 263-267.

Beardsall, K., Ogilvy-Stuart, A. L., Ahluwalia, J., Thompson, M., Dunger, D. B. (2005). The continuous glucose monitoring sensor in neonatal intensive care. *Arch Dis Child Fetal Neonatal Ed* 90(4): F307-310.

Bloom, S. R., Johnston, D. I. (1972). Failure of glucagon release in infants of diabetic mothers. *Br Med J* 4(5838): 453-454.

Bozzetti, P., Ferrari, M. M., Marconi, A. M., Ferrazzi, E., Pardi, G., Makowski, E. L., et al. (1988). The relationship of maternal and fetal glucose concentrations in the human from midgestation until term. *Metabolism* 37(4): 358-363.

Brown, R. J., Wallis P. G. (1963). Hypoglycaemia in the newborn infant. *Lancet* 1(7294): 1278-1282.

Capkova, A., Jirasek J. E. (1968). Glycogen reserves in organs of human foetuses in the first half of pregnancy. *Biol Neonat* 13(3): 129-142.

Carter, P. E., Lloyd, D. J., Duffty, P. (1988). Glucagon for hypoglycaemia in infants small for gestational age. *Arch Dis Child* 63(10): 1264-1266.

Chan, A. Y., Swaminathan, R., Cockram, C. S. (1989). Effectiveness of sodium fluoride as a preservative of glucose in blood. *Clin Chem* 35(2): 315-317.

Chantler, C., Baum, J. D., Norman, D. A. (1967). Dextrostix in the diagnosis of neonatal hypoglycaemia. *Lancet* 2(7531): 1395-1396.

Chiu, N. T., Huang, C. C., Chang, Y. C., Lin, C. H., Yao, W. J., Yu, C. Y. (1998). Technetium-99m-HMPAO brain SPECT in neonates with hypoglycemic encephalopathy. *J Nucl Med* 39(10): 1711-1713.

Collins, J. E., Leonard, J. V., Teale, D., Marks, V., Williams, D. M., Kennedy, C. R., et al. (1990). Hyperinsulinaemic hypoglycaemia in small for dates babies. *Arch Dis Child* 65(10): 1118-1120.

Cornblath, M., Hawdon, J. M., Williams, A. F., Aynsley-Green, A., Ward-Platt, M. P., Schwartz, R., et al. (2000). Controversies regarding definition of neonatal hypoglycemia: suggested operational thresholds. *Pediatrics* 105(5): 1141-1145.

Cornblath, M., Ichord R. (2000). Hypoglycemia in the neonate. *Semin Perinatol* 24(2): 136-149.

Cornblath, M., Schwartz R. (1999). Outcome of neonatal hypoglycaemia. Complete data are needed. *BMJ* 318(7177): 194-195.

Corstjens, A. M., Ligtenberg, J. J., van der Horst, I. C., Spanjersberg, R., Lind, J. S., Tulleken, J. E., et al. (2006). Accuracy and feasibility of point-of-care and continuous blood glucose analysis in critically ill ICU patients. *Crit Care* 10(5): R135.

Cowett, R. M., Howard, G. M., Johnson, J., Vohr, B. (1997). Brain stem auditory-evoked response in relation to neonatal glucose metabolism. *Biol Neonate* 71(1): 31-36.

Critchell, C. D., Savarese, V., Callahan, A., Aboud, C., Jabbour, S., Marik, P. (2007). Accuracy of bedside capillary blood glucose measurements in critically ill patients. *Intensive Care Med* 33(12): 2079-2084.

de Lonlay, P., Cuer, M., Vuillaumier-Barrot, S., Beaune, G., Castelnau, P., Kretz, M., et al. (1999). Hyperinsulinemic hypoglycemia as a presenting sign in phosphomannose isomerase deficiency: A new manifestation of carbohydrate-deficient glycoprotein syndrome treatable with mannose. *J Pediatr* 135(3): 379-383.

de Rooy, L., Hawdon, J. (2002). Nutritional factors that affect the postnatal metabolic adaptation of full-term small- and large-for-gestational-age infants. *Pediatrics* 109(3): E42.

Denne, S. C., Kalhan, S. C. (1986). Glucose carbon recycling and oxidation in human newborns. *Am J Physiol* 251(1 Pt 1): E71-77.

Deshpande, S., Ward Platt, M. (2005). The investigation and management of neonatal hypoglycaemia. *Semin Fetal Neonatal Med* 10(4): 351-361.

Diwakar, K. K., Sasidhar M. V. (2002). Plasma glucose levels in term infants who are appropriate size for gestation and exclusively breast fed. *Arch Dis Child Fetal Neonatal Ed* 87(1): F46-48.

Economides, D. L., Nicolaides, K. H. (1989). Blood glucose and oxygen tension levels in small-for-gestational-age fetuses. *Am J Obstet Gynecol* 160(2): 385-389.

Elimam, A., Horal, M., Bergstrom, M., Marcus, C. (1997). Diagnosis of hypoglycaemia: effects of blood sample handling and evaluation of a glucose photometer in the low glucose range. *Acta Paediatr* 86(5): 474-478.

Ghajar, J. B., Plum, F., Duffy, T. E (1982). Cerebral oxidative metabolism and blood flow during acute hypoglycemia and recovery in unanesthetized rats. *J Neurochem* 38(2): 397-409.

Gibson, G. E., Blass, J. P. (1976). Impaired synthesis of acetylcholine in brain accompanying mild hypoxia and hypoglycemia. *J Neurochem* 27(1): 37-42.

Goossens, A., Gepts, W., Saudubray, J. M., Bonnefont, J. P., Nihoul, Fekete, Heitz, P. U., et al. (1989). Diffuse and focal nesidioblastosis. A clinicopathological study of 24 patients with persistent neonatal hyperinsulinemic hypoglycemia. *Am J Surg Pathol* 13(9): 766-775.

Grazaitis, D. M., Sexson, W. R. (1980). Erroneously high Dextrostix values caused by isopropyl alcohol. *Pediatrics* 66(2): 221-223.

Griffiths, A. D. (1968). Association of hypoglycaemia with symptoms in the newborn. *Arch Dis Child* 43(232): 688-694.

Griffiths, A. D., Bryant, G. M. (1971). Assessment of effects of neonatal hypoglycaemia. A study of 41 cases with matched controls. *Arch Dis Child* 46(250): 819-827.

Harris, D. L., Battin, M. R., Weston, P. J., Harding, J. E., et al. (2010). Continuous glucose monitoring in newborn babies at risk of hypoglycemia. *J Pediatr* 157(2): 198-202 e1.

Hartmann, A. F., Sr., Wohltmann, H. J., Holowach, J., Caldwell, B. M. (1960). Studies in hypoglycemia. *J Pediatr* 56: 211-233.

Hawdon, J. M., Aynsley-Green, A., Bartlett, K., Ward Platt, M. P. (1993a). The role of pancreatic insulin secretion in neonatal glucoregulation. II. Infants with disordered blood glucose homoeostasis. *Arch Dis Child* 68(3 Spec No): 280-285.

Hawdon, J. M., Ward Platt, M. P., Aynsley-Green, A. (1992). Patterns of metabolic adaptation for preterm and term infants in the first neonatal week. *Arch Dis Child* 67(4 Spec No): 357-365.

Hawdon, J. M., Weddell, A., Aynsley-Green, A., Ward Platt, M. P. (1993b). Hormonal and metabolic response to hypoglycaemia in small for gestational age infants. *Arch Dis Child* 68(3 Spec No): 269-273.

Hawdon, J. M., Aynsley-Green, A., Ward Platt, M. P. (1993c). Neonatal blood glucose concentrations: metabolic effects of intravenous glucagon and intragastric medium chain triglyceride. *Arch Dis Child* 68(3 Spec No): 255-261.

Hay, W. W., Jr. Sparks, J. W. (1985). Placental, fetal, and neonatal carbohydrate metabolism. *Clin Obstet Gynecol* 28(3): 473-485.

Heck, L. J. Erenberg, A. (1987). Serum glucose levels in term neonates during the first 48 hours of life. *J Pediatr* 110(1): 119-122.

Ho, H. T., Yeung, W. K., Young, B. W. (2004). Evaluation of "point of care" devices in the measurement of low blood glucose in neonatal practice. *Arch Dis Child Fetal Neonatal Ed* 89(4): F356-359.

Holtrop, P. C., Madison, K. A., Kiechle, F. L., Karcher, R. E., Batton, D. G. (1990). A comparison of chromogen test strip (Chemstrip bG) and serum glucose values in newborns. *Am J Dis Child* 144(2): 183-185.

Hume, R. Burchell, A. (1993). Abnormal expression of glucose-6-phosphatase in preterm infants. *Arch Dis Child* 68(2): 202-204.

Jain, R., Myers, T. F., Kahn, S. E., Zeller, W. P., et al. (1996). How accurate is glucose analysis in the presence of multiple interfering substances in the neonate? (glucose analysis and interfering substances). *J Clin Lab Anal* 10(1): 13-16.

Joosten, K. F., Schellekens, A. P., Waelkens, J. J., Wulffraat, N. M. (1991). [Erroneous diagnosis 'neonatal hypoglycemia' due to incorrect preservation of blood samples]. *Ned Tijdschr Geneeskd* 135(37): 1691-1694.

Kalhan, S. C., Bier, D. M., Savin, S. M., Adam, P. A. (1980). Estimation of glucose turnover and 13C recycling in the human newborn by simultaneous [1-13C]glucose and [6,6-1H2]glucose tracers. *J Clin Endocrinol Metab* 50(3): 456-460.

Kalhan, S. C., D'Angelo, L. J., Savin, S. M., Adam, P. A. (1979). Glucose production in pregnant women at term gestation. Sources of glucose for human fetus. *J Clin Invest* 63(3): 388-394.

Kalhan, S. C., Parimi, P., Van Beek, R., Gilfillan, C., Saker, F., Gruca, L., et al. (2001). Estimation of gluconeogenesis in newborn infants. *Am J Physiol Endocrinol Metab* 281(5): E991-997.

Kalimo, H., Auer, R. N., Siesjo, B. K. (1985). The temporal evolution of hypoglycemic brain damage. III. Light and electron microscopic findings in the rat caudoputamen. *Acta Neuropathol* 67(1-2): 37-50.

Kaplan, M., Blondheim, O., Alon, I., Eylath, U., Trestian, S., Eidelman, A. I.. (1989). Screening for hypoglycemia with plasma in neonatal blood of high hematocrit value. *Crit Care Med* 17(3): 279-282.

Koh, T. H., Aynsley-Green, A., Tarbit, M., Eyre, J. A. (1988). Neural dysfunction during hypoglycaemia. *Arch Dis Child* 63(11): 1353-1358.

Koh, T. H., Eyre, J. A., Aynsley-Green, A. (1988). Neonatal hypoglycaemia--the controversy regarding definition. *Arch Dis Child* 63(11): 1386-1388.

Lehrer, G. M., Bornstein, M. B., Weiss, C., Silides, D. J. (1970). Enzymatic maturation of mouse cerebral neocortex in vitro and in situ. *Exp Neurol* 26(3): 595-606.

Lilien, L. D., Pildes, R. S., Srinivasan, G., Voora, S., Yeh, T. F. (1980). Treatment of neonatal hypoglycemia with minibolus and intraveous glucose infusion. *J Pediatr* 97(2): 295-298.

Lucas, A., Boyes, S., Bloom, S. R., Aynsley-Green, A. (1981). Metabolic and endocrine responses to a milk feed in six-day-old term infants: differences between breast and cow's milk formula feeding. *Acta Paediatr Scand* 70(2): 195-200.

Lucas, A., Morley, R., Cole, T. J. (1988). Adverse neurodevelopmental outcome of moderate neonatal hypoglycaemia. *BMJ* 297(6659): 1304-1308.

Madan, A., Kumar, R., Adams, M. M., Benitz, W. E., Geaghan, S. M. Widness, J. A. (2005). Reduction in red blood cell transfusions using a bedside analyzer in extremely low birth weight infants. *J Perinatol* 25(1): 21-25.

Mantych, G. J., Sotelo-Avila, C., Devaskar, S. U. (1993). The blood-brain barrier glucose transporter is conserved in preterm and term newborn infants. *J Clin Endocrinol Metab* 77(1): 46-49.

Milner, R. D. Wright, A.D. (1967). Plasma glucose, non-esterified fatty acid, insulin and growth hormone response to glucagon in the newborn. *Clin Sci* 32(2): 249-255.

Mitrakou, A., Ryan, C., Veneman, T., Mokan, M., Jenssen, T., Kiss, I., et al. (1991). Hierarchy of glycemic thresholds for counterregulatory hormone secretion, symptoms, and cerebral dysfunction. *Am J Physiol* 260(1 Pt 1): E67-74.

Mujsce, D. J., Christensen, M. A., Vannucci, R. C. (1989). Regional cerebral blood flow and glucose utilization during hypoglycemia in newborn dogs. *Am J Physiol* 256(6 Pt 2): H1659-1666.

Narayan,S., Wazir,S., Mishra, S.(2010). Managemant of Neonatal Hypoglycemia. In *Evidence Based Clinical Practice Guidelines*. Eds. Bhakoo, O.N., Kumar, P., Jain, N., Thakre, R., Murki, S., Venkataseshan, S. National Neonatology Forum, India. Pp63-76.

Nehlig, A. Pereira de Vasconcelos, A. (1993). Glucose and ketone body utilization by the brain of neonatal rats. *Prog Neurobiol* 40(2): 163-221.

Newman, J. D., Pecache, N. S., Barfield, C. P., Balazs, N. D. (2002). Point-of-care testing of blood glucose in the neonatal unit using the AVL Omni 9 analyser. *Ann Clin Biochem* 39(Pt 5): 509-512.

Norberg, K. Siesio, B. K. (1976). Oxidative metabolism of the cerebral cortex of the rat in severe insulin-induced hypoglycaemia. *J Neurochem* 26(2): 345-352.

Otonkoski, T., Kaminen, N., Ustinov, J., Lapatto, R., Meissner, T., Mayatepek, E, et al. (2003). Physical exercise-induced hyperinsulinemic hypoglycemia is an autosomal-dominant trait characterized by abnormal pyruvate-induced insulin release. *Diabetes* 52(1): 199-204.

Pearson, E. R., Boj, S. F., Steele, A. M., Barrett, T., Stals, K., Shield, J. P. et al. (2007). Macrosomia and hyperinsulinaemic hypoglycaemia in patients with heterozygous mutations in the HNF4A gene. *PLoS Med* 4(4): e118.

Pegorier, J. P., Chatelain, F., Thumelin, S., Girard, J. (1998). Role of long-chain fatty acids in the postnatal induction of genes coding for liver mitochondrial beta-oxidative enzymes. *Biochem Soc Trans* 26(2): 113-120.

Persson, B., Settergren, G., Dahlquist, G. (1972). Cerebral arterio-venous difference of acetoacetate and D- -hydroxybutyrate in children. *Acta Paediatr Scand* 61(3): 273-278.

Plecko, B., Stoeckler-Ipsiroglu, S., Schober, E., Harrer, G., Mlynarik, V., Gruber, S., et al. (2002). Oral beta-hydroxybutyrate supplementation in two patients with hyperinsulinemic hypoglycemia: monitoring of beta-hydroxybutyrate levels in blood and cerebrospinal fluid, and in the brain by in vivo magnetic resonance spectroscopy. *Pediatr Res* 52(2): 301-306.

Powers, W. J., Rosenbaum, J. L., Dence, C. S., Markham, J., Videen, T. O. (1998). Cerebral glucose transport and metabolism in preterm human infants. *J Cereb Blood Flow Metab* 18(6): 632-638.

Pryds, O. (1991). Control of cerebral circulation in the high-risk neonate. *Ann Neurol* 30(3): 321-329.

Pryds, O., Christensen, N. J., Friis-Hansen, B. (1990). Increased cerebral blood flow and plasma epinephrine in hypoglycemic, preterm neonates. *Pediatrics* 85(2): 172-176.

Pryds, O., Greisen, G., Friis-Hansen, B. (1988). Compensatory increase of CBF in preterm infants during hypoglycaemia. *Acta Paediatr Scand* 77(5): 632-637.

Rahier, J., Sempoux, C., Fournet, J. C., Poggi, F., Brunelle, F., Nihoul-Fekete, C., et al. (1998). Partial or near-total pancreatectomy for persistent neonatal hyperinsulinaemic hypoglycaemia: the pathologist's role. *Histopathology* 32(1): 15-19.

Reynolds, G. J. Davies, S. (1993). A clinical audit of cotside blood glucose measurement in the detection of neonatal hypoglycaemia. *J Paediatr Child Health* 29(4): 289-291.

Ribeiro, M. J., Boddaert, N., Delzescaux, T., Valayannopoulos, V., Bellanne-Chantelot, C., Jaubert, F., et al. (2007). "Functional imaging of the pancreas: the role of [18F]fluoro-L-DOPA PET in the diagnosis of hyperinsulinism of infancy." *Endocr Dev* 12: 55-66.

Shelley, H. J., Neligan, G. A. (1966). Neonatal hypoglycaemia. *Br Med Bull* 22(1): 34-39.

Shilyansky, J., Fisher, S., Cutz, E., Perlman, K., Filler, R. M. (1997). Is 95% pancreatectomy the procedure of choice for treatment of persistent hyperinsulinemic hypoglycemia of the neonate? *J Pediatr Surg* 32(2): 342-346.

Siesjo, B. K. (1988). Hypoglycemia, brain metabolism, and brain damage. *Diabetes Metab Rev* 4(2): 113-144.

Skov, L. Pryds, O. (1992). Capillary recruitment for preservation of cerebral glucose influx in hypoglycemic, preterm newborns: evidence for a glucose sensor? *Pediatrics* 90(2 Pt 1): 193-195.

Soothill, P. W., Nicolaides, K. H., Campbell, S. (1987). Prenatal asphyxia, hyperlacticaemia, hypoglycaemia, and erythroblastosis in growth retarded fetuses. *Br Med J (Clin Res Ed)* 294(6579): 1051-1053.

Spar, J. A., Lewine, J. D., Orrison, W. W., Jr. (1994). Neonatal hypoglycemia: CT and MR findings. *AJNR Am J Neuroradiol* 15(8): 1477-1478.

Sperling, M. A., DeLamater, P. V., Phelps, D., Fiser, R. H., Oh, W., Fisher, D. A. (1974). Spontaneous and amino acid-stimulated glucagon secretion in the immediate postnatal period. Relation to glucose and insulin. *J Clin Invest* 53(4): 1159-1166.

Srinivasan, G., Pildes, R. S., Cattamanchi, G., Voora, S., Lilien, L. D. (1986). Plasma glucose values in normal neonates: a new look. *J Pediatr* 109(1): 114-117.

Stanley, C. A., Anday, E. K., Baker, L., Delivoria-Papadopolous, M. (1979). Metabolic fuel and hormone responses to fasting in newborn infants. *Pediatrics* 64(5): 613-619

Suh, Aoyama, K., Chen, Y., Garnier, P., Matsumori, Y., Gum, E., et al. (2003). Hypoglycemic neuronal death and cognitive impairment are prevented by poly(ADP-ribose) polymerase inhibitors administered after hypoglycemia. *J Neurosci* 23(33): 10681-10690.

Sunehag, A., Ewald, U., Larsson, A., Gustafsson, J. (1993). Glucose production rate in extremely immature neonates (< 28 weeks) studied by use of deuterated glucose. *Pediatr Res* 33(2): 97-100.

Swenne, I., Ewald, U., Gustafsson, J., Sandberg, E., Ostenson, C. G. (1994). Inter-relationship between serum concentrations of glucose, glucagon and insulin during the first two days of life in healthy newborns. *Acta Paediatr* 83(9): 915-919.

Tang, Z., Du, X., Louie, R. F., Kost, G. J. (2000). Effects of pH on glucose measurements with handheld glucose meters and a portable glucose analyzer for point-of-care testing. *Arch Pathol Lab Med* 124(4): 577-582.

Tang, Z., Lee, J. H., Louie, R. F., Kost, G. J. (2000). Effects of different hematocrit levels on glucose measurements with handheld meters for point-of-care testing. *Arch Pathol Lab Med* 124(8): 1135-1140.

Tang, Z., Louie, R. F., Lee, J. H., Lee, D. M., Miller, E. E., Kost, G. J. (2001). Oxygen effects on glucose meter measurements with glucose dehydrogenase- and oxidase-based test strips for point-of-care testing. *Crit Care Med* 29(5): 1062-1070.

Thornton, P. S., Alter, C. A., Katz, L. E., Baker, L., Stanley, C. A. (1993). Short- and long-term use of octreotide in the treatment of congenital hyperinsulinism. *J Pediatr* 123(4): 637-643.

Togari, H., Oda, M., Wada, Y. (1987). Mechanism of erroneous Dextrostix readings. *Arch Dis Child* 62(4): 408-409.

Vannucci, R. C., Nardis, E. E., Vannucci, S. J., Campbell, P. A. (1981). Cerebral carbohydrate and energy metabolism during hypoglycemia in newborn dogs. *Am J Physiol* 240(3): R192-199.

Vannucci, R. C., Vannucci, S. J. (1978). Cerebral carbohydrate metabolism during hypoglycemia and anoxia in newborn rats. *Ann Neurol* 4(1): 73-79.

Vannucci, R. C., Vannucci, S. J. (2000). Glucose metabolism in the developing brain. *Semin Perinatol* 24(2): 107-115.

Volpe, J. J. (2008). Hypoglycemia and brain injury, In: *Neurology of the newborn*. Volpe, J.J. Ed pp. 591-618, Saunders Elsevier, Philadelphia.

Ward Platt, M., Deshpande, S. (2005). Metabolic adaptation at birth. *Semin Fetal Neonatal Med* 10(4): 341-350.

Whipple, A. O., Frantz, V. K. (1935). Adenoma of Islet Cells with Hyperinsulinism: A Review. *Ann Surg* 101(6): 1299-1335.

Wieloch, T. (1985). Hypoglycemia-induced neuronal damage prevented by an N-methyl-D-aspartate antagonist. *Science* 230(4726): 681-683.

Wieloch, T., Harris, R. J., Symon, L., Siesjo, B. K. (1984). Influence of severe hypoglycemia on brain extracellular calcium and potassium activities, energy, and phospholipid metabolism. *J Neurochem* 43(1): 160-168.

Wilkins, B. H., Kalra, D. (1982). Comparison of blood glucose test strips in the detection of neonatal hypoglycaemia. *Arch Dis Child* 57(12): 948-950.

Williams, A. F. (1997). Hypoglycaemia of the newborn: a review. *Bull World Health Organ* 75(3): 261-290.

Williams, A. F. (2005). Neonatal hypoglycaemia: clinical and legal aspects. *Semin Fetal Neonatal Med* 10(4): 363-368.

Wilson, J. E. (1972). The relationship glycolytic and mitochondrial enzymes in the developing rat brain. *J Neurochem* 19(1): 223-227.

Wu, P. Y., Modanlou, H., Karelitz, M. (1975). Effect of glucagon on blood glucose homeostasis in infants of diabetic mothers. *Acta Paediatr Scand* 64(3): 441-445.

Yan, H., Rivkees S. A. (2006). Hypoglycemia influences oligodendrocyte development and myelin formation. *Neuroreport* 17(1): 55-59.

Part 3

Section C

8

Drug-Induced Hypoglycemia

Kristen Helms and Kristi Kelley
Auburn University, Harrison School of Pharmacy
United States

1. Introduction

Although it is noted throughout the literature that adverse effects occur, one review of safety reporting determined clinical trials only report adverse effects between 29% (laboratory adverse effects) and 39% (clinical adverse effects) (Ioannidis, et al, 2001). It is important to keep these numbers in mind when looking at the number of drug-induced hypoglycemia cases. Seltzer's review of the literature from 1940 to 1989 reveals 1418 documented cases of drug-induced hypoglycemia. Based on estimates of the lack of adverse effect reporting, it is unlikely that these cases were the only incidents of drug-induced hypoglycemia that occurred during this time (Seltzer, 1989).

It is also reasonable to look at estimates of adverse drug effects (ADEs) in hospitalized patients. Such estimates indicate ADEs may account for between 3 and 5% of all hospital admissions (Pandit et al, 1993). In a 2006 study it was determined approximately 22% of admissions attributed to ADEs were due to hypoglycemia at a university hospital versus 23% at a community hospital (Kilbridge et al, 2006). These admissions were related to an overall admission rate attributed to ADEs of 4.4% at the university hospital and 6.2% at a community hospital (Kilbridge et al, 2006). In addition there are estimates that as many as 30% of hospitalized patients experience an ADE while in the hospital (Pandit et al, 1993). Estimates of 3 - 4.5 billion dollars, which is now outdated, just begin to attribute a cost to treating ADEs. However, the cost is probably grossly underestimated since the actual number of ADEs reported is underestimated (Pandit et al, 1993). Not only is the cost of managing an ADEs a significant issue but the risk of mortality must be considered as well. Mortality has been estimated to occur in as many as 140,000 patients each year (Pandit et al, 1993). One study looking at death due to drug-induced hypoglycemia determined a 1.3% mortality rate (Juurlink et al, 2003).

The incidence and impact of drug-induced hypoglycemia should be contrasted with the incidence and impact of hypoglycemia in patients with diabetes mellitus (DM) - type 1 or type 2. For patients with type 1 DM, it is estimated that hypoglycemia, by the numbers (blood glucose less than 50 - 60 mg/dL), occurs 1 in 10 times when patients check their blood glucose (Cryer et al, 2003). While the number of asymptomatic hypoglycemia episodes is undocumented, it is estimated that patients with type 1 DM experience "an average of 2 symptomatic hypoglycemic episodes per week.and an episode of severe, at least temporarily disabling hypoglycaemia once a year" (Cryer et al, 2003). The incidence of hypoglycemia in patients with type 2 DM is more challenging. When comparing the incidence of severe hypoglycemia in patients with type 1 DM versus patients with type 2 DM being treated with insulin, estimates are anywhere from 10% to equal incidence of hypoglycemia (Cryer et al, 2003). Other studies that have tried to quantify the incidence of hypoglycemia in type 2 patients have varied from an overall incidence of 20% in patients taking oral agents to 0.5% episodes of severe hypoglycemia in patients using insulin (Jennings AM et al, 1989 & Miller CD et al, 2001). Unfortunately, as with drug-induced hypoglycemia, hypoglycemia may result in death. One estimate of the rate of death from hypoglycemia is 2 to 4% of patients with type 1 DM, but, as with the incidence of hypoglycemia, there is not a reliable estimate of death attributed to hypoglycemia in patients with type 2 DM (Cryer et al, 2003). However, a 1999 review of cases of hypoglycemic coma provides some perspective on potential morbidity and mortality. In this study, out of 102 reported cases, 5 patients died. (Ben-Ami et al, 1999).

These statistics emphasize the importance of recognizing and treating hypoglycemia as well as ADEs when they occur. The numbers also serve as a reminder to all healthcare providers of their responsibility in the prevention of ADEs, especially drug-induced ADEs. However, in order to prevent ADEs, one must know what patients are at risk for development of an ADE. The risk for drug-induced hypoglycemia, the mechanism of potentially causative agents as well as management and prevention are discussed below in effort to make healthcare providers aware of this potential ADE and how to avoid it.

2. Definition of hypoglycemia

Before determining if a patient is experiencing drug-induced hypoglycemia, the definition of hypoglycemia should be established. Since all patients respond to blood glucose concentrations differently, it is challenging to establish a blood glucose at which every patient will experience symptoms. However, it is widely accepted that most patients will begin to experience symptoms when their blood glucose level is less than 3.3 mmol/l (60 mg/dL). The symptoms patients commonly experience are listed in Table 1 below and can be manifestations of the response by the autonomic nervous system as well as the brain's response to being deprived of glucose (Cryer et al, 2003, White, 2007). Physiologic responses with escalating hypoglycemia are shown in Table 2. Severe episodes of hypoglycemia may be characterized by loss of consciousness and/or seizures and, in instances of sustained hypoglycemia, may result in brain damage or death (Cryer et al, 2003). The blood glucose level at which a patient experiences symptoms of hypoglycemia can be influenced by other factors such as: the frequency of hypoglycemic episodes, which may result in hypoglycemic unawareness; frequent hyperglycemia episodes, and increased caffeine intake (Cryer et al, 1999).

Neurogenic Symptoms of Hypoglycemia	Neuroglycopenic Symptoms of Hypoglycemia	Physical Signs of Hypoglycemia
Anxiety/arousal	Blurry vision	Increased systolic blood pressure
Hunger	Changes in behavior - irritability is often noted	Pallor
Shaky/trembling	Confusion/difficulty thinking	Sweating
	Difficulty speaking	
Parethesias	Dizziness	
Sweating	Emotional lability	Tachycardia
	Fatigue	
	Loss of consciousness	
	seizures	
	Warmth	
	Weakness	

Adapted from Cryer et al, 2003 and White, 2007

Table 1. Common symptoms of hypoglycemia

Blood glucose level	Classification	Physiologic response
70 mg/dl (3.9 mmol/l)	Hypoglycemia	• Glucagon release • Epinephrine release • Growth hormone release • Cortisol release
54 mg/dl (3 mmol/l)	Symptomatic hypoglycemia	• Autonomic symptoms
36 mg/dl (2 mmol/l)	Hypoglycemia affecting brain function (neuroglucopenia)	• Cognitive decline
18 mg/dl (1 mmol/l)	Severe neuroglucopenia	• Coma • Seizures

Adapted from White, 2007

Table 2. Physiologic response based on blood glucose level

It is important to note that monitoring blood glucose levels is the best way to monitor hypoglycemia since hemoglobin A1C (A1C) does not adequately depict hypoglycemia given that A1C provides a measure of average control of blood glucose over the past 2 to 3 months (American Diabetes Association, 2011).

In one technical review of hypoglycemia in patients with diabetes, it was noted that hypoglycemia resulted in "physical morbidity" as evidenced in the physical symptoms and even neurologic impairment patients may experience as well as "psychological morbidity" which were differences in moods and outlook as a result of experiencing hypoglycemia (Cryer PE et al, 2003). Specific manifestations of physical and psychological morbidity are detailed in Table 3. When thinking of these symptoms of hypoglycemia, it should be recognized that they can make patients feel uncomfortable physically as well as socially since experiencing these symptoms may result in patients receiving unwanted attention. It is important to consider that hypoglycemia affects patients both physically, psychologically, and can have a significant impact on a patient's overall sense of well-being. Although the same evidence does not exist for patients that experience drug-induced hypoglycemia, it could be argued that the toll is equally as hard on these individuals and therefore, emphasizes the importance of avoiding drug-induced hypoglycemia.

Examples of Physical Morbidity Associated with Hypoglycemia	**Examples of Psychological Morbidity Associated with Hypoglycemia**
Physical symptoms - anxiety, hunger, palpitations, sweating, hunger Neurologic impairment - changes in behavior, decline in cognitive function, seizures, coma	Fear of experiencing hypoglycemia Guilt related to being fearful of experiencing hypoglycaemia Anxiet overall happiness

Adapted from Cryer PE et al, 2003

Table 3. Physical and psychological morbidity associated with hypoglycemia.

3. Risk factors

Table 4 lists patient characteristics that may increase the risk of drug-induced hypoglycemia. Specific pharmacokinetic and pharmacodynamic drug parameters may affect the level of risk associated with the described patient characteristics.

Risk Factors	Mechanism
Advancing age	Decreased symptoms/decreased awareness, decreased counterregulatory response to low blood glucose
Renal insufficiency	Decreased insulin clearance
Hepatic insufficiency	Decreased gluconeogenesis
Decreased food intake (skipping meals)	Insufficient glucose intake
Excessive alcohol intake	Decreased gluconeogenesis
Polypharmacy	Increased risk of drug interactions resulting in hypoglycemia

Table 4. Risk factors for drug-induced hypoglycemia

It should be noted that the risk factors associated with drug-induced hypoglycemia are similar to the risk factors associated with the development of hypoglycemia in patients with DM. In particular it is known that advanced age, alcohol intake, and polypharmacy are all risk factors for hypoglycemia in patients with type 1 diabetes (Zammitt et al, 2005). As noted above, these are risk factors that may also place patients at risk for drug-induced hypoglycemia. In addition to the risk factors discussed above, risk factors that place patients with type 1 diabetes at risk for hypoglycemia are: caffeine intake; variations in sleep; and physical activity, in particular exercise, in relation to meals and medications (Zammitt et al, 2005). However, it is unknown how these factors affect the risk of hypoglycemia in patients with type 2 diabetes (Zammitt et al, 2005). It is known that patients with type 2 diabetes who have been taking in insulin for more than 10 years are increased risk for experiencing hypoglycemia (Zammitt et al, 2005). Obviously, the greatest concern for the development of drug-induced hypoglycemia becomes when patients have pre-exsiting diabetes and then are placed on a medication that has the potential to cause hypoglycemia.

4. Glucose regulation

Changes in serum glucose levels are a result of the following process: glucose absorption from the gastroinstestinal tract, release of stored glucose through hepatic glycogenolysis, and creation of glucose from non-glucose sources through hepatic gluconeogenesis. Glycogenolysis releases glucose through breakdown of glycogen, the stored form of glucose, and glycogenolysis creates glucose from amino acid and lactate. All three processes affect glucose levels based on proximity to meals. The rate of rise of serum glucose during and after meals is predominantly a result of the rate of gastric emptying. Rate of gastric emptying determines amount of glucose absorbed in gastrointestinal tract. During periods of fasting, glucose levels are regulated by glycogenolysis and gluconeogenesis. Glycogenolysis impacts serum glucose levels in the first 8 to 12 hours of fasting, while gluconeogenesis contributes more to glucose levels after longer periods of fasting (Aronoff et al, 2004).

The processes above are all regulated by glucoregulatory hormones. The hormones, their site of origin, and specific gluco-regulatory actions are listed in table 5. In addition to those listed, blood glucose levels are affected by epinephrine, cortisol, and growth hormones (Aronoff et al, 2004).

Hormone	Site of origin/production	Action
Insulin	Beta (β)-cells of the pancreas	Induces uptake of glucose by cells Inhibits glucagon secretion post-prandially Enhances protein and fat synthesis Stimulates glycogenesis in the liver
Glucagon	Alpha (α)-cells of the pancreas	Stimulates hepatic glycogenolysis, hepatic gluconeogenesis, and hepatic ketogenesis
Amylin	B-cells of the pancreas	Slows gastric emptying Inhibits glucagon secretion post-prandially Decreases food intake
Glucagon-like peptide 1 (GLP-1)	L-cells of the intestine	Slows gastric emptying Stimulates glucose-dependent (prandial) insulin secretion Inhibits glucagon secretion post-prandially Decreases food intake
Glucose-dependent insulinotropic peptide (GIP),	L-cells of the intestine	Stimulates glucose-dependent (prandial) insulin secretion Inhibits glucagon secretion post-prandially

Table 5. Gluco-regulatory hormones

Insulin and glucagon play large roles in the overall regulation of blood glucose (Figure 1). Increases in serum blood glucose stimulate insulin release from the pancreas. The amount of insulin released is dependent on the level of blood glucose. Insulin is not released until blood glucose levels reach 3.3 mmol/l (59.4 mg/dl). Insulin acts to both decrease existing glucose in the blood and to decrease production of further glucose. Insulin binds to receptors on fat, muscle, and liver cells to stimulate glucose uptake. Additional serum glucose is converted to glycogen, the storage form of glucose, through hepatic glycogenesis. Insulin decreases production of glucose from gluconeogenesis and glycogenolysis by inhibiting glucagon release from the pancreas. The combination of these actions results in a decrease in serum blood glucose. Glucagon serves as the hormone that balances the glucose lowering effects of insulin. Glucagon controls fasting levels by stimulating gluconeogenesis and glycogenolysis in the liver. Stimulation of these mechanisms results in release of glucose, increasing serum blood glucose levels. Release of glucagon from the pancreas occurs when serum glucose levels fall below approximately 5 mmol/l (90 mg/dl) (Aronoff et al, 2004).

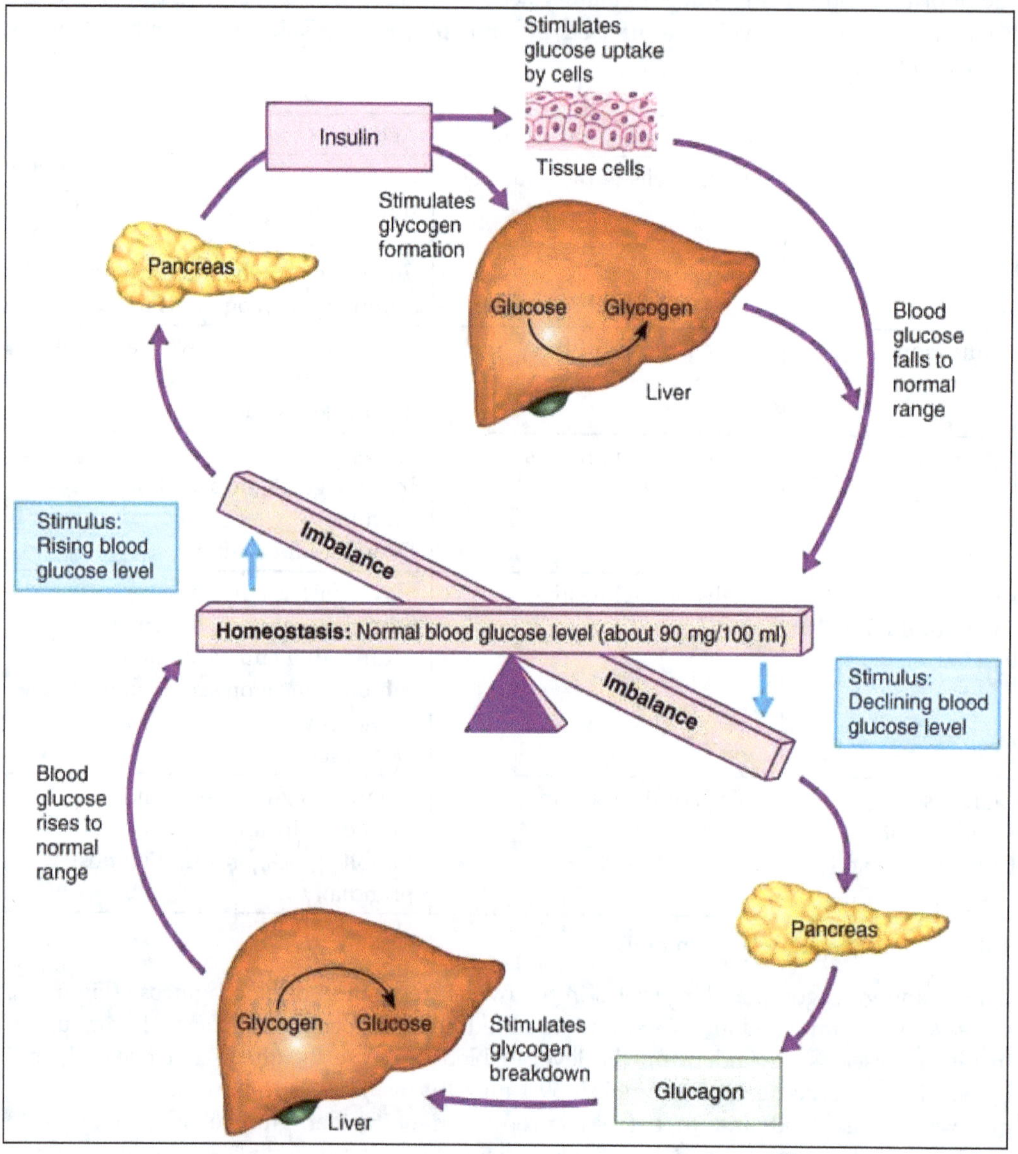

Fig. 1. Glucose regulation (Dugi K, 2009)

5. Causative agents

5.1 There are a number of agents implicated in causing hypoglycemia; however, the level of evidence available varies significantly amongst agents. The most highly documented drug-induced hypoglycemia occurs with medications used to treat hyperglycemia. The specific agents and classes are included in table 6 below.

Anti-diabetic agents
Exenatide
Insulin
Pramlintide
Secratagogues (non-sulfonylurea)
Sitagliptin
Sulfonylureas

Table 6. Anti-diabetic agents with greatest evidence of causing hypoglycaemia

Of potentially greater concern are the agents which are used for indications other than hyperglycemia because the hypoglycemic episodes are often less predictable and/or unexpected. These agents often have very little or no quality evidence to document the frequency and severity of their hypoglycemic effects. This is illustrated in the systematic review of literature through 2007 conducted by The Hypoglycemia Task Force of The Endocrine Society which identified hypoglycemia associated with 164 different medications (Murad et al, 2009). This study found that no individual or class of drugs has high quality evidence supporting its impact on glucose levels, though drugs used to treat hyperglycemia were not included. Table 7 provides a list of the most commonly cited agents in the literature and their level of evidence. Level of evidence was defined by use of the GRADE approach to literature evaluation. Available evidence was evaluated for quality of study design, strength of association of the medication to the reported adverse effects, and quantity of evidence available (Murad et al, 2009).

Moderate Quality Evidence	
Agent/Class	**Mechanism of hypoglycemia**
Fluoroquinolones (gatifloxacin)	Unclear May increase insulin secretion from pancreas
Indomethacin	Increase insulin secretion from pancreas, decrease in insulin clearance, decrease in gluconeogenesis, and increase in glucose uptake in periphery
Pentamadine	Increased insulin secretion from pancreas through cell damage
Quinine	Increased insulin secretion from pancreas
Poor Quality Evidence	
Agent/Class	**Mechanism of hypoglycemia**
Angiotensin Converting Enzyme Inhibitors (ACEIs)	Increase insulin sensitivity
Beta blockers	Mask signs/symptoms of hypoglycemia, increase in glucose uptake in the periphery
Ethanol	Decrease in gluconeogenesis in the liver
Lithium	Unclear
Propoxyphene	Unclear
Sulfamethoxazole	Increase insulin secretion from pancreas

Table 7. Strength of evidence of drug-induced hypoglycemia and proposed mechanisms (Murad, et al, 2009).

Drug-induced hypoglycemia may be a result of direct changes to glucose homeostasis or indirect effects on a patient's ability to recognize onset of hypoglycemia. Changes that affect glucose homeostasis include direct increase in insulin secretion from the pancreas, indirect increase in insulin secretion through decreased degradation of incretin hormones (GLP-1 and GIP), cytotoxic effects on pancreatic cells leading to increase insulin release, decrease in gluconeogenesis, increase in glucose utilization and storage, decrease in glucagon release from the pancreatic α cells, and decreased gastric emptying (Pandit et al, 1993). Many agents affect glucose homeostasis through a combination of these mechanisms. Location of mechanism is exhibited in table 8.

Pancreas	Liver	Periphery	Kidney	Gut
• Pentamidine • Fluoroquinolones • Sulfamethoxazole • Quinine • Indomethacin • Exenatide • Sulfonylureas • Non-sulfonylurea secretagogues • Sitagliptin	• Ethanol • Indomethacin • Exenatide Pramlintide • Sitagliptin	• Beta adrenergic antagonists • Angiotensin converting enzyme (ACE) inhibitors • Indomethacin • Insulin	• Indomethacin	• Pramlintide

Table 8. Location of action of agents implicated in drug-induced hypoglycemia

5.2 Specific agents

Specific agents, including risk factors and frequency of hypoglycemic events, are discussed below.

5.2.1 Fluoroquinolones

Fluoroquinolones are antibiotics which exhibit their antimicrobial activity through inhibition of DNA gyrase and topoisomerase IV, enzymes involved in bacterial cell division (Product Information: Tequin, 2006). The class includes the following agents: ciprofloxacin, gatifloxacin, levofloxacin, moxifloxacin, norfloxacin, ofloxacin, and rofloxacin. Though there are reports of hypoglycemia with most agents in this class, a majority of the evidence with fluoroquinolone-induced hypoglycemia is with gatifloxacin (Murad et al, 2009). The exact mechanism of this hypoglycemic effect is not clear; however, it is proposed that fluoroquinolones increase insulin secretion from the pancreas and may have a pharmacokinetic or pharmacodynamic interaction with various antidiabetic agents, including sulfonylureas. The adverse effect does not appear dose-related and presents typically within the first three days of therapy for less severe hypoglycemia (Frothingham, 2005; Gajjar, et al, 2000; Park-Wyllie et al, 2006; Product Information: Tequin, 2006). More severe episodes, specifically those requiring hospitalization or prolonged hospitalization, are more common after three days of therapy. Hypoglycemia has been reported with intravenous and oral therapies in both outpatient and inpatient settings, and discontinuation of the medication is often required to resolve the glucose abnormalities (Murad et al, 2009). Though new onset diabetes has been reported, risk factors for patients who are more likely to experience hypoglycemic episodes are: pre-existing diabetes, concomitant use of hypoglycemic medications, advanced age, and decreased renal function (Frothingham, 2005; Product Information: Tequin, 2006; Yip & Lee, 2006).

5.2.2 Indomethacin

Indomethacin belongs to the class of agents called non-steroidal anti-inflammatory drugs (NSAIDs). Anti-inflammatory agents, including salicylates, are all thought to increase risk of hypoglycemia, with indomethacin having the greatest evidence, likely due to the population being treated. Though often used for osteoarthritis and other inflammatory conditions, indomethacin may also be used to close a patent ductus arteriosis in neonates, often in those born prematurely. Increases in pancreatic insulin secretion, decreases in insulin clearance, increases in glucose utilization in the periphery, and decreases in gluconeogenesis all appear to contribute to the hypoglycemic effects of these drugs. Less than three per cent of neonates exposed to therapeutic levels of intravenous indomethacin for patent ductus arteriosis experience hypoglycemia (Product Information: Indocin, 2010). Whether this effect is dose-related is unclear; however, the risk may be significantly decreased by use of a concomitant infusion of intravenous glucose (Hosono, 1999).

5.2.3 Pentamidine

Pentamidine is an anti-fungal agent which exhibits its effects through inhibition of microbial nuclear metabolism. Direct cytotoxic effects on beta cells of the pancreas results in increased secretion of insulin. This early release of insulin is due to the lytic effects on the cell which result in cell death. This can ultimately result in insulin-dependent diabetes as a result of this cell loss (Pandit et al, 1993). Pentamidine is associated with a 6-40% risk of hypoglycemia in patients receiving intravenous or intramuscular administration. Hypoglycemia is most commonly seen in patients with acquired immune deficiency syndrome (AIDS) treated for *Pneumocystis carinii* (Murad et al, 2009 & Product Information: Pentin, 2008) (Product Information: Pentam, 2008 & Product Information: Nebupent, 2008). The risk of hypoglycemia and resultant pancreatic damage associated with pentamidine is greater with higher doses, higher cumulative doses, and prolonged use (Pandit et al, 1993). There also appears to be increased risk with use of pentamidine mesylate compared to pentamidine isothionate (Waskin, 1996).

5.2.4 Quinine

Quinine is an anti-malarial agent used acutely for systemic and cerebral disease. More than 300 cases of hypoglycemia have been reported with quinine therapy and 30 clinical studies have demonstrated similar findings (Murad et al, 2009). The crux of the hypoglycemic effects of quinine appear to be the result of increased insulin secretion from beta cells. Though this is most common in patients infected with malaria, there are reports of quinine-induced hypoglycemia in patients without malaria. Patients with malaria often exhibit more severe or sustained hypoglycemia since the organism responsible for malaria, *Plasmodium falciparum,* independently lowers glucose levels. There is also an increased risk of hypoglycemia with higher doses of quinine and with infusion times of intravenous doses of less than one hour. Manufacturers recommend intravenous infusions occur over four hours to minimize risk of hypoglycemia (Product Information: Qualaquin, 2010). Quinine-induced hypoglycemia can be resistant to traditional therapy with glucose and glucagon; however, treatment with octreotide has been shown to be beneficial (Pandit et al, 1993).

5.2.5 Beta blockers

Non-selective beta-adrenergic antagonists, also known as beta blockers, are vasodilators which are often used to treat hypertension and cardiac disease. A list of non-selective beta blockers is provided in table 9 below. These agents have been linked with hypoglycemic effects in patients with and without diabetes (Murad et al, 2009). Oral formulations are most commonly the culprit; however, hypoglycemia associated with topical formulations is documented (Pandit et al, 1993). Though there are numerous reports of hypoglycemia associated with beta blockers , the quality of the data is limited. Murad, et al, theorizes that the high numbers of reports are a representation of the frequency of use of these agents more than the frequency of the actual hypoglycemic events (Murad et al, 2009).

There are two proposed mechanisms for this hypoglycemic effect in beta blockers. First, there is a blunting of the signs and symptoms of hypoglycemia (White, 2007). The exception to this blunting effect is sweating, an important educational point for all patients (Product Information: Innopran XL, 2010). The second mechanism is a direct potentiation of the effects of insulin. This heightened insulin effect increases glucose utilization in the periphery and inhibits lipolysis. Further, there is a diminished physiologic response to hypoglycemia in patient receiving beta blockers, specifically a decrease in glycogenolysis and gluconeogenesis (Pandit et al, 1993 & White, 2007). Patients at greatest risk for hypoglycemia with beta blockers include patients with hepatic disease, patients on hemodialysis, neonates, and patients with type 1 diabetes (Product Information: Innopran XL, 2010). Use of selective beta blockers, such as atenolol, metoprolol, and bisoprolol are thought to have a decreased risk of hypoglycaemia and may be a reasonable alternative to patients unable to tolerate non-selective agents (Pandit et al, 1993).

Non-selective beta-adrenergic antagonists
Alprenolol Bucindolol Carteolol Nadolol Penbutolol Pindolol Propranolol Sotalol Timolol
Non-selective beta-adrenergic antagonists with additional alpha antagonism:
Carvedilol Labetalol

Table 9. Non-selective beta-adrenergic antagonists (beta blockers)

5.2.6 ACE inhibitors

Angiotensin converting enzyme (ACE) inhibitors are a class of drugs that are typically used for hypertension and cardiovascular disease. Eleven studies document the potential for ACEI inhibitor-associated hypoglycemia, and a majority of these are with the use of captopril (Murad et al, 2009; Herings et al, 1995). All members of this class are listed in table 10 below. Though the mechanism for this drug-induced hypoglycaemia is not well defined, it is proposed that the increase in bradykinins associated with ACE inhibitor use may cause an increase in insulin sensitivity (Pandit et al, 1993; Vuorinen-Markkola & Yki-Jarvinen, 1995). One study by Pollare, et al, suggests that captopril increases glucose utilization in the periphery compared to use of hydrochlorothiazide (Pollare et al, 1989); however, Wiggam, et al, demonstrates in one study that ACE inhibitors have no impact on hepatic or peripheral insulin sensitivity (Wiggam et al, 1998). Because of the contradicting information available, the actual impact of ACE inhibitors on blood glucose is not clear. ACE inhibitor therapy is a mainstay of hypertension, diabetes, and cardiovascular disease management. To date, there is insufficient evidence available to warrant discontinuation of this therapy in patients at risk for hypoglycemia with these disease states; however, in patients with suspected captopril-induced hypoglycemia, switching to another ACE inhibitor is a reasonable recommendation.

ACE Inhibitors
Benazepril
Captopril
Enalapril
Fosinopril
Lisinopril
Moexipril
Perindopril
Quinapril
Ramipril
Trandolapril

Table 10. Angiotensin Converting Enzyme (ACE) Inhibitors

5.2.7 Ethanol

Despite the poor level of evidence, ethanol has been touted as one of the most common causes of drug-induced hypoglycaemia in the United States (Pandit et al, 1993). The proposed mechanism is a direct suppression of gluconeogenesis in the liver, a process that typically occurs in more long-standing fasting states. Some studies suggest that this hypoglycemic potential is present in both occasional and chronic alcohol consumers and is more common with use of non-carbohydrate laden drinks (Pandit et al, 1993). Because of this, patients at greater risk for hypoglycemia should avoid consuming alcohol.

6. Prevention

One easy way to prevent drug-induced hypoglycemia is to avoid the medication that poses the potential for drug-induced hypoglycemia in patients that are at high risk for drug-induced hypoglycemia. Unfortunately, it may not be practical to avoid certain medications that may cause drug-induced hypoglycemia. As when deciding to use any medication, weigh the benefit of using the medication versus risk, in this case drug-induced hypoglycemia.

If avoiding the agent is not possible, attempt to minimize the risk of hypoglycemia by keeping in mind the following restrictions. Use extended-release/sustained-released products if that is an option for the medication needed (Pandit et al, 1993). Reinforce with patients the need to avoid alcohol intake (Pandit et al, 1993). Minimizing the lenth of time and dose of an offending agent may also be beneficial. Since hypoglycemia awareness is largely reliant on patient perception of the signs and symptoms of hypoglycemia, education is key (Cryer et al, 2003). Therefore, it is important to review the signs and symptoms of hypoglycemia with patients and caregivers. One way to monitor patients for evidence of hypoglycemia is to monitor their blood glucose concentrations, which is especially in important in patients with pre-existing diabetes. Blood glucose should be carefully monitored with initiation, dose changes, or discontinuation of any medication in patients with diabetes. It is usually recommended for patients to regularly check their fasting blood glucose readings during the initiation of a medication that can cause drug-induced hypoglycemia. The healthcare provider can make patient specific recommendations on how often to monitor blood glucose based on the patient's underlying risk for hypoglycemia (e.g. patients already taking 1 or more agents that can cause drug-induced hypoglycemia or those patients with a diagnosis of diabetes) as well as any manufacturer recommendations. In addition to instructing the patient to monitor and record their blood glucose levels at home, it is helpful for a healthcare provider to review the history of the patient's blood glucose levels at every visit and ask about signs and symptoms of hypoglycemia. Tracking the patient's weight and reviewing the trend over the time the patient is taking a potentially offending agent may also provide insight into whether the patient is experiencing asymptomatic hypoglycemia, especially when reviewed with the patient's fasting blood glucose levels. When at all possible, patients should not be taking multiple agents that may cause drug-induced hypoglycemia. Healthcare providers should also be diligent to review a patient's medication profile for drug interactions, pharmacokinetics and pharmacodynamic, with potentially offending hypoglycemic agents. Tables 11 and 12 provide a summary of points to remember when prescribing medications with a potential for drug-induced hypoglycemia.

Prescribing Considerations
Use extended or sustained release products when possible
Avoid alcohol intake
Minimize the length of time on an offending agent
Utilize the lowest effective dose of the offending agent
Avoid having multiple medications in the patient's profile that can cause hypoglycemia
Screen the patients medication profile for drug interactions - pharmacokinetic and pharmacodynamic

Table 11. Specific Prescribing Considerations When Prescribing Medications with a Potential to Cause Drug-Induced Hypoglycemia

Prescriber Considerations	Patient Education Points
Monitor blood glucose levels at clinic visits	Demonstration of self-monitoring of blood glucose Discussion of timing of blood glucose monitoring and target levels
Inquire about experiences with hypoglycemia, including specific signs/symptoms	Monitor for signs/symptoms of hypoglycemia Review appropriate treatment of hypoglycemia
Weigh the patient at clinic visits and review the trend	

Table 12. Monitoring Points When Patients Are Taking Medications with a Potential to Cause Drug-Induced Hypoglycemia

7. Management

When measures to prevent drug-induced hypoglycemia do not work or when appropriate prevention measures were not able to be undertaken, hypoglycemia, especially symptomatic hypoglycemia, must be treated. Specific, evidence-based recommendations for management of drug-induced hypoglycemia are not readily available. In the absence of guidelines for drug-induced hypoglycemia, patients who experience this should be treated according to readily accepted guidelines for managing hypoglycemia in patients with diabetes (Cryer et al, 2009, American Diabetes Association, 2011).

7.1 Signs and symptoms of hypoglycemia

As described in the section "Defining Hypoglycemia," patients may experience a variety of nonspecific symptoms (neurogenic symptoms and neuroglycopenic symptoms) as well as physical signs than can be attributed to hypoglycemia. Since there are not clear distinctions in hypoglycemic symptoms that occur regardless of the source of the symptom - drug-induced, diabetes mellitus, or another disease state, it is important that patients and caregivers be knowledgeable of the signs and symptoms of hypoglycemia. Sometimes friends and family members are the ones that recognize the patient is experiencing symptoms that can be attributed to hypoglycemia (Cryer et al, 2003). In particular they may notice changes in the patient's behavior, mood, speech, or train of thought as the patient is trying to communicate with them.

7.2 Differential diagnosis

When hypoglycemia is suspected it is important to recognize that the signs and symptoms a patient may complain of or present with are nonspecific and often other causes of the signs and symptoms must be ruled out. In 2009 the Endocrine Society released a clinical practice guideline specifying a workup strategy for patients who experience hypoglycemia in the absence of DM (Cryer, et al, 2009). The guidelines instruct the healthcare provider to review the patient's past medical history, physical exam, review of systems, laboratory data, and medications - current and past. These guidelines detail additional workup to undertake if the cause of hypoglycemia is not apparent (Cryer, et al, 2009). However, the guidelines are very specific in stating that patients should be confirmed to have Whipple's triad- documented by signs and/or symptoms of hypoglycemia along with a low blood glucose concentration and recovery of the patient/resolution of the hypoglycemic signs/symptoms when the patient's blood glucose is raised – before the additional workup is pursued (Cryer, et al, 2009).

7.3 Treatment of hypoglycemia

While it is important to determine the cause of a patient's hypoglycemia, once signs and symptoms of hypoglycemia are recognized it is imperative to quickly treat the patient's hypoglycemia. Since there are no guidelines that are specific to managing drug-induced hypoglycemia, the current recommendations for managing hypoglycemia in patients with DM should be followed. Regardless of the cause of hypoglycemia, patients that are conscious should be given 15 – 20 g of glucose or any carbohydrate that contains glucose (American Diabetes Association, 2011). See Table 13 for specific examples of 15 – 20 g carbohydrate sources (National Diabetes Information Clearinghouse, 2008). The patient's blood glucose should be monitored in 15 minutes and they should continue to receive 15 – 20 g of glucose until their blood glucose level is greater than 70 mg/dl (3.9 mmol/l). Once the patient's blood glucose is above 70 mg/dl (3.9 mmol/l), the patient should eat something more substantial (a meal or snack) to maintain their blood glucose in a normal range, usually 70 -130 mg/dl (3.9 – 7.2 mmol/l) (American Diabetes Association, 2011).

Product	**1 serving = 15 g carbohydrates**
Glucose Products	3 – 4 tablets
	1 serving of glucose gel
Beverages	4 oz. = ½ cup of fruit juice
	4 oz = ½ cup of non-diet soft drink
	8 oz = 1 cup of milk
Hard Candy	5 – 6 pieces
Sugar or honey	1 tablespoon

Adapted from National Diabetes Information Clearinghouse, 2008.

Table 13. Quick Sources of Glucose

Hypoglycemia is defined as **severe** when a patient cannot treat their hypoglycemia on their own due to loss of consciousness. In cases of severe hypoglycemia, caregivers should administer glucagon (American Diabetes Association, 2011). It should be noted that glucagon is a prescription medication, available as a glucagon kit, whereas the glucose products routinely used for mild to moderate hypoglycemia are available without a prescription. Caregivers should be trained on glucagon administration since it requires preparation of the dose and intramuscular administration (Lilly, 2005). It is also important for patient and caregivers to routinely check the expiration date on the glucagon kit to ensure it is still in date (American Diabetes Association, 2011). Although there are numbers indicating the occurrence of hypoglycemia, it is unclear how often drug-induced hypoglycemia is severe. Therefore, it will be up to the healthcare provider to determine the patient's risk for severe hypoglycemia. If a patient is taking multiple agents that can alter their blood glucose or if they have multiple risk factors for hypoglycemia then it would be reasonable for the patient to be provided with a prescription for a glucagon kit and for their caregiver(s) to receive appropriate training. If the patient's hypoglycemia is severe enough to warrant attention of emergency personnel, then additional measures to raise their blood glucose may include the administration of intravenous dextrose sources.

In addition to quickly trying to reverse the patient's hypoglycemia once it has occurred, a plan should be developed to prevent future episodes of hypoglycemia. As discussed in the "Prevention" section in Table 12, prescribing of the medication suspected to be causing hypoglycemia should be continued under close supervision. Providers should recognize that if offending drugs must be continued that there may need to be decreases in the dose, duration, or timing of administration. Once an episode of hypoglycemia has occurred, afterwards is an appropriate time to re-visit how the situation was managed and to make sure there is an action plan for any future episodes. A summary of general principles of the management of drug-induced hypoglycemic episodes are found below in Table 14.

Initial Treatment of Hypoglycemia
Recognition of signs and symptoms of hypoglycemia - differentiation between mild - moderate versus severe
Appropriate treatment of hypoglycemia - patient-treated with a quick acting glucose source versus caregiver assisted with glucagon or healthcare provider treatment with dextrose
Plan for Prevention of Future Episodes of Hypoglycemia
Evaluation of offending medication for adjustment in dosage and length of therapy
Consider of timing of administration of medication with meals
Consistent intake of meals/snacks
Institute blood glucose monitoring

Table 14. General Management of Drug-Induced Hypoglycemia

7.4 Resolution of hypoglycemia

Once a patient has experienced a hypoglycemic episode, the patient and healthcare providers will be anxious for it be resolved. Since the mechanism by which each offending medication causes hypoglycemia is different, the time to resolution of hypoglycaemia will vary accounting for both pharmacokinetic and pharmacodynamic properties of the offending medication as well as any other interfering medications. The mechanism by which hypoglycemia occurs will also determine whether the effects are reversible. In the case of pentamidine, the beta cell loss that may occur is not reversible (Pandit et al, 1993).

8. Discussion

When evaluating drug-induced hypoglycemia in comparison to what is reported in the literature, it is important to remember that the cases reported in the literature could be a result of publication bias. Many of the cases denoted patients with hospitalization and morbidity indicating patients were experiencing severe hypoglycemia (Murad et al, 2009).

Mild cases of hypoglycemia, even potentially asymptomatic cases, have not necessarily been documented in the literature, reinforcing the under-reporting of drug-induced hypoglycemia (Murad et al, 2009). In the most recent systematic review conducted, the reviewers noted that cases in the literature were patients who were taking medications at their recommended doses; however, the patients still experienced severe, symptomatic hypoglycemic episodes (Murad et al, 2009). This systematic review did reinforce the risk factors for drug-induced hypoglycemia that had been reported in earlier literature. Cases identified for the review were often patients of advanced age and who were experiencing renal and/or hepatic insufficiency. However, one additional patient risk factor that was identified was severe systemic disease (Murad et al, 2009). The drugs most often implicated in the reported cases were anti-diabetic agents, specifically insulin and sulfonylureas, as denoted in Table 6 (Murad et al, 2009).

9. Conclusion

Hypoglycemia is a potentially common and underreported complication of medication use which can result in significant morbidity and mortality. Patients must be educated on common signs and symptoms of hypoglycemia, especially when specific symptoms may be masked by medications. Specific characteristics, including renal insufficiency, hepatic insufficiency, and advancing age, may predispose patients to development of drug-induced hypoglycemia. Patient evaluation may help the clinician identify patients at greatest risk and avoid complications associated with the more commonly associated drugs. Preventative strategies include drug avoidance, minimizing time or dose of offending agents, using controlled-release formulations where available, limiting use of the medication or multiple medications which may cause hypoglycemia, and frequent, proactive blood glucose monitoring. Though these strategies may not prevent all occurrences, they may limit the number or severity of those that do happen. In the case of a hypoglyemic episode, management strategies should include those used in managing hypoglycemia of non-drug-induced origin.

10. References

American Diabetes Association (2011). Standards of medical care. *Diabetes Care*, Vol. 34., Suppl. 1, (January 2011), pp. S11-S61.

Aronoff S, Berkowitz K, Shreiner B, Shreiner B, & Want L (2004). Glucose metabolism and regulation: beyond insulin and glucagon. *Diabetes Spectrum*, Vol. 15, No. 3, (2004), pp. 183-190.

Ben-Ami H, Nagachandran P, Mendelson A, & Edoute Y (1999). Drug-induced hypoglycemic coma in 102 diabetic patients. *Arch Intern Med*, Vol. 159, No. 3, (February 1999), pp. 281-284, ISSN 0003-9926.

Cryer PE, Axelrod L, Grossman AB, et al (2009). Evaluation and management of adult hypoglycemic disorders: an endocrine society clinical practice guideline. *J Clin Endocrinol Metab*, Vol. 94, No. 3, (March 2009), pp. 709-728, ISSN 1945-7197.

Cryer PE, Davis SN, & Shamoon H (2003). Hypoglycemia in diabetes. *Diabetes Care*, Vol. 26, No. 3, (June 2003), pp. 1902 – 12.

Dugi, K. (2006). Title, In: *Science in School*, 5/17/2011, Available from: http://recreationalpharmacy.tumblr.com/

Frothingham R (2005). Glucose homeostasis abnormalities associated with use of gatifloxacin. *Clin Infect Dis*, Vol. 41, No. 9, (Nov 2005), pp.1269-1276, ISSN 1537-6591.

Gajjar D, LaCreta F, Kollia G, Stolz G, Berger R, Smith S, Swingle W, & Grasela D (2000). Effect of multiple-dose gatifloxacin or ciprofloxacin on glucose homeostasis and insulin production in patients with noninsulin-dependent diabetes mellitus maintained with diet and exercise. *Pharmacotherapy*, Vol. 20, No. 6, (June 2000), pp. 76S-86S, ISSN 0277-0008.

Herings R, de Boer A, Stricker B, Leufkens H, & Porsius A (1995). Hypoglycaemia associated with use of inhibitors of angiotensin converting enzyme. *Lancet*, Vol. 345, No. 8959, (September 1995), pp. (1195-1198), ISSN 0140-6736.

Hosono S, Ohno T, Kimoto H, Nagoshi R, Shimizu M, & Nozawa W (1999). Reduction in blood glucose values following indomethacin therapy for patent ductus arteriosus. *Pediatr Int*. Vol. 41, No. 5, (October 1999), pp. 525-528, ISSN 1328-8067.

Ioannidis JP & Lau J (2001). Completeness of safety reporting in randomized trials: an evaluation of 7 medical areas. *JAMA*, Vol. 285, No. 4, (January, 2001), pp. 437-443, ISSN 0098-7484.

Jennings AM, Wilson RM, & Ward JD (1989). Symptomatic hypoglycemia in NIDDM patients treated with oral hypoglycemic agents. *Diabetes Care*, Vol.12, No. 3, (March 1989), pp. 203-207, ISSN 0149-5992.

Juurlink DN, Mamdani M, Kopp A, Laupacis A, & Redelmeier DA (2003). Drug-drug interactions among elderly patients hospitalized for drug toxicity. *JAMA*, Vol. 289, No. 13, (April 2003), pp. 1652-1658, ISSN 0098-7484.

Kilbridge PM, Campbell UC, Cozart HB, & Mojarrad MC (2006). Automated surveillance for adverse drug events at a community hospital and an academic medical center. *J Am Med Inform Assoc*, Vol. 13, No. 4, (Jul-Aug 2006), pp.372-377, ISSN 1067-5027.

LeBlanc M, Belanger C, & Cossette P (2004). Severe and resistant hypoglycemia associated with concomitant gatifloxacin and glyburide therapy. *Pharmacotherapy*, Vol. 24, No. 7, (July 2004), pp. 926-931, ISSN 0227-0008.

Lilly (2005). Glucagon, In: Humalog - How to use glucagon tutorial, 5/23/11, Available from: http://www.humalog.com/Documents/pdf/HI62334_GlucagonBrochure.pdf

Miller CD, Philips LS, Ziemer DC, Gallina DL, Cook CB, & El-Kebbi IM (2001). Hypoglycemia in patients with type 2 diabetes mellitus. *Arch Intern Med*, Vol. 161, No. 9 (July 2001), pp. 1653-1659, ISSN 0003-9926.

Murad M, Coto-Yglesias F, Wang A, Sheidaee N, Mullan R, Elamin M, Erwin P, & Montori V (2009). Drug-induced hypoglycemia: a systematic review. *J Clin Endocrinol Metab*, Vol. 94, No. 3, (March 2009), pp. (741-745), ISSN 1945-7197.

National Diabetes Information Clearinghouse. (October 2008) Hypoglycemia (NIH Publication No. 09–3926), In: Diabetes home , 5/23/11, Available from: http://diabetes.niddk.nih.gov/dm/pubs/hypoglycemia/#prevention

Pandit M, Burke J, Gustafson A, Minocha A, & Peiris A (1993). Drug-induced disorders of glucose tolerance. *Annalsof Internal Medicine*, Vol. 118, No. 7, (April 1993), pp. 529-539, ISSN 0003-4819.

Park-Wyllie L, Juurlink D, Kopp A, Shah B, Stukel T, Stumpo C, Dreser L, Low D, & Mamdani M (2006). Outpatient gatifloxacin therapy and dysglycemia in older adults. *N Engl J Med*, Vol 354, No. 25, (June 2006), pp. 1352 - 1361, ISSN 1533-4406.

Pollare T, Little H, & Berne C (1989). A comiparison of the effects of hydrochlorothiazide and captoptil on glucose and lipid metabolism in patients with hypertension. *N Eng J Med*, Vol 321, No. 13, (September 1989), pp. 868-873. ISSN

Product Information: Indocin intravenous injection, indomethacin intravenous injection. (2010). In: *Lundbeck Inc.* 4/10/2011, Available from: http://www.lundbeckinc.com/USA/products/hospital/indocin/usa_ind_pi_temp.pdf

Product Information: InnoPran XL oral capsules, propranolol hydrochloride oral capsules. (2010). In: *GlaxoSmithKline*, 4/10/2011, Available from: http://us.gsk.com/products/assets/us_innopran-xl.pdf

Product Information: Nebupent inhalation solution, pentamidine isethionate inhalation solution. (2008). In: *American Pharmaceutical Partners*, 4/10/2011, Available from: http://editor.apppharma.com/PIs/NebuPent_45847C_Feb_08.pdf.

Product Information: Pentam 300 IV, IM injection, pentamidine isethionate IV, IM injection. (2008). In: *American Pharmaceutical Partners, LLC*, 4/10/2011, Available from: http://editor.apppharma.com/PIs/Pentam_for_Inj_45851C_Mar_08.pdf.

Product Information: Qualaquin oral capsules, quinine sulfate oral capsules (2010), In: *AR Scientific, Inc.*, 4/10/2011, Available from http://www.urlpharma.com/Files/QUALAQUIN_6_10(Rev14).pdf

Product Information: Tequin oral tablets, injection, gatifloxacin oral tablets, injection. (2006), In: *Bristol-Myers Squibb Company*, 4/10/2011, Available from: http://www.onlinepharmacycatalog.com/drugs-medications/antibiotics/gatifloxacin/tequin-prescribing-information.pdf

Seltzer HS (1989). Drug-induced hypoglycemia. A review of 1418 cases. *Endocrinol Metab Clin North Am*, Vol. 18, No. 1, (March, 1989), pp. 163-183, ISSN 0889-8529.

Vuorinen-Markkola H, & Yki-Jarvinen H (1995). Antihypertensive therapy with enalapril improves glucose storage and insulin sensitivity in hypertensive patients with non insulin-dependent diabetes mellitus. *Metabolism,* Vol. 44, No. 1, (January 1995), pp. (85-89), ISSN 0026-0495.

Waskin H, Stehr-Green J, Helmick C, & Sattler F (1986). Risk factors for hypoglycemia associated with pentamidine therapy for pneumocystis pneumonia. *JAMA*. Vol. 260, No. 3, (July 1986), pp. 2383-2385, ISSN 0098-7484.

White J (2007). The contribution of medications to hypoglycemia unawareness. *Diabetes Spectrum*. Vol. 20, No. 2, (2007), pp. 77-80.

Wiggam M, Hunter S, Atkinson A, Ennis C, Henry J, Browne J, Sherida B, & Bell P (1998). Captopril does not improve insulin action in essential hypertension: A double-blind placebo-controlled study. *J Hypertens*, Vol. 16, No. 11, (November 1998), pp. 1651-1657, ISSN 0263-6352.

Yip C & Lee AJ (2006). Gatifloxacin - induced hyperglycemia: a case report and summary of the current literature . *Clin Ther*, Vol 28, No. 11, (Nov 2006), pp. 1857 - 1866, ISSN 0149-2918.

Zammit NN & Frier BM (2005). Hypoglycemia in type 2 diabetes. Pathophysiology, frequency, and effects of different treatment modalities. *Diabetes Care*, Vol. 28, No. 12, (December 2005), pp. 2948-61, ISSN 0149-5992.

9

Drugs and Hypoglycemia

Marek Pytliak, Viola Vargová and Viola Mechírová
Medical Faculty of the University of P.J. Safarik, Košice, Slovakia

1. Introduction

Manifested hypoglycemia is relatively frequent cause of out-patient office visit at general practitioner, diabetologist and in severe cases represents emergent situation requiring transport to hospital and hospitalization. Severe and untreated hypoglycemia can even lead to death. The aetiology of hypoglycemia is variable, and includes drugs, insulinoma, liver failure, renal failure, hormonal deficiencies, alcohol abuse and reactive hypoglycemia. The medication history is an integral part in the evaluation of a patient with hypoglycemia. A variety of medications have been associated with hypoglycemia, and the list of these medications is expanding (Comi, 1993). The common causes of acute hypoglycemia are related to therapy for diabetes mellitus – insulin and its analogues or oral antidiabetic drugs (OAD). Determining the aetiology of hypoglycemia poses little difficulty in patients known to be taking parenteral or oral hypoglycaemic agents. Severe hypoglycemia, associated with coma or requiring assistance of another person for reversal occurs at least once a year in 10% of patients treated with insulin, with a mortality of 2-4%. There is difficulty assessing the absolute rates but the frequency of iatrogenic hypoglycemia is substantially lower in type 2 than in type 1 diabetes. Thus, the rates of severe hypoglycemia in type 2 diabetes are approximately 10% of those in type 1 diabetes even during aggressive insulin therapy (Marks, 1981).

Episodes of hypoglycemia may occur also in patients without diabetes mellitus, insulin or OAD therapy. In these patients, hypoglycemia absents often among diagnostic concerns what might worsen subsequently their prognosis. It is necessary to consider the possibility of drug induced hypoglycemia after excluding its organic aetiology (endocrinopathies, malnutrition, cancer etc.). There are various groups of drugs with provable hypoglycemic effects that may potentiate diabetes mellitus treatment or lead to hypoglycemia in nondiabetic patients as well (Table 1). Some prospective studies carried out in last decade

• Insulin and its analogues	• Trimetoprim/sulfametoxazol
• Sulfonylurea derivates	• Tetracyclins
• Betablockers	• Disopyramide
• Salicylates	• Pentamidine
• Chinine and chinidine	• Ethanol

Table 1. The most common drugs with hypoglycemic effects

find that hypoglycemia is present in 12% patients with beta-blocker poisoning and in 30.9% patients with salicylate poisoning. Among drug-induced hypoglycemias in non-diabetic subjects, alcohol represents the most frequent cause, followed by beta-blockers, and salicylates (Guettier & Gorden, 2006).

2. Most common drugs leading to hypoglycemia

2.1 Insulin and its analogues

Insulin is a hormone central to regulating carbohydrate and fat metabolism in the body. Insulin causes cells in the liver, muscle, and fat tissue to take up glucose from the blood, storing it as glycogen in the liver and muscle. cells. Insulin also influences other body functions, such as vascular compliance and cognition. Once insulin enters the human brain, it enhances learning and memory and benefits verbal memory in particular. Enhancing brain insulin signalling by means of intranasal insulin administration also enhances the acute thermoregulatory and glucoregulatory response to food intake, suggesting central nervous insulin contributes to the control of whole-body energy homeostasis in humans. Insulin is a peptide hormone composed of 51 amino acids and has a molecular weight of 5808 Da (Fig. 1). It is produced in the islets of Langerhans in the pancreas (Chang et al., 1997).

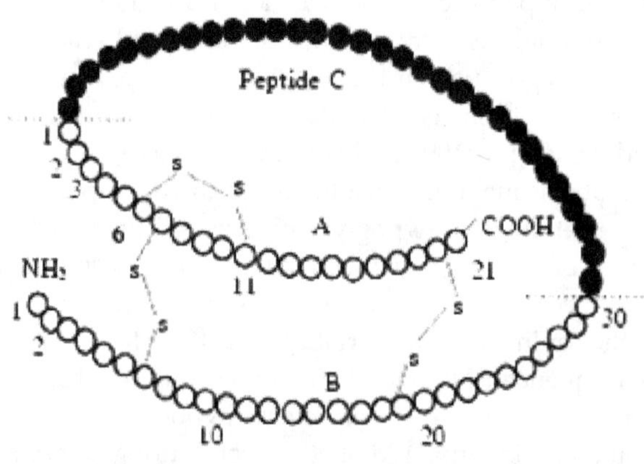

Fig. 1. Pro-insuline with C-peptide.

Insulin replacement therapy has witnessed several major developments since its inception in the early 20th century, allowing for treatment approaches that seek to mimic normal insulin physiology and achieve tight glycemic control. Hypoglycemia can hinder these efforts as the glycemic control trials in both type 1 and type 2 diabetes have shown (UK Hypoglycaemia Study Group, 2007).

The data on the frequency of hypoglycemia in diabetic subjects is uncertain. Depending on the severity of the hypoglycemic event, hypoglycemia is defined as asymptomatic, mild or severe. While there is much more information on the frequency of severe hypoglycemia, little is known on the real frequency of asymptomatic and mild hypoglycemia. (MacLeod et al., 1993)

Insulin resistance with hyperinsulinemia is a prominent feature in the early stages of the disease. Thus, type 2 diabetics benefit from measures to improve insulin sensitivity, such as caloric restriction, exercise and weight management, early in their disease. With progression of type 2 diabetes, there is ultimately a progressive loss of pancreatic b-cell function and endogenous insulin secretion. At this stage, most patients require exogenous insulin therapy to achieve optimal glucose control (Abraira et al, 1995).

A relative or absolute excess in insulin mainly occurs in excessive dose of insulin or when an incorrect dose is given at the wrong time. Hypoglycemia also occurs during prolonged fasting, after exercise, in renal or liver failure. The risk of severe hypoglycemia in insulin-requiring patients with type 2 diabetes has consistently been reported to be significantly reduced compared with the risk in type 1 diabetic patients undergoing intensive insulin therapy. The lower incidence of severe hypoglycemia in type 2 diabetes may result from insulin resistance. In the randomized Diabetes Control and Complications Trial (DCCT), hypoglycemia occurred approximately once per week in the standard insulin treatment group (under 3 doses of insulin daily) and approximately twice per week in the intensive treatment group (3 and more doses of insulin daily). Most patients with type 1 diabetes lose their ability to secrete glucagon in response to hypoglycemia shortly after developing diabetes, and thus the incremental secretion of epinephrine assumes a primary role in the hormonal response to hypoglycemia in this disease (DCCT Research Group, 1993). Basdevant et al. reported that during a one-year period of observation, 17% of patients with type 1 diabetes mellitus on the intensive insulin treatment had a severe hypoglycemic reaction. Because the ability to secrete epinephrine is also impaired in approximately 25% of patients with longstanding type 1 diabetes mellitus, such patients may manifest the syndrome of "hypoglycemic unawareness", resulting in a tendency to develop frequent, severe and prolonged hypoglycemia (Basdevant et al, 1982).

In the DCCT study 9.8% of subjects in the standard treatment diabetic group had severe hypoglycemia during the 12 months of study. In the same study, subjects the intensive treatment group had a threefold increase in the incidence of serious hypoglycemia compared with those in the standard treatment group. Other authors have also noted an increased risk of hypoglycemia in patients with diabetes controlled very rigidly (DCCT Research Group, 1993).

On the other side, tight glycemic control has been shown to reduce mortality in surgical intensive care patients and in long-term medical intensive care patients. But, the high incidence of hypoglycemia may override the potential beneficial effects of intensive insulin therapy. In the studies by van den Berghe et al., the proportion of patients experiencing severe hypoglycemia in the intensive treatment group was 5.1% in surgical and 18.7% in medical patients, whereas in the conventionally treated group the incidences were 0.8% and 3.1%, respectively (Van den Berghe et al., 2001).

2.2 Sulfonylurea derivates

Sulfonylureas were introduced into medical practice in 1955 for the treatment of diabetes and other conditions, and have been used by both diabetic and nondiabetic subjects.

Sulfonylureas bind to an ATP-dependent K^+ (K^+ATP) channel on the cell membrane of pancreatic beta cells. This inhibits a tonic, hyperpolarizing efflux of potassium, thus causing the electric potential over the membrane to become more positive. This depolarization opens voltage-gated Ca^{2+} channels. The rise in intracellular Ca^{2+} leads to increased fusion of insulin granulae with the cell membrane, and therefore increased secretion of pro-insulin. The structure of sulfonlyureas is on the fig. 2.

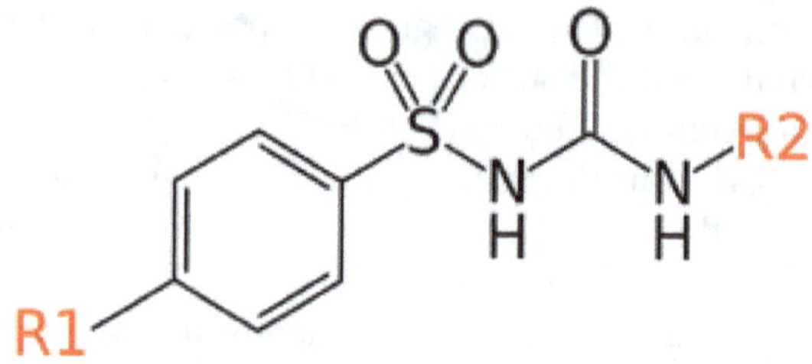

Fig. 2. Structure of the sulfonylureas

Sulfonylureas also sensitize β-cells to glucose, and hey limit glucose production in the liver,, they decrease lipolysis,, and decrease clearance of insulin by the liver. Sulfonylureas produce hypoglycemia by releasing preformed insulin from b-cells by a direct action, and possiblyby sensitizing them to the action of certain endogenous insulinotrophs such as leucine (Kunte H et al, 2007).

The sulfonylureas resemble one another more than they differ, and the greatest differences are found in their blood glucose-lowering potencies and in the way in which they are eliminated from the body . The hypoglycemic potency of an individual agent is a function of the biological half-life of the drug itself and its active metabolites.

Sulfonylureas, as opposed to metformin, the thiazolidinediones, exenatide, symlin and other newer treatment agents may induce hypoglycemia as a result of excesses in insulin production and release. This typically occurs if the dose is too high, and the patient is fasting. Some people attempt to change eating habits to prevent this, however it can be counter productive. Like insulin, sulfonylureas can induce weight gain, mainly as a result of their effect to increase insulin levels.

Sulfonylureas are potentially teratogenic and cannot be used in pregnancy or in woman who may become pregnant. Impairment of liver or kidney function increases the risk of hypoglycemia, and are contraindications for the use of sulfonylureas (Campbell, 1985).

Second-generation sulfonylureas have increased potency by weight, compared to first-generation sulfonylureas. All sulfonylureas carry an FDA-required warning about increased risk of cardiovascular death. The ADVANCE trial (Action in Diabetes and Vascular Disease), found no benefit from tight control with gliclazide for the outcomes of heart attack (myocardial infarction), cardiovascular death, or all-cause death (Patel et al, 2005).

Similarly, ACCORD (Action to Control Cardiovascular Risk in Diabetes) and the VADT (Veterans Affairs Diabetes Trial) studies showed no reduction in heart attack or death in patients assigned to tight glucose control with various drugs (Gerstein et al., 2007; Reaven et al., 2004).

Various sulfonylureas have different pharmacokinetics. The choice depends on the propensity of the patient to develop hypoglycemia. Long-acting sulfonylureas with active metabolites can induce prolonged hypoglycemia. The shorter-acting agents may not control blood sugar levels adequately, but the hypoglycemia does not last so long.

Due to varying half-life, some drugs have to be taken twice or three times a day rather than once. The short-acting agents may have to be taken about 30 minutes before the meal, to ascertain maximum efficacy when the food leads to increased blood glucose levels.

Some sulfonylureas are metabolised by liver metabolic enzymes and inducers of this enzyme system (e.g rifampicin) can therefore increase the clearance of sulfonylureas. In addition, because some sulfonylureas are bound to plasma proteins, use of drugs that also

bind to plasma proteins can release the sulfonylureas from their binding places, leading to increased clearance.
Mild sulfonylurea-induced hypoglycemia produces only few symptoms and mostly they are of a subacute neuroglycopenic variety. Although mild hypoglycemia causes unpleasant symptoms and disrupts patients daily activities, severe hypoglycemia can result in coma, seizures and death (Herbel & Boyle, 2000)
Hypoglycemia due to ingestion of sulfonylures has been documented as a accidental ingestion and also when ingested in a suicide attempt leading to death. Sulfonylurea compounds have also been reported to cause severe hypoglycemia when prescribed simultaneously with either a second blood glucose-lowering agent or a nonhypoglycemic drug that prolongs the activity of the sulfonylurea. The different drugs which were involved include phenformin or buformin, salicylate, alcohol, phenylbutazone, sulfadimidine or sulfamethoxazole for urinary tract infection (Bandyopadhyay, 2004).

2.3 β-blockers

Beta blockers block the action of endogenous catecholamines (adrenaline and noradrenaline) on β-adrenergic receptors. There are three known types of beta receptor, designated β1, β2 and β3 receptors. β1-adrenergic receptors are located mainly in the heart and in the kidneys. β2-adrenergic receptors are located mainly in the lungs, gastrointestinal tract, liver, uterus, vascular smooth muscle, and skeletal muscle. β3-adrenergic receptors are located in fat cells. Stimulation of β2 receptors induces smooth muscle relaxation induces tremor in skeletal muscle, and increases glycogenolysis in the liver and skeletal muscle. Stimulation of β3 receptors induces lipolysis.
Spontaneous hypoglycemia may occur in diabetic and nondiabetic patients receiving β-adrenoceptor antagonists. This complication of treatment with β-blockers was first described by Kotler et al. in 1966. Mechanism of β-blocker-induced hypoglycemia includes inhibition of hepatic gluconeogenesis, which is normally potentiated by the sympathetic nervous system. Reduction of lipolysis with decreased plasma concentrations of nonesterified fatty acid increase β-blockers the glucose uptake of skeletal muscles. Non-selective β-blockers, which are currently used only in a limited way, may intensify hypoglycemia-induced hypoglycemic therapy or delay and suppress clinical manifestations of hypoglycemia (tachycardia, tremor) (Abramson et al, 1965). Sweating as a symptom of hypoglycemia remains preserved even when taking β-blockers, therefore, attention or this symtome should be given in the absence of other symptoms of hypoglycemia and neuroglycopenia. In addition, β-adrenergic antagonists block the effect of adrenaline as a counter-regulatory mechanism, resulting in a reduction in glycogenolysis. However, cases of severe hypoglycemia were also described with the use of therapeutic doses of cardioselective beta-blockers (Miller et al., 2001).
At risk of hypoglycemia are particularly insulin-dependent diabetics, but severe hypoglycemia while taking β-blockers have been described as well in non-diabetic hemodialysated patients during dialysis (Murata et al., 1981). The literature has described the emergence of severe hypoglycemia in the treatment of glaucoma with eye drops containing timolol in patients with diabetes mellitus type 1 (Angelo-Nielsen, 1980).

2.4 ACE inhibitors

Angiotensin converting enzyme inhibitors (ACEI) are potent antihypertensive agents with multiple pleiotropic effects, which are used for the treatment of hypertension, heart failure or in patients after myocardial infarction. ACE inhibitors block the conversion of angiotensin I to angiotensin II. Under normal conditions, angiotensin II will have the following effects:

- vasoconstriction, which lead hypertension
- constriction of the efferent arterioles of the kidney, leading to increased perfusion pressure in the glomeruli
- contribute to ventricular remodeling and ventricular hypertrophy of the heart
- stimulation of the adrenal cortex to release aldosterone, with sodium retention.
- stimulation of the posterior pituitary to release vasopressin (anti-diuretic hormone - ADH), which acts on the kidneys to increase water retention.
- decrease renal protein kinase C (Acharya et al, 2003)

With ACE inhibitor use, the effects of angiotensin II are prevented.

Unlike other groups of drugs they have a relatively low incidence of adverse effects. Hypertension, chronic heart failure and coronary heart disease in diabetics are very frequent co morbidities and ACEI are due they indifferent effect on the metabolism of glucose and lipids and proven renoprotective effect in these patients the drugs of first choice. The association between use of ACE inhibitors and episodes of hypoglycemia in patients with diabetes mellitus is controversial. Were the cases illustrated the need to reduce doses of insulin or oral hypoglycemic agents failure after initiation of ACEI therapy and few cases of ACEI-associated hypoglycemia, although it has been reported particularly in patients with the presence of severe co-morbidities - heart failure, chronic kidney disease and the like (Herings et al., 1995)

Possible mechanism of the hypoglycemic effect of ACEI is not yet well understood, may involve increased insulin sensitivity of peripheral tissues, blocking of angiotensiogen II as one of the counter-regulatory hormones with similar effects as adrenaline, speeding up absorption of subcutaneous insulin etc. (Buchanan et al., 1993).

Nevertheless, it appears that some episodes of hypoglycemia associated with ACEI use were the result of potentiation of hypoglycemic effects of other drugs and ACE inhibitors remain a safe choice for treatment of patients with diabetes mellitus (Seghieri et al., 1992).

2.5 Salicylates

Salicylic acid is a monohydroxybenzoic acid, a type of phenolic acid and a beta hydroxy acid. It is derived from the metabolism of salicin. This colorless crystalline organic acid is widely used in organic synthesis and functions as a plant hormone. The salts and esters of salicylic acid are known as salicylates.

Salicylates in the past short period of use as hypoglycemic drugs, but to achieve the hypoglycemic effect, administration of high doses was necessary, which had many adverse effects (Baron, 1982). Since diabetics are at increased incidence of coronary heart disease, myocardial infarction or cerebrovascular diseases, today we meet with frequent use of antiplatelet drugs in this population, especially acetylsalicylic acid, which is used in the primary and secondary prevention of cardiovascular events. Symptomatic hypoglycemia was described in many cases of the use of salicylates, especially in young children. Salicylates in therapeutic doses have the hypoglycemic potential similar to some sulphonylurea agent or metformin (Micossi et al, 1978). On the other hand, lotions containing salicylates are used to treat certain skin disorders, and the drug can be absorbed through the skin and has been associated with life-threatening complications. A case of

severe refractory hypoglycemia in a man with terminal kidney disease using a salicylate lotion for treatment of psoriasis has been described in the literature (Raschke et al, 1991). Intentional salicylate overdose usually occurs predominantly in adolescents and young adults. Overdoses in children are usually accidental and in the elderly they occur as therapeutic misadventures. Elderly patients with chronic salicylate overdose tend to present with nonspecific findings such as deterioration of cognition, or self care, pulmonary edema or failure to thrive. Important clinical clues may be tachypnea, hyperpnea and an unexplained positive ion gap metabolic acidosis (Marks & Teale , 1999)
The mechanism of the hypoglycemic effect of salicylates is not precisely known, yet. Possible mechanisms include a reduction of hepatic gluconeogenesis and increase of insulin secretion, increases glucose utilization in peripheral tissues due to disconnection of oxidative phosphorylation or reduction of the concentration of circulating nonesterified fatty acid by suppression of lipolysis. Meanwhile organic acids (pyruvate and lactate) accumulate in the periphery because ATP is no longer being generated through the Krebs cycle, as several of the Krebs cycle enzymes are blocked by excess salicylate. The body becomes increasingly dependent on the less efficient anaerobic energy pathways by way of which more energy is dissipated as heat. This produces fever and increased utilization of glucose. This inhibition of glucose oxidative metabolism is particularly hazardous to the brain because of the inability of neuronal tissue to employ fatty acids. The resulting lipolysis increases production of ketones and organic acids culminating in metabolic acidosis when the body's buffering capacity becomes sufficiently depleted. These metabolic changes eventually lead to renal depletion of fluid and electrolytes, hypoglycemia, hypokalemia and a mixed picture of respiratory and metabolic alkalosis coupled with metabolic acidosis (Rumore & Kim, 2010).

2.6 Paracetamol

Paracetamol (acetaminophen - fig.3) intoxication, most frequently in suicidal intent, may lead to liver necrosis with severe hypoglycemia. Paracetamol toxicity is one of the most common causes of poisoning worldwide. In the United States and the United Kingdom it is the most common cause of acute liver failure (Khashab et al, 2007).

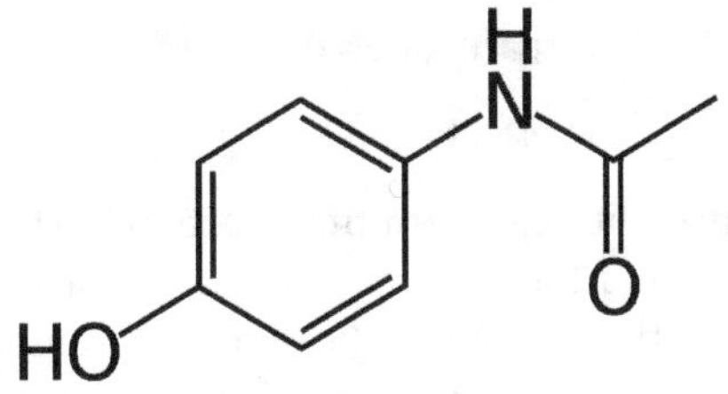

Fig. 3. Structure of the paracetamol (acetaminophen)

Hypoglycemia while taking paracetamol in the usual therapeutic doses has been described in a child, but also had documented hypoglycemia after salicylates. Two case reports of patients with anion gap metabolic lactic acidosis and hypoglycemia were presented in literature. Both patients subsequently died of acute liver failure secondary to paracetamol hepatotoxicity. The development of lactic acidosis with hypoglycemia might have been caused by a deficit in gluconeogenesis secondary to severe hepatic failure and/or a toxic metabolite of paracetamol (Bandyopadhyay, 2004).

2.7 Antibiotics and chemotherapeutics

2.7.1 Trimethoprim-sulfamethoxazole

Trimethoprim-sulfamethoxazole or Co-trimoxazole is a sulfonamide antibiotic combination of trimethoprim and sulfamethoxazole, in the ratio of 1 to 5, used in the treatment of a variety of bacterial infections. The synergy between trimethoprim and sulfamethoxazole was first described in a series of in vitro and in vivo experiments published in the late 1960´s. Trimethoprim and sulfamethoxazole have a greater effect when given together than when given separately, because they inhibit successive steps in the folate synthesis pathway. Sulfamethoxazole acts as a false-substrate inhibitor of dihydropteroate synthetase. Sulfonamides such as sulfamethoxazole are analogues of para-aminobenzoic acid (PABA) and are competitive inhibitors of the dihydropteroate-synthetase, and, thus, inhibiting the production of dihydropteroic acid. Trimethoprim acts by interfering with the action of bacterial dihydrofolate reductase, inhibiting synthesis of tetrahydrofolic acid. Folic acid is an essential precursor in the de novo synthesis of the DNA nucleosides (fig. 4) (Brumfitt & Hamilton-Miller, 1993).

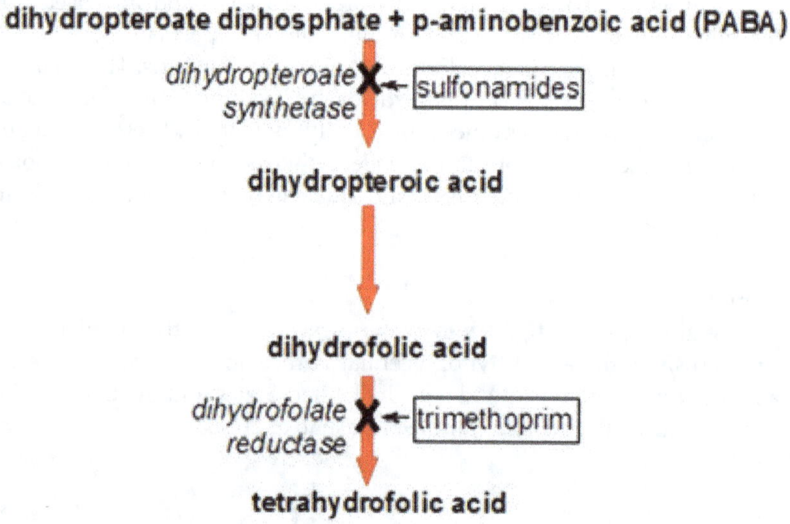

Fig. 4. Mechanism of co-trimoxazole effects

Bacteria are unable to take up folic acid from the infection host and, thus, are dependent on their own synthesis. Inhibition of the enzyme starves the bacteria of two bases (thymidine and uridine) which are necessary for DNA replication and transcription.

Sulfonamide antibiotics may potentiate the hypoglycaemic effect of sulphonylureas, but can also cause hypoglycemia in patients not taking this type of OAD. Several cases of severe and fatal hypoglycemia especially in combination of sulfamethoxazole with older types of sulphonylureas have been described (Hekimsoy et al., 1997). For structural similarity of sulfamethoxazole and sulphonylureas it is assumed to have the similar mechanism of action on pancreatic cell, namely that in the perceptive group of patients there is an increased release of insulin due to the modification of K^+ channel of the β-cells (Mihic et al., 1975). Hyperinsulinemic hypoglycemia associated with trimethoprim-sulfamethoxazole has generally been reported in adults who had renal impairment or in patients with AIDS using high dose of trimethoprim-sulfamethoxazole. High insulin and C-peptide levels were documented at the time of hypoglycemia (Rosinini et al. 2008).

2.7.2 Ciprofloxacin and other fluoroquinolons

Ciprofloxacin is a synthetic chemotherapeutic antibiotic of the fluoroquinolone drug class. It is a second-generation fluoroquinolone antibacterial. It functions by inhibiting DNA gyrase, a type II topoisomerase, and topoisomerase IV, enzymes necessary to separate bacterial DNA, thereby inhibiting cell division. Thus, it kills bacteria by interfering with the enzymes that cause DNA to rewind after being copied, which stops synthesis of DNA and of proteins (Kawahara, 1998).

Ciprofloxacin is one of the most commonly used fluoroquinolones in clinical practice. Hypoglycemia after its administration has been described only in isolated cases so far, especially in patients concomitantly receiving older types of sulphonylureas. Fluoroquinolones are widely associated with dysglycemias, particularly in diabetic patients receiving hypoglycemic agents. Renal insufficiency has been also implicated to precipitate hypoglycemia after fluoroquinolones combinated with sulfonylureas. The cellular mechanisms by which sulfonylureas and ciprofloxacin interact to produce hypoglycemia are poorly described but likely to be complex and multifactorial. Mechanisms might include interactions at one or more of the P450 isoenzymes or ciprofloxacin-related blockage of ATP-potassium channels that are responsible for insulin control (Roberge et al., 2000). Since the bounding of the ciprofloxacin to plasma proteins is relatively weak, probably it does not interact with OAD at that level. Sulfonylurea-induced hypoglycemia after using of ciprofloxacin can be serious and refractory to traditional therapy. In the report by Roberge et al, the patient developed hypoglycemia after treatment with ciprofloxacin for one week (Roberge et al., 2000). On the other hand, in the case report of Lin et al,, a 68-year-old man with a history of coronary artery disease, atrial fibrillation, and type 2 diabetes on OAD therapy (glyburide) developed significant hypoglycemia after one dose of ciprofloxacin (Lin et al., 2004).

Other fluoroquinolones can also induce severe hypoglycemia, especially in the combination with sulfonylurea derivates. Sporadic published case reports have linked administration of fluoroquinolone antibiotics, in particular gatifloxacin, with early-onset hypoglycemia in patients with diabetes. Most reported patients were aged over 65 years and were concomitantly receiving the sulfonyureas. fluoroquinolones have been demonstrated to augment insulin release in a dose-dependent manner from isolated pancreatic islet cells and to increase insulin levels in patients with type 2 diabetes mellitus. Gatifloxacin therapy is associated with a higher incidence of hypoglycemia than therapy with non-fluoroquinolones in the group of older patients (LeBlanc et al 2004; Baker & Hangii , 2002).

2.7.3 Tetracyclines

Tetracyclines are broad-spectrum polyketide antibiotics. Tetracyclin alone is produced by the Streptomyces genus of Actinobacteria. They are protein synthesis inhibitors. Tetracyclines bind to the 30S subunit of microbial ribosomes. They inhibit protein synthesis by blocking the attachment of charged aminoacyl-tRNA. Thus, they prevent introduction of new amino acids to the nascent peptide chain. The action is usually inhibitory and reversible after withdrawal of the drug (Olson et al., 2006).

The mechanism of tetracyclins-induced hypoglycemia is still not clear. Increased sensitivity to insulin and decreased clearance if insulin were implicated. Miller reported ocytetracyclininduced hypoglycemia in a patient with diabetes with initially uncontrolled glycemia because of glandular fever (Miller, 1966). In the case report of Basaria et al., severe hypoglycemia occurred in young non-diabetic man with Marphan´s syndrome with doxycyklin therapy due to acne (Basaria et al, 2002). Moreover, severe hypoglycemia occurred in non-diabetic patient after intrapleural administration of tetracycline, for the purpose of pleurodesis.

2.7.4 Pentamidine

Pentamidine is a biguanide, which was originally used in the treatment of trypanosomiasis. However, in recent decades, it is also often used to treat pneumocystis pneumonia (PCP) caused by Pneumocystis jirovecii (formerly known as Pneumocystis carinii), predominantly in patients with HIV infection. Pentamidine is also used as a prophylactic against PCP in patients receiving chemotherapy, as they also have a depressed immune system as a direct side-effect of the drugs used. Additionally, pentamidine has good clinical activity in treating leishmaniasis, and yeast infections caused by Candida albicans (Nguewa et al.). Hypoglycemia occurs in about 10-40% of patients treated with pentamidine at higher doses and is considered the most common metabolic abnormality associated with this treatment (Waskin et al., 1988). The prevalence of hypoglycemia is more common in patients with AIDS infection than in other patients treated with pentamidine. Hypoglycemic reaction is usually seen after several days from the start of the treatment. However, several cases of hypoglycemia were described after several hours of pentamidine treatment. Episodes of hypoglycemia can be frequent, severe and can lead to irreversible damage of central nervous system (Satler & Waskin, 1987). The mechanism of hypoglycemia includes mainly cytolytic response of pancreatic cells with subsequent release of insulin. Prolonged treatment with pentamidine may lead to destruction of pancreatic cells and the onset of insulin-dependent diabetes mellitus. Hypoglycemia have also been reported after pentamidine aerosol therapy (Hauser et al., 1991).

2.7.5 Quinine and quinidine

Quinine (fig. 5) is a natural white crystalline alkaloid having antipyretic, antimalarial, analgesic and anti-inflammatory properties. Though it has been synthesized in the laboratory, the bark of the cinchona tree is the only known natural source of quinine. Quinine was the first effective treatment for malaria caused by Plasmodium falciparum, appearing in therapeutics in the 17th century. It remained the antimalarial drug of choice until the 1940s, when other drugs replaced it. Since then, many effective antimalarials have been introduced, although quinine is still used to treat the disease in certain critical situations. As of 2006, quinine is no longer recommended by the WHO as first line treatment for malaria and should be used only when artemisinins are not available. It is sometimes also used in the treatment of lupus erythematodes and rheumatoid arthritis (Kaufman & Rúveda, 2005).

Quinine-induced hypoglycemia is dose-dependent and, several fatal cases of hypoglycemia by the treatment of tropical malaria were reported. Quinine sulfate causes hypoglycemia also in nondiabetic patients, particular by increasing insulin release. Quinine is excreted by the kidneys, so the presence of chronic kidney disease increases the risk of quinine-induced hypoglycemia (Harats et al, 1984).

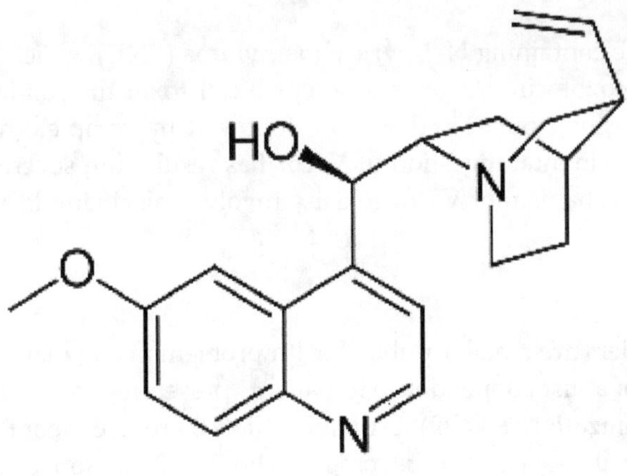

Fig. 5. Structure of quinine

Quinidine is a stereoisomer of quinine, and it acts as a class I antiarrhythmic agent in the heart. Quinidine primarily works by blocking the fast inward sodium influx (I_{Na}). Quinidine's effect on I_{Na} is known as a use dependent block - at higher heart rates, the block increases, while at lower heart rates the block decreases. The effect of blocking the fast inward sodium influx causes decrease of the cardiac action potential in the phase 0 of the heart depolarization (Jones et al., 1986).

2.8 Disopyramide

Disopyramide, group I antiarrhythmic drug, is mainly used for the treatment of ventricular and supraventricular rhythm disturbances. Commonest side effects result from disopyramide's anticholinergic activity. It is also used in ventricular arrhythmia and supraventricular arrhythmia that might follow myocardial infarctions. It has no effect on alpha or beta adrenergic receptors. Disopyramide is an analogue of quinidine and hence has similar effects, that means, it stimulates insulin secretion and may lead to hyperinsulinemic hypoglycemia. It is excreted by the kidneys, therefore older patients and patients with chronic kidney disease using this drug are at risk of hypoglycemic episodes (Cacoub et al., 1989).

2.9 Sertraline

Unlike other groups of antidepressants from the selective serotonin reuptake inhibitors (SSRI) group, sertraline has linear pharmacokinetics, so an increase in dose leads to a proportional increase in its plasma concentrations. Sertraline is primarily used to treat major depression in adult outpatients as well as obsessive-compulsive, panic, and social anxiety disorders in both adults and children. In 2007, it was the most prescribed antidepressant on the U.S. retail market. Hypoglycemia has been described in several cases, mostly in diabetic patients stabilized on long-term treatment of OAD, in which treatment with sertraline was added. The most likely mechanism of potentiating effect of antidiabetic agents is inhibition of cytochrome P-450. Although the mechanism of action of SSRIs is usually thought to involve an increase of the synaptic concentration of serotonin secondary to blockade of its reuptake by nerve terminals, it is also possible that nonneuronal mechanisms contribute. Sertraline treatment may have potentiated hypoglycemia-induced epinephrine secretion by a direct action in the adrenal medulla (Pollak et al., 2001).

2.10 Vacor

Vacor is a rodenticide containing N-3-pyridylmethylurea (PNU), which is chemically related to alloxan and streptozotocin. Vacor is a potent b-cell toxin that initially produces severe hypoglycemia by washing out stored insulin, followed by complete destruction of b-cells and fatal diabetes. Accidental ingestion of Vacor has resulted in severe hypoglycemia. It is suggested that the mechanism of Vacor toxicity involves niacinamide antagonism (Johnson et al, 1980)

2.11 Ethanol

Substance use disorders are a major public health problem facing many countries. The most common substance of abuse/dependence in patients presenting for treatment is alcohol. The World Health Organization (WHO) estimates that there are about 2 milliards people worldwide who consume alcoholic beverages, about 140 million people throughout the world suffer from alcohol dependence, and 76.3 million patients with diagnosable alcohol use disorders. Alcohol causes 1.8 million deaths (3.2% of total) and a loss of 58.3 million (4% of total) of Disability-Adjusted Life Years (DALY). Unintentional injuries alone account for about one third of deaths, while neuropsychiatric conditions account for approximately 40% of the 58.3 million DALYs. Alcohol consumption is the leading risk factor for disease burden in low mortality developing countries and the third largest risk factor in developed countries (White et al., 1993). Generally, the WHO European Region has the highest proportion in the world of total ill health and premature death due to alcohol. At a societal level, the European Union is the heaviest-drinking region in the world, with over one fifth of the European population aged 15 years and above reporting heavy episodic drinking (five or more drinks on an occasion, or 50g alcohol) at least once a week (Fig 6).

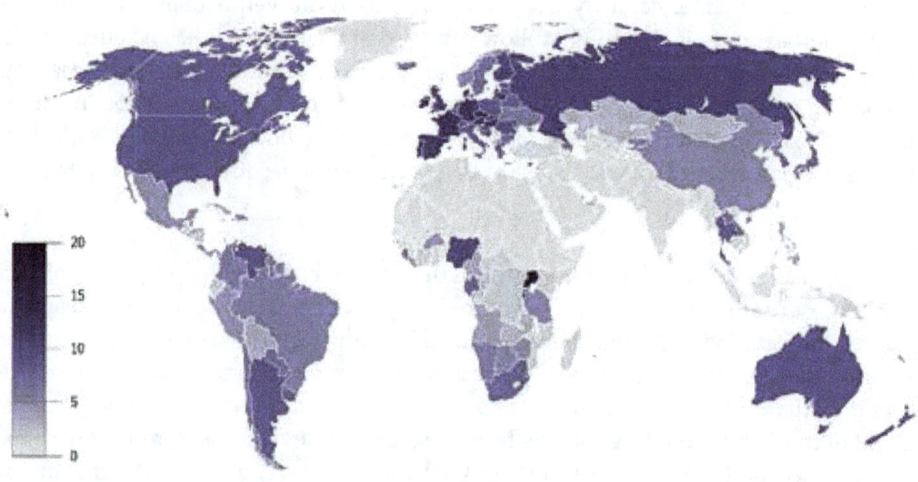

Fig. 6. Alcohol consumption in the world (litres per capita)

Heavy episodic drinking is widespread across all ages and all of Europe, and not only among young people or those from northern Europe. Alcohol consumption has health and social consequences via intoxication (drunkenness), alcohol dependence, and other biochemical effects of alcohol. Overall there is a causal relationship between alcohol consumption and more than 60 types of disease and injury. Alcohol is estimated to cause about 20–30% of oesophageal cancer, liver cancer, cirrhosis of the liver, homicide, epileptic seizures, and motor vehicle accidents worldwide. The risk of death from a chronic alcohol-related condition is found to increase linearly from zero consumption in a dose–response manner with the volume of alcohol consumed (WHO Global Status Report on Alcohol, 2004).

Although alcoholism is a very common condition, alcohol related hypoglycemia is a relative rare complication of alcohol abuse. In one older clinical study authors proved that alcohol associated hypoglycemia at an emergency department constituted only 0.9% of ethanol detectable cases over 3-month period. On the other hand, only a few hypoglycemic clinical features are exhibited other like coma, and many symptoms and signs of hypoglycemia are identical to those of alcohol intake. Thus, hypoglycemia in these patients could be unrecognised even by first aid or emergency physician. Assessment of plasma glucose is cheap, quick and reproducible and prolongated hypoglycemia may lead to irreversible brain damage or death. Alcohol related hypoglycemia often develops slowly and probably accounts for some deaths of chronic alcohol abusers and drunks who are confined in police cells to sober up overnight. That's why the assessment of plasma glucose level is necessary in chronic abusers admitted to emergencies (Fishbain & Rotundo).

In healthy individuals 2-3 days of fasting are necessary for depletion of hepatic glycogen reserve. Alcohol-related fasting hypoglycemia results from depletion of glycogen storage by starvation, and impairment of gluconeogenesis in liver cells. Thus, in chronically malnutricient patient it could develop within 6-36 hours after ingestion of a moderate to high dose of alcohol. In addition, suppression of counter-regulatory mechanisms (e.g. glucagon, growth hormone or epinephrine secretion) is also contributing to development of hypoglycemia (Chen & Ng, 2003).

Alcohol-related reactive hypoglycemia often occurs after drinking alcohol with some calories rich beverages (gin-tonic, rum-cola). This combination can lead to profound hypoglycemia 3-4 hours afterward, probably due to attenuation of counter-regulatory mechanism. Acute and sustained alcohol use can suppress growth hormone release in response to insulin-induced hypoglycemia. At night, acute and chronic alcohol administration is associated with a 75% reduction in the usual night time sleep-related release of growth hormone (Flanagan et al, 1998).

Many drugs interact with alcohol resulting in undesirable outcomes. There are two types of alcohol-drug interactions: pharmacokinetic and pharmacodynamic. Acute alcohol use increases the risk of severe hypoglycemia in patients with 2. type diabetes mellitus treated with derivates of sulfonylurea. Alcohol may prolong glipizide's effect on blood glucose by delaying glipizide absorption and elimination. In addition, alcohol enhanced glucose-lowering action of insulin Weathermon & Crabb , 1999).

3. Conclusion

The most common cause of medication-induced hypoglycemia is improper management of diabetes. Missing meals, overexertion, and intentional or unintentional overdose of medications used to treat the condition can all cause blood glucose levels to drop.

Cases of hypoglycemia were also described for other pharmaceuticals, but rather of sporadic outbreaks which do not meet very often in clinical practice. It should be noted that any quantitative disturbance of consciousness or sudden change in behavior in patients with diabetes mellitus with far offset the amount of glucose patterns, or an elderly patient with polypolymorbid possibly with chronic kidney disease may be caused by the effect of hypoglycemic drugs. In the clinical practice, it is necessary to think about this eventuality and carry out blood glucose testing for each suspected hypoglycemia. Acute treatment of dru-induced hypoglycemia is different from the treatment of hypoglycemia from other causes. When relapse hypoglycemia after discontinuation of the suspect drug it is necessary to revise the diagnosis and rule out organic causes of hypoglycemia (endocrinopathy, malignancy, insulinoma, etc.). Table 2 summarised the most common drugs with hypoglycemic effects.

Drug	Mechanism of Action	Clinical Significance
Alcohol (ethanol)	Impairs gluconeogenesis and increases insulin secretion.	+++
Pentamidine	Cytolytic response in pancreas accompanied by insulin release.	+++
Triazole antifungals	Enhance the effect of sulfonylureas.	+++
Case Series		
β-Adrenergic antagonists	Inhibit glycogenolysis; attenuate signs and symptoms of hypoglycemia.	++
Chloramphenicol	May inhibit metabolism of sulfonylureas.	++
Chloroquine	Unknown (hypoglycemia leading to death has been reported in overdose).	++
Disopyramide	Unknown; appears to result from endogenous insulin secretion.	++
Phenylbutazone	Reduces clearance of sulfonylureas.	++
Salicylates	Increase insulin secretion and sensitivity; may alter pharmacokinetic disposition of sulfonylureas.	++
Case reports		
Anabolic steroids	Decrease glucose tolerance.	+
Angiotensin-converting enzyme inhibitors	May improve insulin sensitivity, particularly in skeletal muscle.	+
Clofibrate	Unknown.	+
Gatifloxacin	Unknown.	+
Monoamine oxidase inhibitors	May increase insulin release and decrease sympathetic response to hypoglycemia.	+
Saquinavir	Unknown.	+
Sulfonamides	Alter clearance of sulfonylureas.	+

Table 2. Most common hypoglycemic pharmaceuticals and their clinical significance.

4. References

Abraira C, Colwell JA, Nuttall FQ, et al. Veterans Affairs Cooperative Study on glycemic control and complications in type II diabetes (VA CSDM). Results of the feasibility trial. Veterans Affairs Cooperative Study in type II diabetes. *Diabetes Care,* 1995, 18, pp. 1113–23.

Abramson EA, Arky RA, Woeber KA. Effects of propranolol on the hormonal and metabolic responses to insulin-induced hypoglycaemia. *Lancet*, 1966; 2, pp. 1386-92.

Acharya KR, Sturrock ED, Riodan JK, Ehlers MR. ACE revisited: A New Target for Structure-Based Dug Design. *Nature Reviews*, 2003, 2 (11), pp. 891–902.

Angelo-Nielsen, K. Timolol topically and diabetes mellitus. *JAMA*,1980, 244, pp. 2263-67

Baker SE, Hangii MC. Possible gatifloxacin-induced hypoglycemia. *Ann Pharmacoth*, 2002, 36, pp. 1722-1726.

Bandyopadhyay P. Drug-induced hypoglycemia. *Drugs of the Future*, 2004, 29(6), pp. 581-607

Baron S.H. Salicylates as hypoglycaemic agents. *Diabetes Care*, 1982, 5, pp. 64-71

Basaria S, Braga M, Moore WT. Doxycycline-Induced Hypoglycemia in a Nondiabetic Young Man. South Med J, 2002, 95(11), pp. 45-9.

Basdevant A, Costagliola D, Lanöe JL, Goldgewicht C, Triomphe A, Metz F, Denys H, Eschwege E, Fardeau M, Tchobroutsky G. The risk of diabetic control: a comparison of hospital versus general practice supervision. *Diabetologia*, 1982, 22(5), pp. 309–314.

Brumfitt W, Hamilton-Miller JM . Limitations of and indications for the use of co-trimoxazole. *J Chemother*, 1993, 6 (1), pp. 3–11.

Buchanan TA, Thawani H, Kade W. et al. Angiotensin II increases glucose utilisation during acute hyperinsulinaemia via a haemodyanamic mechanism. *J Clin Invest*, 1993, 92, pp. 720-6.

Cacoub P, Deray G, Baumelou A, Grimaldi A, Soubrie C, Jacobs C. Disopyramide-induced hypoglycaemia: Case report and review of the literature. *Fundam Clin Pharmacol*, 1989, 3, pp. 527-35.

Campbell, I.W. Metformin and the sulfonylureas: The comparative risk. In: Hormone and Metabolic Research. Supplement series, Vol. 15. Pfeiffer, E.F., Lipsett, M.B. (Eds.). Georg Thieme Verlag, New York 1985, pp. 105-11.

Comi, R.J. Approach to acute hypoglycaemia. *Endocrinol Metab Clin North Am* 1993, 22, pp. 247-62.

Fishbain DA, Rotundo D. Frequency of hypoglycaemic delirium in a psychiatric emergency service. *Psychosomatics* 1988, 29, pp. 346-8

Flanagan D, Wood P, Sherwin R, Debrah K, Kerr D. Gin and Tonic and Reactive Hypoglycemia: What Is Important–the Gin, the Tonic, or Both? *J Clin Endocrinol Metab*, 1998, 83, pp. 796-800.

Gerstein HC, Riddle MC, Kendall DM for the ACCORD Study Group. Glycemia Treatment Strategies in the Action to Control Cardiovascular Risk in Diabetes (ACCORD) Trial. *Am J Cardiol*, 2007, 99, S34-S43,

Guettier J-M, Gorden P. Hypoglycemia. *Endocrinol Metab Clin N Am* 2006;35, pp. 753–66.

Harats N, Ackerman Z, Shalit M. Quinine-related hypoglycaemia. *New Engl J Med*, 1984, 310, pp. 1331-37

Hauser L, Sheehan P, Simpkins H. Pancreatic pathology in pentamidine-induced diabetes in acquired immunodeficiency syndrome patients. *Hum Pathol,* 1991, 22, pp. 926-9.

Hekimsoy Z, Biberoglu S, Comlekci A, Tarhan O, Mermut C, Biberoglu K. Trimethoprim/sulfamethoxazole induced hypoglycaemia in a malnourished patient with severe infection. *Eur J Endocrinol,* 1997, 136, 304-6.

Herbel, G., Boyle, P.J. Hypoglycaemia: Pathophysiology and treatment. *Endocrinol Metab Clin North Am,* 2000, 29, pp. 725-43.

Herings RM, de Boer A, Stricker BH, Leufkens HG, Porsius A. Hypoglycaemia associated with the use of inhibitors of angiotensin-converting enzyme. *Lancet,* 1995, 345, pp. 1195-8.

Chang X, Jorgensen AM, Bardrum P, Led JJ. Solution structures of the R6 human insulin hexamer. *Biochemistry* 1997, 36 (31), pp. 9409–22.

Chen CC, Ng KC. Alcohol-induced fasting hypoglycemia. *Mid Taiwan J Med,* 2003, 8, pp. 174-8.

Johnson D, Kubic P, Levitt C. Accidental ingestion of Vacor rodenticide: The symptoms and sequelae in a 25-monthold child. *Am J Dis Child* ,1980, 134, pp. 161-4.

Jones RG, Sue-Ling HM, Kear C, Wiles PG, Quirke P. Severe symptomatic hypoglycaemia due to quinine therapy. *J R Soc Med,* 1986, 79, pp. 426-8.

Kaufman TS, Rúveda EA. Die Jagd auf Chinin: Etappenerfolge und Gesamtsiege. *Angewandte Chemie, Int. Ed.,* 2005, 117 (6), pp. 876–907.

Kawahara, S. Chemotherapeutic agents under study. *Nippon Rinsho,* 1998, 56 (12), pp. 3096–9.

Khashab M, Tector AJ, Kwo PY. Epidemiology of acute liver failure. *Curr Gastroenterol Rep,* 2007, 9 (1), pp. 66–73

Kunte H, Schmidt S, Eliasziw M, del Zoppo GJ, Simard JM, Masuhr F, Weih M, Dirnagl U. Sulfonylureas improve outcome in patients with type 2 diabetes and acute ischemic stroke. *Stroke,* 2007, 38 (9), pp. 2526–30.

LeBlanc M, Bélanger C, Cossette P. Severe and resistant hypoglycemia associated with concomitant gatifloxacin and glyburide therapy. *Pharmacotherapy,* 2004, 24(7), pp. 926-31.

Lin G, Hays DP, Spillane L. Refractory hypoglycemia from ciprofloxacin and glyburide interaction. *J Toxicol Clin Toxicol,* 2004, 42(3), pp. 295-7.

MacLeod KM, Hepburn DA, Frier BM. Frequency and morbidity of severe hypoglycaemia in insulin-treated diabetic patients. *Diabet Med* 1993, 10, pp. 238–45.

Marks V, Teale JD. Hypoglycemia: factitious and felonious. *Endocrinol Metab Clin North Am,* 1999, 28, pp. 579–601.

Marks, V. Drug-induced hypoglycaemia. In: *Hypoglycaemia,* 2nd Ed. Marks, V., Rose, F.C. (Eds.). Blackwell Scientific Publications: Oxford 1981, 357.

Micossi P, Pantiroli AE, Baron SH et al. Aspirin stimulates insulin and glucagon secretion and increases glucose tolerance in normal and diabetic subjects. Diabetes, 1978, 27, pp. 1196-204

Mihic M, Mautner LS, Feness JZ, Grant K. Effect of trimethoprim-sulfamethoxazole on blood insulin and glucose concentrations of diabetics. *Can Med Assoc J,* 1975, 112, pp. 80-2.

Miller CD, Phillips LS, Ziemer DC, Gallina DL, Cook CB, El-Kebbi IM. Hypoglycaemia in patients with type 2 diabetes mellitus. *Arch Intern Med,* 2001, 161, pp. 1653-9.

Miller JB. Hypoglycaemic effect of oxytetracycline. *Br Med J*, 1966, 2, pp. 1007-12

Murata, T., Matsumoto, J., Umemura, S. et al. b-Blocker induced hypoglycaemia in three non-diabetic patients under long-term dialysis treatment. *Nippon Jinzo Gakkai Shi*,1981, 23, pp. 751-9.

Nguewa PA, Fuertes MA, Cepeda V, et al. Pentamidine is an antiparasitic and apoptotic drug that selectively modifies ubiquitin. *Chem. Biodivers*, 2005, 2 (10), pp. 1387–400.

Olson MW, Ruzin A, Feyfant E, Rush TS, O'Connell J, Bradford PA. Functional, biophysical, and structural bases for antibacterial activity of tigecycline. *Antimicrobial agents and chemotherapy, 2006,* 50 (6), pp. 2156–66

Patel A, Chalmers J, Poulter N. ADVANCE: action in diabetes and vascular disease. *J Hum Hyperten*, 2005, 19, S27–S32.

Pollak PT, Mukherjee SD, Fraser AD. Sertraline-induced hypoglycaemia. *Ann Pharmacother*, 2001, 35(11), pp. 1371-4.

Raschke R, Arnold-Capell PA., Richeson R, Curry SC. Refractory hypoglycemia secondary to topical salicylate intoxication. Archives of Internal Medicine, 1991, 37, pp. 56-9

Reaven PD, Sacks J, VADT Investigators: Reduced coronary and abdominal artery calcification in Hispanics with type 2 diabetes. *Diabetes Care*, 2004, 27, pp. 1115-1120,

Roberge RJ, Kaplan R, Frank R, Fore C. Glyburideciprofloxacin interaction with resistant hypoglycaemia. *Ann Emerg Med* ,2000, 36, pp. 160-3

Rosini JM, Martinez E, Jain R. Severe Hypoglycemia Associated with Use of Trimethoprim/Sulfamethoxazole in a Patient with Chronic Renal Insufficiency. *Ann Pharmacoth*, 2008, 42, pp. 593-594.

Rumore MM, Kim KS. Potential Role of Salicylates in Type 2 Diabetes. *Ann Pharmacother*, 2010, 44, pp. 1207-1221

Sattler FR, Waskin H. Pentamidine and fatal hypoglycaemia. *Ann Intern Med*, 1987, 107, pp. 789-90.

Seghieri G, Yin W, Boni C. et al. Effect of chronic ACE inhibition on glucose tolerance and insulin sensitivity in hypertensive type 2 diabetic patients. *Diabetes Med*, 1992, 9, pp. 732-8.

The Diabetes Control and Complications Trial Research Group. The effect of intensive treatment of diabetes on the development and progression of long-term complications in insulin-dependent diabetes mellitus. *N Engl J Med*, 1993, 329(14), pp. 977-86

United Kingdom Hypoglycaemia Study Group. Risk of hypoglycaemia in types 1 and 2 diabetes: effects of treatment modalities and their duration. *Diabetologia,* 2007, 50, pp. 1140–47.

Van den Berghe G, Wouters P, Weekers F, Verwaest C, Bruyninckx F, Schetz M, Vlasselaers D, Ferdindande P, Lauwers P, Bouillon R. Intensive insulin therapy in critically ill patients. *N Engl J Med,* 2001, 345, pp. 1359–67.

Waskin H, Stehr-Green JK, Helmick CG, Sattler AR. Risk factors for hypoglycaemia associated with pentamidine therapy for Pneumocystis pneumonia. *JAMA* , 1988, 260, pp. 345-7

Weathermon R, Crabb DW. Alcohol and medication interactions. Alcohol Res Health, 1999, 23, pp. 40-54

White JR, Hartman J, Campbell RK. Drug interactions in diabetic patients: The risk of losing glycaemic control. *Postgrad Med*, 1993, 93, pp. 131-9.

WHO Global Status Report on Alcohol 2004. World Health Organization, 2004.

Part 4

Section D

10

Pancreatogenous Hypoglycemic Syndrome - Insulinoma or Non-Insulinoma Origin (NIPHS)

Chen-Hsen Lee, Justin Ging-Shing Won and Hsiao-Shan Tseng
Departments of Surgery, Internal Medicine and Radiology
National Yang-Ming University and Taipei
Veterans General Hospital, Taipei,
Taiwan

1. Introduction

Pancreatogenous hypoglycemic syndrome (PHS) is a heterogeneous disorder that occurs as a consequence of inappropriate and unregulated secretion of insulin by pancreatic β-cell tumors (insulinomas) or by nesidiodysplastic β-cells presenting as non-insulinoma pancreatogenous hypoglycemic syndrome (NIPHS). NIPHS, formerly termed adult nesidioblastosis, is characterized by postprandial hypoglycemia and negative prolonged fasts, and yields negative perioperative localization studies for insulinoma but positive intra-arterial calcium stimulation (IACS) tests as well as nesidioblastosis in the gradient-guided resected pancreas (Service et al., 1999a; Won et al., 2006). NIPHS is an increasingly recognized entity and appears to develop much more frequently in patients who have undergone either a Billroth II operation for peptic ulcer diseases or a Roux-en-Y gastric bypass procedure for medically complicated obesity (Service et al., 2005; Patti et al., 2005). Even though the histology of the resected pancreatic tissues from those patients resemble some of the histologic features observed in patients of congenital hyperinsulinism (CHI), in which genetic mutations in the 2 subunits (Kir6.2 and SUR 1) of the pancreatic β-cell ATP-sensitive potassium channel (K_{ATP}) are observed (Kapoor et al., 2006), screening for similar mutations in those patients has proven unsuccessful (Service et al., 1999; Patti et al., 2005). Although the existence of post-gastric bypass NIPHS as a discrete entity has been strongly questioned (Meier et al., 2006), several lines of evidence—the neuroglycopenic nature of spells, the usual unresponsiveness to dietary modification, and the very high recurrence rate (up to 87%) after gradient-guided pancreatectomy (Vanderveen et al., 2010)—suggest functional as well as structural abnormalities of the disorder.

Traditionally, PHS in adults is most commonly caused by circumscribed solitary or multiple insulinomas, while in 0.5-5% of patients, localized or diffuse proliferation of islet cells budding from pancreatic ducts (nesidioblastosis) has been defined (Fajans & Vinik 1989). With increasing utilization of IACS test, however, evidence shows that NIPHS has been found to account for 40-50% of all the patients with PHS (Starke et al., 2006; Thompson 2007). In our hospital, we routinely performed IACS tests for patients with documented hyperinsulinemic hypoglycemia, and during the past 15 years we found roughly an equal incidence of insulinoma and NIPHS (Won et al., 2006), among the latter one-third had had gastric bypass surgery that was not bariatric-related.

2. Clinical presentations

The hypoglycemic symptoms are usually divided into adrenergic and neuroglycopenic symptoms. The sympathetic adrenergic symptoms include tachycardia, palpitations, sweating, tremor, and anxiety. The glucose deprivation of central nervous system (CNS) results in neuroglycopenic symptoms including behavioral changes, confusion, weakness, fatigue, loss of consciousness, amnesia, dizziness, blurry vision, diplopia, paresthesia, seizures, and coma (Fajans & Vinik 1989). These symptoms can occur during fasting, after exercise, or postprandially (3-5 hours after meal). Although the adrenergic symptoms are not unique to hypoglycemia, the possibility of neuroglycopenia should always be suspected in patients whose adrenergic symptoms are followed by spells of disturbed CNS functions, patients whose symptoms occur in the setting of a documented absolute hypoglycemia (plasma glucose ≤ 45 mg/dl; 2.8 mmol/l), and patients whose symptoms are relieved by glucose administration. A detailed history to ascertain the type of symptoms, the frequency of spells and its relationship to meals, and history of gastric bypass surgery should be obtained. Furthermore, clinical evidence of neuroglycopenia should be highly suggestive of organic hyperinsulinism, such as PHS, and warrants meticulous attentiveness and further testing until proven otherwise (Dizon et al., 1999). Approximately one-fourth of patients with insulinoma develop only neuroglycopenic symptoms (Fajans & Vinik 1989; Dizon et al., 1999).

Insulinoma is typically associated with fasting hypoglycemia, but may occur during both fasting and in postprandial states or even exclusively postprandially (Placzkowski et al., 2009). In contrast, NIPHS is often manifested as postprandial hypoglycemia, although fasting hypoglycemia can also occur. In a few of our NIPHS patients, persistent hypoglycemia during both fasting and postprandial periods requiring continuous infusion of dextrose to prevent neuroglycopenia was observed.

3. Diagnosis

The diagnosis of PHS requires biochemical confirmation of inappropriately elevated plasma insulin concentrations in the settings of absolute hypoglycemia, which may occur spontaneously or can be provoked (Service 1999). The diagnostic criteria for hyperinsulinemia consist of a plasma insulin level ≥ 6 μU/ml (36 pmol/l), a plasma C-peptide ≥ 0.6 ng/ml (200 pmol/l), or a plasma proinsulin ≥ 5 pmol/l, and a plasma β-hydroxybutyrate ≤ 2.7 mmol/l at the time of hypoglycemia (plasma glucose ≤ 45 mg/dl or less) (Service 1999b). Nevertheless, with the development of the more sensitive and highly specific assay for insulin, the immunochemiluminometric assay (ICMA), an insulin level of ≥ 3 μU/ml (18 pmol/l) has been suggested as the criterion for hyperinsulinemia (Service 1999b). It is therefore crucial to measure, in addition to insulin, the concentrations of plasma C-peptide (a marker of endogenous insulin production), proinsulin, and ketone body (an indicator of insulin action) concurrently during a symptomatic hypoglycemia, as occasional insulinoma cases have reported persistent low serum insulin levels as determined by ICMA, despite the elevated C-peptide and/or proinsulin concentrations (Chia & Saudek 2003; Coelho et al., 2009). Also, it is prudent to measure the level of insulin secretagogues (i.e., sulfonylureas and glinides), if available, to differentiate the factitious hypoglycemia;and insulin autoantibody to identify and exclude the insulin autoimmune syndrome, a rare disorder reported to occur primarily among persons of Japanese ancestry (Comi 1993) . Our experience shows that, during hypoglycemic spells, the insulin levels tend to be higher in patients with insulinoma than in patients with NIPHS, in whom the detected insulin concentration may be a little higher than the aforementioned diagnostic criteria.

4. Laboratory tests

4.1 72 h fast

The 72 h supervised fast remains the gold standard for the diagnosis of insulinoma as the test enables the clinical demonstration of Whipple's triad: symptoms and signs consistent with hypoglycemia, a concomitant plasma glucose level of 45 mg/dl or less, and reversibility of symptoms with administration of glucose (Service & Natt 2000). In addition, the test provides biochemical confirmation of unsuppressed insulin secretion in the settings of hypoglycemia by measuring plasma insulin, C-peptide, proinsulin, and β-hydroxybutyrate concentrations simultaneously, as aforementioned. In most reports, one-third of patients with insulinoma develop symptoms within 12 hours, two-thirds within 24 hours, 95% in 48 hours, and 99% in 72 hours (Service & Natt 2000). A recent study suggests that a 48-h fast may be an alternative, with a sensitivity rate of 95% (Hirshberg et al., 2000). In our hospital, we routinely perform the 48-h prolonged fast. As expected, most patients with NIPHS, by definition, do not develop hypoglycemia during a 72 h prolonged fast.

4.2 The 5-hour oral glucose tolerance test (OGTT)

In contrast to the 72 h fast testing, the OGTT test may offer biochemical evidence of postprandial hypoglycemia associated with clinical symptoms and signs of neuroglycopenia, which may be missed in the supervised 72 h fast, though an abnormal OGTT is not helpful in the diagnosis or differential diagnosis of organic hyperinsulinism (Service 1999a). Interestingly, very few cases of insulinoma show signs of glucose-induced hypoglycemia alone (Wiesli et al., 2002; Kar et al., 2006).

4.3 Insulin/glucose (I/G) ratio or amended I/G ratio

These measurements are no longer applied to the diagnosis of organic hyperinsulinism as currently most insulin assays have been replaced by the more specific ICMA technique worldwide.

5. Image studies

Because of the small size (90% tumors usually less than 2 cm in size), potential multiplicity, and possible throughout the whole pancreas, preoperative localization of tumors is very important and essential in determining prognosis and appropriate surgical intervention. There are a variety of preoperative imaging modalities for the detection of insulinomas. However, no single one imaging examination could localize tumors in all patients. Most experienced endocrine surgeons obtain one or more localization tests before treatment is performed. In choosing the localization technique, specific tumor characteristics need to be considered.

a. Most insulinomas are vascular and visualized in arterial phase imaging.
b. Most tumors are intrapancreatic.
c. 80 - 90% are solitary and 80% less than 2 cm in diameter.
d. Distributed equally within the head, body and tail of the pancreas.
e. Multiple tumors are found in only 8% of patients associated with MEN-1.

5.1 Preoperative transabdominal ultrasound

Just like other abdominal diseases, transabdominal ultrasound is the most convenient imaging modality to examine the pancreatic insulinomas. It is noninvasive, radiation free, and readily available. However, the pancreas is deeply located in the abdomen and most patients with insulinoma are obese due to frequent snacking to resolve hypoglycemic symptoms. To fully investigate the whole pancreas demands meticulous technique. Besides the usual supine position, placing the patient in recumbent or upright oblique position may be necessary. Using the fluid-filled stomach or the spleen as acoustic window is also useful to examine the body and tail of pancreas (Galiber et al.,1988; Gorman et al., 1986).

Usually, insulinoma is detected as a solitary, rounded, well-defined, hypoechoic mass with smooth outlines (Galiber et al.,1988). Gorman and colleagues reported 10% insulinoma either isoechoic or hyperechoic to surrounding parenchyma that may be due to normal pancreatic parenchyma. It is less echogenic in younger patients than in older ones (Gorman et al., 1986).

The ultrasound is operator dependent; thus, different detection rates were reported. Guettier and colleagues reported only a 14% accurate localization rate, a 72% false negative and a 14% false positive rates (Guettier et al., 1986). Grant reported their Mayo Clinic experience from July 1982 through October 2004 with a 65% sensitivity and a 91% positive predictive value (Grant, 2005). Not surprisingly, the bigger the tumor ,the easier it is to be detected. Böttger and colleagues reported a sensitivity of 43% for tumors less than 1 cm in diameter, 67% for tumors between 1 and 1.5 cm, and 80% for tumors larger than 1.5 cm (Böttger et al., 1990). Kuzin and colleagues reported rates of 10%, 21.4% and 53.8% for tumors less then 1 cm,1 to 2 cm and larger than 2 cm, respectively (Kuzin et al., 1998). They also found tumor location may affect the sensitivity of this test, with a 50% detection rate for tumor at pancreatic body, 16.7% for head and 23% for tail (Kuzin et al., 1998).

5.2 Endoscopic ultrasound (EUS)

Compared with transabdominal ultrasound, EUS is close to pancreas and can use high-frequency probe that improves the image resolution and increases the detection rate of insulinoma. The appearance of insulinomas in EUS is similar to that in transabdominal ultrasound. Most published series reported high sensitivity. Rösch and colleagues described a sensitivity of 82% (Rösch et al., 1992). Nikfarjam and colleagues reported 92% (Nikfarjam et al., 2008). But Druce and colleagues reported only 65.4% (Druce et al., 2010). This discrepancy implies the importance of expertise to carry out the procedure. Tumor location is another important factor. To detect an insulinoma in the pancreatic head portion is easier than one in the tail. Schumacher et al. had a 83% sensitivity for tumors at the head and 37% at the tail (Schumacher et al., 1996).

5.3 Computed tomography (CT)

CT is widely used to scan the pancreatic insulinoma. The reported sensitivity rate varied with different techniques. The conventional CT scan had low sensitivity with a range of 16 - 72% (Chatziioannou et al., 2001). There are at least two reasons to account for the low detection rate. First, most insulinomas are small that conventional CT may skip the tumors. Second, small insulinomas appear similar density as normal parenchyma in pre-contrast and post-contrast delayed scan of conventional CT. With modern multidetector CT with dynamic contrast study, the above mentioned problems can be solved. After taking non-contrast study with thick slices (5–8 mm), biphasic images are taken after intravenous injection of 120–150 ml non-ionic contrast medium at the rate of 3-5 ml/sec with power injector. The arterial phase is taken about 30 seconds after injection and venous phase at 70 seconds. Thin slices and reformatted images may help to demonstrate smaller lesions (Chung et al., 1997). Nikfarjam and colleagues found the sensitivity rate increased from 24% before 1997 to 80% between 1994 and 2007 (Nikfarjam et al., 2008). Most insulinomas show isodensity nodule in pre-contrast scan and high density in the arterial phase images. Atypical CT appearances of insulinomas include a high density mass in pre-contrast CT scan, low density mass in post contrast scan, cystic or calcified mass (Chatziioannou et al., 2001).

5.4 Magnetic resonance imaging (MRI)

Modern MRI provides a high sensitive test in the localization of insulinoma. High field (1.5 T or 3 T) magnet combined with torso phased-array coil is used. Antiperistaltic agents may be used to decrease artifact caused by bowel movement. The protocol includes axial T1 and spin echo image with and without fat suppression, and spoiled gradient-echo (GRE) image before and after intravenous administration of gadolinium (Thoeni et al., 2000). Insulinomas usually show a low signal intensity in T1-weighted image and high in T2-weighted image, and marked enhancement after intravenous gadolinium administration. With modern MRI, the detection rates of 70% (Nikfarjam et al., 2008), 75% (Druce et al., 2010), and 85% (Thoeni et al., 2000) had been reported. The MRI technique is in constant evolution. Recently, the diffusion weighted image technique is applied to examine the abdomen. It may improve the detection of pancreatic insulinomas (Lee et al., 2008).

5.5 Angiography

Though angiography was considered also sensitive to localize insulinomas, it was rarely performed alone today in this hospital, and usually was combined with hepatic venous sampling. To perform angiography, a catheter is advanced through femoral artery and selected into the arteries that supplying the pancreas, including the celiac, superior mesenteric, splenic and gastroduodenal arteries. Modern angiographic suite is armamentarium with digital subtraction technique that will improve the sensitivity of this test. However, antiperistaltic agents may be necessary to suppress bowel movement which causes motion artifact (Jackson, 2005). Besides, different projections are mandatory to avoid overlapping with other organ, such as the spleen, that may interfere with the blush of insulinoma. Classical angiographic picture of an insulinoma is a well defined blushing appearing in early arterial phase and persist to venous phase. But hypovascular insulinomas are not uncommon because of their small sizes. Fulton and colleagues reported 9 of 24 insulinomas were hypovascular (Fulton et al., 1975). The reported detection rate of angiography ranged from 35% (Doherty et al., 1991) to 100% (Geoghegan et al., 1994).

5.6 Percutaneous transhepatic portal venous sampling (PTPVS)

The concept of PTPVS is that insulinomas secrete insulin which would be drained into adjacent venous system. The closer to the insulinoma, the higher the concentration of insulin would be detected. After puncturing the branch of right portal vein, a catheter with side-hole at tip was advanced into the splenic vein and superior mesenteric vein. Venography was taken first as a map. Then, samplings were taken along the splenic, superior and inferior mesenteric veins as well as the portal trunk at 1 to 1.5 cm intervals. Pancreatic veins were also sampled when possible (Cho et al., 1982). PTPVS was highly accurate and considered to be the gold standard for this purpose (Nikfarjam et al., 2008; Vinik et al., 1991). However, severe complications, which mainly related to catheterizing the portal vein, are not infrequent. Miller and colleagues reported a rate of 6% severe complications (Miller et al., 1992). For this reason and the development of other less invasive modality, i.e. selective intra-arterial calcium stimulation with hepatic venous sampling, PTPVS is rarely performed nowadays.

5.7 Selective intra-arterial calcium stimulation (IACS) with hepatic venous sampling

In 1987, Imamura and colleagues described a novel method of intra-arterial injection of secretin and then sampling blood from hepatic vein to localize gastrinoma in patients with Zollinger-Ellisson Syndrome (Imamura et al., 1987). In 1991, Doppman and colleagues adopted the concept but using calcium as secretagogue to localize insulinoma in four cases (Doppman et al. 1991). To perform IACS, a catheter with side-hole at the tip is threaded through femoral vein into right hepatic vein. After selective angiography, 10% calcium gluconate diluted with saline to equivalent to 0.0125 mmol/kg (0.025 mEq/kg) is injected as quickly as possible but not spilled into adjacent vessles to avoid bias. In obese patients, the dose is adjusted to 0.005mmol/kg. Blood samples are obtained from the right hepatic vein before and 30, 60, 90, 120, and 180 seconds after injection of calcium. All the arteries supplying pancreas should be studied that including superior mesenteric, gastroduodenal, and splenic arteries. Sometimes, dorsal pancreatic artery is also studied if it is large enough to be catheterized safely. A two-fold or greater increase of insulin above baseline indicates a positive result. A positive result in superior mesenteric artery or gastroduodenal artery means the lesion at pancreatic head or uncinate process, while in splenic artery means pancreatic body or tail. To further differentiate tumor location in body or tail, two sets of splenic artery samplings are collected. One is at proximal injection, another is distal to the pancreatic magna artery. If both are positive, the lesion is at pancreatic tail. If only proximal one is positive, the lesion is at pancreatic body. Besides the above mentioned arteries, proper hepatic artery is also studied to search the possibility of liver metastasis. The time between two calcium injections should be at least 5 minutes apart to allow the possible stimulated elevation of insulin level to return to its baseline (Jackson, 2005). Since its development, IACS is considered the most reliable preoperative localization modality for insulinoma. In most reported series, successful rates were more than 90% (Jackson, 2005) .Diazoxide that is used to treat hyperinsulinemia should be suspended before IACS test as it may affect the result of the test (Doppman et al., 1991).

Besides insulinomas, beta-cell hyperfunction, the so-called nesidioblastosis, is another important cause of PHS. Since most nesidioblastosis did not form discrete nodule, the non-invasive image studies are usually negative (Raffel et al., 2007; Service et al., 1999a; Starke et al., 2006). But the IACS test always shows positive result and is an important clue to the diagnosis of nesidioblastosis. Meanwhile, if surgical treatment is to be performed, the gradient-guided resection according to the results of IACS test is mandatory (Thompson et al., 2000; Tseng et al., 2007).

5.8 Somatostatin receptor scintigraphy (SRS)

The somatostatin receptor scintigraphy (OctreoscanTM), which uses Indium-111 pentetreotide as a traceable somatostatin analog that predominantly binds to receptor subtypes, sst2 and sst5 (Bertherat et al., 2003), serves as a functional imaging modality for neuroendocrine tumors and some non-neuroendocrine tumors which contain somatostatin receptors.

The diagnostic accuracy of the SRS is affected by the size and presence of different receptor subtypes of the tumors. The sensitivity of SRS in detecting insulinoma is reported to be as low as 50-60% (Balon et al., 2001; Mirallie et al., 2002), but the positive predictive value is high (Proye et al., 1998).

The SRS serves as a complementary role in the localization of an insulinoma when the diagnosis is established but undetectable or equivocal on CT or MRI.

6. Treatment

6.1 Medical treatment

For the insulinoma patients surgery is not amenable or is contraindicated, and for those with unresectable disease, medical treatment with diazoxide, a β-cell K_{ATP} channel agonist to inhibit insulin secretion, can be used with a reported effective rate of 97% (Gill et al., 1997). The usual dosage range is 150 to 450 mg daily, given orally twice or thrice a day. Side effects include nausea, hypertrichosis, and sodium retention. The addition of a benzothiadiazine diuretics, such as chlorothiazide, can combat the edema and potentiate the hyperglycemic effect of diazoxide (Fajans & Vinik 1989). Octreotide, a long-acting somatostatin analog that acts mainly via the somatostatin receptor subtype 2, is sometimes effective (Vezzosi et al., 2005).

Once the diagnosis of NIPHS in the patient is confirmed by IACS, medical treatment with diazoxide should be tried first. Our limited experience found that almost all the patients, with or without a previous gastric bypass surgery, responded satisfactorily, with alleviation of neuroglycopenic episodes presumably in those with intact function of β-cell K_{ATP} channel, which the action of diazoxide requires (Won et al., 2006). Whether octreotide or the newer analog, pasireotide (SOM230), is effective in patients with NIPHS is unclear and requires further study.

6.2 Surgical treatment

Surgical resection remains the treatment of choice for insulinomas. Usually, the successful rate of surgical treatment is over 90% in experienced hands. However, over resection of the pancreas may lead to diabetes which causes another problem affecting the patients' quality of life .With the advancement in imaging technology, increase in knowledge as well as improvement in surgical technique, blind resection for an unlocalized insulinoma is no more acceptable. Various modalities of resection are available for the surgical treatment of insulinomas. Enunciation is usually employed for an insulinoma superficially located and away from the main pancreatic duct either in the head or body portion of the pancreas. The postoperative occurrence rate of pancreatic fistula varied from 18 to 57%. Enucleation of the pancreatic tail insulinomas is also feasible in selective conditions such as a pedunculated or a small bulging tumor from pancreatic surface; or a clearly visible image of 2 to 3 mm distance between the tumor and main pancreatic duct. In the author's opinion, enucleation is always first considered and evaluated before a resection of pancreas. If feasible, it causes less damage, avoids sacrificing islets in the pancreatic tail and saves time for operation. A distal pancreatectomy (40% distal pancreas resection) is done for multiple or big insulinomas ; or the tumor is attached to the pancreatic duct. The spleen should be preserved as possible; A Whipple's operation is rarely necessary for pancreatic head insulinoma unless it is big, deep or located near the main duct; Subtotal pancreatectomy (60~85% distal pancreatctomy) with enucleation of tumors in the head was advised for MEN-1 associated insulinomas because of its multiple and diffuse lesions before the IACS test was popular (Thompson 1995). Our recent experiences showed that a solitary insulinoma disease may exist in MEN-1 patients, and distal pancreatectomy achieved euglycemia for more than 10 years. Individualized judgment according to the IACS insulin gradients is mandatory to avoid over resections and ensuing sequellae, although in the published large series (Tonelli et al., 2005; Bartsch et al., 2005; Norton et al., 2006) most patients needed an extended distal pancreatectomy and enucleation of tumors in the head.

With repeated emphasis on the management of hypoglycemia in medical education as well as increased alertness of physicians at emergency department, more and more patients had diagnosis of spontaneous pancreatogenous hypoglycemia at its early presentation. It is our recommendation that image studies are done to localize the lesion instead of screening for diagnosis. However, despite the advancement in imaging technology, up to 25% of insulinomas remain occult preoperatively (Norton 1989). An occult insulinoma is defined as biochemically proven tumor with indeterminate anatomical site before operation. It should not prohibite the physicians from referring to surgery because intraoperative ultrasonography(IOUS) and palpation (96~100% sensitivity) by experienced surgeon may help to find out the tumor. A preoperative IACS test is helpful to indicate the region the tumor is located. It is especially useful in re-do operations or in patients with previous episodes of pancreatitis. In both situations dense peripancreatic adhesion usually exists and causes difficulties in dissection. Following the guidance of IACS test, a limited regional exploration may help to save operation time and prevent post-operative pancreatitis due to over manipulation (Tseng et al., 2007).

In case, IOUS and palpation failed to find the lesion, we recommend a regional resection of pancreatic tail (40%) or tail and body (80-85%) as suggested by the insulin gradients in the splenic artery alone or plus SMA. This is different from a blind resection and is helpful in the surgical treatment of adult NIPHS. Our previous report has shown its advantage over a subtotal pancreatectomy in terms of post-operative diabetes (Lee et al., 2002). However, long-term follow up is needed to observe any recurrence.

In summary, the goal of surgical treatment for PHS should aim at post-operative euglycemia and long term recurrence free. A blind distal pancreatectomy or an improper extensive subtotal pancreatectomy should not be performed. The IACS test plus IOUS is a good resection guide in the treatment of PHS. Surgical intervention for NIPHS is reserved for those refractory to medical treatment.

7. Conclusion

Spontaneous pancreatogenous hypoglycemic syndrome is a rare disease. With typical clinical presentation and compatible laboratory tests, it is not difficult for early diagnosis.

With pre-operative localization and intra-operative palpation as well as the use of intraoperative ultrasonography, blind resection of the distal pancreas is no more accepted. The cure rate of surgical treatment for insulinomas is usually more than 90%. Medical treatment is for those with high operation risk, previous failure of pre-operative and intra-operative localization or diffuse islet cell hyperplasia as indicated in the selective intra-arterial calcium stimulation test.

8. References

Balon, H.R.; Goldsmith, S.J.; Siegel, B.A.; Silberstein, E.B.; Krenning, E.P.; Lang, O. & Donohoe, K.J. (2001). Procedure Guideline for Somatostatin Receptor Scintigraphy with ^{111}In-Pentetreotide. *The Journal of Nuclear Medicine,* Vol..42, No.7, (July), pp. 1134-1138.

Bartsch, D. K.; Fendrich, V.; Langer, P. Celik I;Kann P.H. & Rothmund M., (2005). Outcome of Duodenopancreatic Resections in Patients with Multiple Endocrine Neoplasia Type 1. *Annals of Surgery,* Vol.242, No.6, (December), pp. 757-766.

Bertherat, J.; Tenenbaum, F.; Perlemoine, K.; Videau, C.; Alberini, J.L.; Richard, B.; Dousset, B.; Bertagna, X. & Epelbaum, J. (2003). Somatostatin Receptors 2 and 5 are the Major Somatostatin Receptors in Insulinomas: an in Vivo and in Vitro Study. *The Journal of Clinical Endocrinology & Metabolism,* Vol.88, No.11, (November), PP. 5353-5360.

Böttger, T.C.; Weber, W.; Beyer, J. & Jungineger, T. (1990). Value of Tumor Localizaton in Patients with Insulinoma. *World Journal of Surgery,* Vol.14, No.1, (January-February), pp. 107-114, ISSN 0364-2313.

Chatziioannou, A.; Kehagias, D.; Mourikis, D.; Antoniou, A.; Limouris, G.; Kaponis, A.; Kavatzas, N.; Tseleni, S. & Vlachos, L. (2001). Imagining and Localization of Pancreatic Insulinomas. *Clinical Imaging,* Vol.25, No.4, (July-August), pp. 275-283.

Chia, C. W. & Saudek, C. D. (2003). The Diagnosis of Fasting Hypoglycemia Due To an Islet-Cell Tumor Obscured by a Highly Specific Insulin Assay. *The Journal of Clinical Endocrinology & Metabolism,* Vol.88, No.4, (April), pp. 1464-1467.

Cho, K.J.; Vinik, A.I.; Thompson N.W.; Porter D.J.; Brady, T.M.; Cadavid, G. & Fajans, S.S. (1982). Localzation of the Source of Hyperinsulinism: Percutaneous Transhepatic Portal and Pancreatic Vein Catheterization with Hormone Assay. *American Journal of Roentgenology,* Vol.139, No.2, (August), pp. 237-245.

Chung, M.J.; Choi, B.I.; Han, J.K.; Chung, J.W.; Han, M.C. & Bae, S.H. (1997). Functioning Islet Cell Tumor of the Pancreas. Localization with Dynamic Spiral CT. *Acta Radiologica,* Vol.38, No.1, (January), pp. 135-138, ISSN 0284-1851.

Coelho, C.; Druce, M. R. & Grossman, A. B. (2009). Diagnosis of Insulinoma in a Patient with Hypoglycemia without Obvious Hyperinsulinemia. Nature Review of Endocrinology Vol.5, No.11, (November), pp. 628-631.

Comi, R. J. (1993). Approach to Acute Hypoglycemia. *Endocrinology and Metabolism Clinics of North America,* Vol. 22, No 2, (June), pp. 247-262.

Dizon, A. M.; Kowalyk, S.& Hoogwerf, B. J. (1999). Neuroglycopenic and Other Symptoms in Patients with Insulinomas. *The America Journal of Medicine*, Vol.106, No.3, (March), pp. 307-310.

Doherty, G.M.; Doppman, J.L.; Shawker, T.H.; Miller, D.L.; Eastman, R.C.; Gorden, P. & Norton, J.A. (1991). Reults of a Prospective Strategy to Diagnose, Localize, and Resect Insulinomas. *Surgery*, Vol.110, No.6, (December), pp. 989-997.

Doppman, J.L.; Miller, D.L.; Chang, R.; Shawker, T.H.; Gorden, P. & Norton, J.A. (1991). Insulinomas: Localization with Selective Intra-arterial Injection of Calcium. *Radiology*, Vol.178, No.1, (January), pp. 237-241.

Druce, M.R.; Muthuppalaniappan, V.M.; O'Leary, B.; Chew, S.L.; Drake, W.M.; Monson, J.P.; Akker, S.A.; Besser, M.; Sahdev, A.; Rockall, A.; Vyas, S.; Bhattacharya, S.; Matson, M.; Berney, D. & Grossman, A.B. (2010). Diagnosis and Localization of Insulinoma: the Value of Modern Magnetic Resonance Imaging in Conjuction with Calcium Stimulation Catheterization. *European Journal of Endocrinology*, Vol.162, No.5, (May), pp. 971-978.

Fajans, S. S. & Vinik, A. I. (1989). Insulin-producing Islet Cell Tumors. *Endocrinology and Metabolism Clinics of North America*, Vol.18, No.1, (March), pp. 45-74.

Fulton, R.E.; Sheedy, P.F.; McIlrath, D.C. & Ferris, D.O. (1975). Preoperative Angiographic Localization of Insulin-producing Tumors of the Pancreas. *American Journal of Roentgenology*, Vol. 123, No.2, (February), pp. 367-377

Galiber, A.K.; Reading, C.C.; Charboneau J.W.; James, E.M.; Gorman, B.; Grant, C.S.; van Heerden, J.A. & Telander,R.L. (1988). Localization of Pancreatic Insulinoma: Comparison of Pre- and Intraoperative US with CT and Angiography. *Radiology*, Vol.166, No.2, (February), pp. 405-408.

Geoghegan, J.G.; Jackson, J.E.; Lewis, M.P.N.; Owen, E.R.T.C.; Bloom, S.R.; Lynn, J.A. & Williamson, R.C.N. (1994). Localization and Surgical Management of Insulinoma. *British Journal of Surgery*, Vol.81, No.7, (July), pp. 1025-1028.

Gill, G. V.; Rauf, O. & MacFarlane, I. A. (1997). Diazoxide Treatment for Insulinomas: A national UK survey. *Postgraduate Medical Journal*, Vol.73, No.864, (October), pp. 640-641.

Gorman, B.; Charboneau J.W.; James, E.M.; Reading, C.C.; Galiber, A.K.; Grant, C.S.; van Heerden, J.A.; Telander, R.L. & Service F.J. (1986). Benign Pancreatic Insulinoma: Preoperative and Intraoperative Sonographic Localization. *American Journal of Roentgenology*, Vol.147, No.5, (November), pp. 929-934.

Grant, C.S. (2005). Insulinoma. *Best Practice & Research Clinical Gastroenterology*, Vol.19, No.5, (October 2005), pp. 783-798.

Guettier, J.M.; Kam, A.; Chang, R.; Skarulis, M.C.; Skarulis, M.C.; Cochran, C.; Alexander, H.R.; Libutti, S.K.; Pingpank, J.F. & Gorden, P. (2009). Localization of Insulinomas to Regions of Pancreas by Intraarterial Calcium Stimulation: The NIH Experience. *The Journal of Clinical Endocrinology & Metabolism*, Vol.94,pp.1074-1080.

Hirshberg, B.; Livi, A.; Bartlett, D. L.; Libutti, S. K.; Alexander, H. R.; Doppman, J.L., Skarulis, M. C. & Gorden, P. (2000). Forty-Eight-Hour Fast: the Diagnostic Test for Insulinoma. *The Journal of Clinical Endocrinology & Metabolism*, Vol.85, No.9, (Semptember), pp. 3222-3226.

Imamura, M.; Takahashi, K.; Adachi, H.; Minematsu, S.; Shimada, Y.; Naito, M.; Suzuki, T.; Tobe, T. & Azuma, T. (1987). Usefulness of Selective Arterial Secretin Injection Test for Localization of Gastrinoma in the Zollinger-Ellison Syndrome. *Annals of Surgery,* Vol.205, No.3, (March), pp. 230-239.

Jackson, J.E. (2005). Angiography and Arterial Stimulation Venous Sampling in the Localization of Pancreatic Neuroendocrine Tumours. *Best Practice & Research Clinical Endocrinology & Metabolism,* Vol.19, No.2, (June), pp. 229-239.

Kapoor, R. R.; James, C. & Hussain, K. (2009). Advances in the Diagnosis and Management of Hyperinsulinemic Hypoglycemia. *Nature Clinical Practice of Endocrinology & Metabolism,* Vol.5, No.2, (February), pp. 101-112.

Kar, P.; Price, P.; Sawers, S.; Bhattacharya, S.; Reznek, R. H. & Grossman, A. B. (2006). Insulinomas May Present with Normoglycemia after Prolonged Fasting but Glucose-stimulated Hypoglycemia. *The Jounal of Clinical Endocrinology & Metabolism,* Vol.91, No.12, (December), pp. 4733-4736.

Kuzin, N.M.; Egorov, A.V.; Kondrashin, S.A.; Lotov, A.N.; Kuznetzov, N.S. & Majorova, J.B. (1998). Preoerative and Intraoperative Topographic Diagnosis of Insulinomas. *World Journal of Surgery,* Vol.22, No.6, (June), pp. 593-597, ISSN 0364-2313.

Lee, C.H.; Wong, J.G. & Chiang, J.H. (2002).Benign Diffuse Islet Cell Disease in Adults: A comparison of the results from distal and arterial stimulated venous sampling - guided pancreatectomies. Chinese Medical Journal(Taipei). Vol.65, No.1, pp. 111-118.

Lee, S.S.; Byun, J.H.; Park, B.J.; Park, S.H.; Kim, N.; Park, B.; Kim, J.K. & Lee, M. (2008). Quantitative Anaslysis of Diffusion-Weighted Magnetic Resonance Imaging of The Pancreas: Usefulness in Characterizing Solid Pancreatic Masses. *Journal of Magnetic Resonance Imaging,* Vol.28, No.4, (October), pp. 928-936.

Meier, J. J.; Nauck, M. A. & Butler, P. C. (2006). Comment to: Patti ME, McMahon G, Mun EC et al. (2005) Severe Hypoglycaemia Post-gastric Bypass Requiring Partial Pancreatectomy: evidence for inappropriate insulin secretion and pancreatic islet hyperplasia. *Diabetologia* Vol.48, pp. 2236-2240. *Diabetologia,* Vol.49, No.3, (March), pp. 607-608.

Miller, D.L.; Doppman, J.L.; Metz, D.C.; Maton, P.N.; Norton, J.A. & Jensen, R.T. (1992). Zollinger-Ellison Syndrome: Technique, Results, and Complications of Portal Venous Sampling. *Radiology,* Vol.182, No.1, (January), pp. 235-241.

Mirallie, E.; Pattou, F.; Malvaux, P.; Filoche, B.; Godchaux, J.M.; Maunoury, V.; Palazzo, L.; Lefebvre, J.; Huglo, D.; Paris J.C.; Carnaille, B. & Proye, C. (2002). Value of Endoscopic Ultrasonography and Somatostatin Receptor Scintigraphy in the Preoperative Localization of Insulinomas and Gastrinomas. Experience of 54 cases. *Gastroenterologie clinique et biologique,* Vol.26, No.4, (April), pp. 360-366.

Nikfarjam, M.; Warshaw A.L.; Axelrod, L.; Deshpande, V.; Thayer, S.P.; Ferrone, C.R. & Castillo, C.F. (2008). Improved Contemporary Surgical Management of Insulinomas. A 25-year Experience at the Massachusetts General Hospital. *Annals of Surgery,* Vol.247, No.1, (January), pp. 165-172, ISSN 0003-4932/08/24701-0165.

Norton, J. A.; Cromack D. T. ; Shawker T. H.;Doppman J.L.; Comi R.; Gorden P.; Maton P.N.; Gardner J.D. & Jensen R.T. (1988). Intraoperative ultrasonographic localization of islet cell tumors. A prospective Comparison to Palpation. *Annals of Surgery*, Vol.207, No.2, (February), pp. 160-168.

Norton, J. A.; Fang, T. D. & Jensen, R. T. (2006). Surgery for Gastrinoma and Insulinoma in Multiple Endocrine Neoplasia Type 1. *The Journal of the National Comprehensive Cancer Network*, Vol.4, pp. 148-153.

Patti, M. E.; McMahon, G.; Mun, E. C.; Bitton, A.; Holst, J. J.; Goldsmith, J.; Hanto, D. W.; Callery, M.; Arky, R.; Nose, V.; Bonner-Weir, S. & Goldfine, A. B. (2005). Severe Hypoglycaemia Post-gastric Bypass Requiring Partial Pancreatectomy: Evidence for inappropriate insulin secretion and pancreatic islet hyperplasia. *Diabetologia*, Vol.48, No.11, (November), pp. 2236-2240.

Placzkowski, K. A.; Vella, A.; Thompson, G. B.; Grant, C. S.; Reading, C. C.; Charboneau, J. W.; Andrews, J. C.; Lloyd, R. V. & Service, F. J. (2009). Secular Trends in the Presentation and Management of Functioning Insulinoma at the Mayo Clinic, 1987-2007. *The Journal of Clincal Endocrinology & Metabolism*, Vol.94, No.4, (April), pp. 1069-1073.

Proye, C.; Malvaux, P.; Pattou, F.; Filoche, B.; Godchaux, J.M.; Maunoury, V.; Palazzo, L.; Huglo, Damien.; Lefebvre, J.& Paris, J.C. (1998). Noninvasive Imaging of Insulinomas and Gastrinomas with Endoscopic Ultrasonography and Somatostatin Receptor Scintigraphy. *Surgery*, Vol.124, No.6, (December), pp. 1134-1144.

Raffel, A.; Krausch, M.; Anlauf, M.; Wieben, D.; Braunstein, S.; Klöppel, G.; Röher, H. & Knoefel, W.T. (2007). Diffuse Nesidioblastosis as a Cause of Hyperinsulinemic Hypoglycemia in Adults: a Diagnosis and Therapeutic Challenge. *Surgery*, Vol.141, No.2, (February), pp. 179-184.

Rösch, T.; Lightdale, C.J.; Botet, J.F.; Boyce, G.A.; Sivak, M.V.; Yasuda, K.; Heyder, N.; Palazzo, L.; Dancygier, H.; Schusdziarra, V. & Classen, M. (1992). Localization of Pancreatic Neuroendocrine Tumours by Endoscopic Ultrasonogprahy. *The New England Journal of Medicine*, Vol.326, No.26, (June), pp. 1721-1726.

Schumacher, B.; Lübke, H.J., Frieling T.; Strohmeyer, G. & Starke A.A.R. (1996). Prospective Study on the Detection of Insulinomas by Endoscopic Ultrasonography. *Endoscopy*, Vol.28, No.3, (March), pp. 273-276.

Service, F.J.; Natt, N.; Thompson, G.B.; Grant, C.S.; van Heerden, J.A.; Andrews, J.C.; Lorenz, E.; Terzic, A. & Lloyd, R.V. (1999a). Noninsulinoma Pancreatogenous Hypoglycemia: a Novel Syndrome of Hyperinsulinemic Hypoglycemia in Adults Independent of Mutations in Kir6.2 and SUR1 Genes. *The Journal of Clinical Endocrinology & Metabolism*, Vol.84, No.5, (May), pp. 1582-1589.

Service, F.J. (1999b). Diagnostic Approach to Adults with Hypoglycemic Disorders. *Endocrinology and Metabolism Clinics of North America*, Vol.28, No.3, (September), pp. 519-532.

Service, F.J. & Natt, N. (2000). The Prolonged Fast. *The Journal of Clincal Endocrinology & Metabolism*, Vol.85, No.11, (November), pp. 3973-3974.

Service, G. J.; Thompson, G. B. & Service, F. J.; Andrews, J.C; Collazo-Clavell, M. L & Lloyd, R.V. (2005). Hyperinsulinemic Hypoglycemia with Nesidioblastosis after Gastric-bypass Surgery. *The New England Journal of Medicine*, Vol.353, No.3, (July), pp. 249-254.

Starke, A.; Saddig, C.; Kirch, B.; Tschahargane, C. & Goretzki, P. (2006). Islet Hyperplasia in Adults: Challenge to Preoperatively Diagnose Non-Insulinoma Pancreatogenic Hypoglycemia Syndrome. *World Journal of Surgery*, Vol.30, No.5, (May), pp. 670-679, ISSN 0364-2313.

Thoeni, R.F.; Mueller-Lisse, U.G.; Chan, R.; Do, N.K. & Shyn, P.B. (2000). Detection of Small, Functional Islet Cell Tumors in the Pancreas: Selection of MR Imaging Sequences for Optimal Sensitivity. Radiology, Vol.214, No.2, (February 2000), pp. 483-490.

Thompson, G. B. (2007). Invited commentary: On Diffuse Nesidioblastosis As a Cause of Hyperinsulinemic Hypoglycemia in Adults: A diagnostic and therapeutic challenge. *Surgery*, Vol.141, No.2, (February), pp. 185-186.

Thompson, G.B.; Service F.J.; Andrews, J.C.; Lloyd, R.V.; Natt, N.; von Heerden J.A. & Grant C.S. (2000). Noninsulinoma Pancreatogenous Hypoglycemia Syndrome: an Update in 10 Surgically Treated Patients. *Surgery*, Vol.128, No.6, (December), pp. 937-945.

Thompson, N. W.(1995). The Surgical Management of Hyperparathyroidism and Endocrine Diseases of the Pancreas in the Multiple Endocrine Neoplasia Type 1 Patient. *Journal of Internal Medicine*, Vol.238, No.3, (August), pp269-280.

Tonelli, F. ; Fratini, G.; Falchetti, A., Nesi G. & Brandi M.L., (2004). Surgery for Gastroenteropancreatic Tumours in Multiple Endocrine Neoplasia Type 1: Review and personal experience. *Journal of Internal Medicine*, Vol.257, No.1, (December), pp38-49.

Tseng, L.M.; Chen, J.Y.; Won, J.G.; Tseng, H.S.; Yan, A.H.; Wang, S.E. & Lee, C.H. (2007). The Role of Intra-Arterial Calcium Stimulation Test with Hepatic Venous Smapling (IACS) in the Management of Occult Insulinomas. *Annals of Surgical Oncology*, Vol.14, No.7, (July), pp. 2121-2127.

Vanderveen, K. A.; Grant, C. S.; Thompson, G. B.; Farley, D. R.; Richards, M. L.; Vella, A.; Vollrath, B. & Service, F. J. (2010). Outcomes and Quality of Life after Partial Pancreatectomy for Noninsulinoma Pancreatogenous Hypoglycemia from Diffuse Islet Cell Disease. *Surgery*, Vol.148, No.6, (December), pp. 1237-1246.

Vezzosi, D.; Bennet, A.; Rochaix, P.; Courbon, F.; Selves, J.; Pradere, B.; Buscail, L; Susini, C. & Caron, P. (2005). Octreotide in Insulinoma Patients: Efficacy on hypoglycemia, relationships with Octreoscanscintigraphy and immunostaining with anti-sst2A and anti-sst5 antibodies. *European Journal of Endocrinology*, Vol.152, No.5, (May), pp. 757-767.

Vinik, A.I.; Delbridge, L.; Moattari, R.; Cho, K. & Thompson, N. (1991). Transhepatic Portal Vein Catheterization for Localization of Insulinomas: a Ten-Year Experience. *Surgery*, Vol.109, No.1, (January), pp. 1-11.

Wiesli, P.; Spinas, G. A.; Pfammatter, T.; Krahenbuhl, L. & Schmid, C. (2002). Glucose-Induced Hypoglycaemia. *The Lancet*, Vol.360, No.9344, (November), pp. 1476.

Won, J. G. S.; Tseng, H. S.; Yang, A. H.; Tang, K. T.; Jap, T. S.; Lee, C. H.; Lin, H.D.; Burcus, N.; Pittenger, G. & Vinik, A. (2006). Clinical Features and Morphological Characterization of 10 Patients with Noninsulinoma Pancreatogenous Hypoglycaemia syndrome (NIPHS). *Clincal Endocrinology*, Vol.65, No.5, (November), pp. 566-578.

11

Insulinoma – Diagnosis and Treatment

Jan Škrha[1,4], Jaroslava Dušková[2], Jan Šváb[3],
Jiřina Hilgertová[4], Josef Hořejš[5] and Radan Keil[6]
[1,4]*Charles University, 1stFaculty of Medicine, 3rdDepartment of Internal Medicine,*
[2]*Institute of Pathology,*
[3] *1stDepartment of Surgery,*
[4]*Laboratory for Endocrinology and Metabolism,*
[5]*Department of Radiology*
[6] *2ndFaculty of Medicine, Department of Internal Medicine,Prague,*
Czech Republic

1. Introduction

1.1 Epidemiology and basic characteristics

Endogenous hyperinsulinism is characterized by repeated hypoglycemic episodes caused by autonomous hypersecretion of insulin produced by adenoma or multiple microadenomatosis originating in the beta-cells of the pancreas. The process is either localized into one or less frequently few solid tumors or is more diffuse within the islets of Langerhans. Endogenous hyperinsulinism is not regulated by plasma glucose and therefore clinical signs of hypoglycemia manifest whenever during the day. The term „organic hyperinsulinism" is sometimes used showing that real endocrine pancreatic disease may be present in comparison with „functional hyperinsulinism" characterized by reactive changes in a consequence of eating habits.

Insulinoma (ICD-08151/1, ICD-08151/3) together with gastrinoma, VIPoma, somatostatinoma, glucagonoma and PPoma are members of nesidioma family which are recognized as neuroendocrine tumors of the pancreas. Some of them produce one hormone only and may therefore cause typical clinical symptoms. However, combined production of hormones may be also found and clinical diagnosis could be difficult when different symptoms would be combined. Positive but weak staining for gastrin or other hormones besides insulin may be sometimes present without any symptoms. On the other hand, neuroendocrine tumor in the pancreas can be described by histological examination in patients without typical clinical symptoms and malignant tumors are then confirmed.

Insulinoma has incidence of 0.05-0.1 cases per 100 000 inhabitants in the Czech Republic (Škrha, 2001) but slightly more (0.4 per 100 000) has been described at the Mayo clinic register (Service et al., 1991). Data may depend on the database availability in different countries. It is predominantly present in women as compared to men. The proportion of insulinoma was around 60 % in women at Mayo clinic whereas our register involves 75 % of women (Service et al., 1991, Škrha et al., 2009). Insulin-producing tumors occur in more than 50 % of neuroendocrine tumors of the pancreas followed by gastrinomas in 30 %, VIPomas in 10-15 % and by others in less than 10 % (Perry & Vinik, 1995).

Solitary adenoma usually occurs in more than 80 % of patients but few adenomas may be sometimes found in different size and stage of development and thus they have not been removed during the first operation (Service et al., 1991). Repeated surgical treatment is then necessary. Multiple adenoma is more frequently present in patients with multiple endocrine neoplasia (MEN I) (Demeure et al., 1991, Fabbri et al., 2010). However, in only few percents of adults the hypoglycemic syndrome has been associated with hyperplasia of the beta-cells (Harrison et al., 1984, Service et al., 1999, Stefanini et al., 1974). It may be caused by neodifferentiation of islet cells from ductal epithelium in the exocrine pancreas. Previously, nesidioblastosis was described in histological finding, more frequently found in newborns or children than in adults (Stefanini et al., 1974). It was suggested to use the term „**hyperplasia of islet cells**" instead of nesidioblastosis because heterogenous descriptions exist (Weinstock et al., 1986). It is supposed that insulinoma and diffuse hyperplasia are two edge variants of hyperfunctional syndrome and some forms exist in between. The genetic background contributing to different histological findings has not been elucidated yet. The above heterogeneity confirms that histological finding need not always correspond with hormonal activity and clinical symptoms. In addition, beta cell hyperplasia contributes to persistent hyperinsulinemic hypoglycemia of infancy, caused by mutations in the islet ATP-sensitive potassium channel, and to non-insulinoma pancreatogenous hypoglycemia in adults (Ouyang et al., 2011).

Insulinoma is usually localized within the pancreas, extrapancreatic tumors (e.g. in duodenum or small intestine) are extremly rare (Service et al., 1991, Škrha, 2001). One case report describes the insulin producing carcinoid of ovary (Morgello et al., 1988). The most of insulinoma cases are benign whereas malignant forms have been described in 5 to 10 % of patients (Perry & Vinik, 1995, Service et al. 1991). However, various forms have been found by histological examination when different stages of angioinvasion were combined with the presence or absence of micrometastases in lymphnodes. It may strongly influence further decision on chemotherapy and follow-up treatment.

2. Diagnosis of insulinoma

The patients with unregulated insulin overproduction develop clinical symptoms associated with hypoglycemia. Two main tasks may be arised to establish proper diagnosis of insulinoma. Firstly, to evaluate correctly clinical picture suspicious from hypoglycemia and, secondly, to prove the association of typical symptoms with low blood glucose concentration. The diagnosis is therefore based on clinical and biochemical finding still before imaging of the process.

2.1 Clinical symptoms

Hypoglycemia may be associated with either neurogenic (adrenergic) or neuroglycopenic symptoms (Dizon et al., 1999) (Table 1). Symptoms are dependent on depth and duration of hypoglycemia. Slightly decreased plasma glucose to 3.0-3.6 mmol/l stimulates catecholamine secretion explaining neurogenic symptoms. They are rare in patients with insulinoma although they may be solely present in up to 10-15 % of patients (Fajans & Vinik, 1989). On contrary, neuroglycopenic symptoms develop when glucose supply to central nervous system is significantly reduced. Manifested symptoms may frequently induce a suspicion of neurologic or psychiatric disorders and the patient admitted to the appropriate department may be treated not seldom like primary neurological or psychiatric disease.

Unsuccessful treatment with psychiatric or neurologic drugs with persisting symptoms needs to be reevaluated and when fasting hypoglycemia is confirmed a suspicion on endogenous hyperinsulinism may be arised.

Symptoms
Neurogenic (autonomous) sweatting, tremor, palpitation, tachycardia, anxiety **Neuroglycopenic** confusion, dizziness, weakness, unconsciousness, blurred vision, amnesia, dysartria, somnolence, cramps, headache, diplopy, parestesia, coma

Table 1. Hypoglycemic symptoms

Hypoglycemic symptoms develop in the fasting state, several hours after the last meal. This is typically in the morning after the overnight fast when neuroglycopenic symptoms may be present. Their manifestation with proven hypoglycemia and improvement after a sweet meal, formerly described as Whipple trias, are great support for clinical diagnosis of autonomous (endogenous) insulin oversecretion. It does not exclude symptoms developing just after the meal ingestion when overstimulation of insulin secretion especially by sugars exists (Del Sindaco et al., 1997, Service et al., 1999). In such cases functional hyperinsulinism may be falsely diagnosed and proper differentiation between functional and endogenous hyperinsulinism needs to be decided (see 3. Differential diagnosis).
Certain neuroglycopenic symptoms are repeated by the single patient during hypoglycemic episodes although they offer very different picture. It has not been explained yet why the same symptoms are always present in the same patient. They may differentiate one patient from the other. On the other hand, the patient can describe if the frequency of episodes would be increased or if their expression would be strenghten. Such information may help to clinician in decision of further examination and treatment. The severity of symptoms correspond to sensitivity of the central nervous system to hypoglycemia but not exactly to hyperinsulinemia which was significantly different in the patients.
Neuroglycopenic symptoms are the crucial point in diagnosis of insulinoma and their careful analysis is considered as the basis for following steps. Their evaluation cannot be substituted by other examination including imagining of the pancreas.

2.2 Laboratory examinations

The estimation of biochemical variables involving plasma glucose and insulin concentrations during development of clinical symptoms may support not only diagnosis, but it may further characterize the severity of the process and therefore the importance of surgical treatment. Severe hypoglycemia and high serum insulin levels should indicate operation without any delay because profound hypoglycemia is dangerous to the patient. In addition, randomly confirmed hypoglycemia during development of clinical symptoms in patient examined by neurologist or psychiatrist may be the only one impuls to send the patient to endocrinologist. When blood glucose is not determined, the patient can be treated on epilepsy or psychiatric disorders several months or even years without significant success and the proper diagnosis of insulinoma is delayed.
Blood glucose concentration associated with neuroglycopenic symptoms can be often found below 2.5 mmol/l in insulinoma patients whereas neurogenic symptoms associated with blood glucose around 3.5 mmol/l frequently exist by functional (reactive) hyperinsulinemia.

However, hypoglycemia was rarely reported without any clinical symptoms when insulinoma was later confirmed (Service, 1995).

Suspicion on insulinoma suggested from clinical symptoms of neuroglycopenia and hypoglycemia needs to be further confirmed. This first step in diagnosis of endogenous hyperinsulinism may be done by GPs as well as by specialists in neurology, psychiatry, internal medicine or endocrinology/diabetology. Diagnostic process is then simplified if the patient would be sent immediately to appropriate center specialised in endocrine disorders.

2.2.1 Fasting test

Patient with a suspicion on insulinoma is admitted to hospital to confirm the autonomous hypersecretion of insulin as a typical feature of insulinoma. The best option for this purpose is to use the test inhibiting insulin secretion because the absence of insulin inhibition confirmes dysregulation of the hormone secretion by autonomous process. This may be proved by prolonged fasting when the patient drinks only water and blood samples for glucose, insulin and C-peptide determinations are drawn in regular interval (every 4-6 hours). Plasma glucose drops down during the test and when clinical symptoms develop, the last blood sample is drawn and the fasting is stopped. Some delay of clinical symptoms following the lowest plasma glucose concentration may be sometimes present. It is elucidated by later decline of intracellular glucose in the brain in comparison with the changes in plasma glucose concentration. Due to activated contrainsulary hormones by hypoglycemia blood glucose concentration goes already up when symptoms develop in a consequence of the lowest intracellular glucose concentration.

The fasting test may be performed up to 72 hours but in the most of patients it is stopped within 24 hours. At our department we could stop the test within 24 hrs in more than 80 % of patients with insulinoma (Škrha et al., 2009). In some very rare insulinoma cases no neuroglycopenic symptoms have been observed still after 72 hrs (Jordan & Kammel, 1976). The patients with insulinoma are adapted on low glucose concentration and symptoms are therefore weak. Typical picture of hypoglycemia unawereness develops (Mitrakou et al., 1993). Plasma glucose and insulin concentrations are always used in clinical practice in diagnosis of insulinoma but sometimes the ratio of serum insulin/glucose concentration may further support diagnosis of endogenous hyperinsulinism. The results may be more expressive when the patient would add the physical training during the fasting. In subjects with insulinoma plasma glucose concentration drops whereas in those with functional hypoglycemia the glucose concentration may arise (Fajans & Vinik, 1989). Our results obtained in 114 patients with endogenous hyperinsulinism are shown in Table 2.

Laboratory variable	Before fasting	End of fasting
Duration of fasting (h)	-	18 (2-60)
Plasma glucose (mmol/l)	3.4±1.4	1.7±0.4
Seum insulin (mU/l)	54±37	56±47
Insulin/glucose ratio (mU/mmol)	18.5±15.3	34.0±30.3
C-peptide (nmol/l)	1.13±0.61	1.16±0.73

Table 2. Biochemical variables in insulinoma patients before and at the end of fasting test. The results are expressed as the means ± SD.

Glucose and insulin in the fasting test

The patients with endogenous hyperinsulinism have plasma glucose concentration at the end of the fasting test below 2.5 mmol/l but in some cases slightly higher levels may be seen, especially when the lowest level was reached still before developed neuroglycopenic symptoms. In about 7 % of normal population plasma glucose concentration after 72 hrs of fasting may be below 2.7 mmol/l (Service et al., 1999). Evaluation of both glucose concentration and clinical symptoms is therefore recommended.

Majority of patients with insulinoma has increased serum insulin concentration when fasting is stopped. However, in some patients the insulin concentration remains within the normal limits and it brings difficulties to confirm diagnosis of hyperinsulinism (Škrha et al., 2009). Evaluation of all insulin concentrations and their oscillations during the fasting is necessary. In our group of insulinoma patients the insulin concentration below 20 mU/l were found in 12 of 114 patients (10 %) at the end of the test.

The insulin/glucose ratio is also sensitive parameter although it reflects the fluctuations of both biochemical variables. Their dynamic changes causing stepwise increase of this ratio during the fasting test differ from obese patients with hyperinsulinemia who have the ratio increased at the beginning but its decreasing value may be found during the test. Numerical value of the ratio has to be compared with clinical finding during the test. The normal values in our population when glucose is expressed in mmol/l and insulin in mU/l are below 6,0 mU/mmol. We found borderline values of this ratio in 5 of 114 patients with insulinoma.

According to our experience, the most important for the diagnosis of insulinoma is time development of plasma glucose concentrations associated with neuroglycopenic symptoms manifesting during the fasting test.

C-peptide and proinsulin

Serum C-peptide concentration is increased in insulinoma but the basal values cannot be distinguished from those found in obese persons. Its concentration decreases with fasting in healthy persons but it remains high in patient with insulinoma. C-peptide values may provide better information at the end of fasting than at basal state. In addition, C-peptide has to be used when suspicion on hypoglycemia factitia has been arised (see 3. Differential diagnosis).

Higher plasma proinsulin concentration depending on the greater proinsulin release from the beta cells is sometimes determined in insulinoma patients. It may be usefull especially in cases with normal insulin concentration. Proinsulin is not routinelly used for diagnosis of insulinoma and it cannot distinguish benign and malign forms of insulinoma (Fajans & Vinik, 1989).

2.2.2 Suppressive and stimulating tests

Different tests either suppressing insulin secretion or stimulating insulin release and consequently changing plasma glucose concentrations have been used (C-peptide suppressive test, tolbutamide test, calcium test etc.) previously mainly for the research purposes (Fajans & Vinik, 1989, Service et al., 1992). However, they do not significantly improve the diagnosis in routine clinical practice.

In conclusion, diagnosis of endogenous (autonomous) hyperinsulinism has to be done from clinical symptoms and biochemical results. If any doubts would exist, repeated fasting test may bring better data for proper diagnosis than the other tests. The evaluation should also respond key question concerning the treatment. Insulinoma should be treated by surgical removal of the tumor and this procedure needs to localise the tumor before the surgery.

2.2.3 Insulin sensitivity

Repeated attempts have been made to elucidate the estimation of insulin sensitivity in diagnosis of insulinoma (Gin et al., 1987, Nauck et al., 1990, Škrha et al., 1996). Hyperinsulinemic clamp technique enabled to study insulin action both in the hormonal hyperactivity and following the removal of the tumor (Škrha et al., 1993). The amount of glucose infused during the clamp and maintaining the plasma glucose at constant level by exogenous insulin infusion was found increased in insulinoma patients as compared to healthy persons (Gin et al., 1998). The amount of glucose infused dropped down after removal of the tumor. Constant infusion of insulin during the clamp resembles C-peptide suppressive test causing a decrease of endogenous insulin and C-peptide secretion. Impaired suppressibility of C-peptide was found in insulinoma patients compared to healthy controls (Yki-Järvinen et al., 1984).

However, similar non-suppressibility of C-peptide was found in obese Type 2 diabetic patients (Škrha et al., 1996). Insulin resistance was found in insulinoma patients by clamp technique (Del Prato et al., 1993, Nankervis et al., 1985, Škrha et al., 1989, de Kreutzenberg et al., 1995). Decreased insulin clearance and decreased glucose production in the liver contributing to fasting hypoglycemia were observed in insulinoma patients (Škrha et al., 1989, Del Prato et al., 1993). However, we found in some of insulinoma patients nearly normal insulin action and we concluded that this parameter depends on concomitant obesity which may strongly impair the insulin sensitivity (Škrha et al., 1996). Decreased insulin sensitivity cannot be used as reliable sign of insulinoma. Hyperinsulinemic clamp technique can differentiate between patients responding and non-responding to diazoxide treatment (Škrha et al. 1989).

2.3 Localization techniques

Several techniques involving non-invasive and invasive tests may be used to localize the insulinoma with different sensitivity and specificity. They have both advantages and disadvantages. Significant development of imaging technique during the past twenty years has contributed to better localization of insulinoma and thus to preoperative decisions.

Simple **transabdominal ultrasonography** does not bring useful information because of the great number of negative data. Although it is noninvasive and simply performing its low sensitivity, mainly due to minimal discrimination of the small size tumor tissue from the surrounding tissue, it cannot be used for localization of the tumor. Only up to one third of the tumors may be found by this imaging (Bottger et al., 1990).

Computer tomography is very popular but large differences exist between the centers (Pasieka et al., 1992, Vinik et al., 1991). Positive results may be obtained in 25-60 % depending on the experience of radiologists. Similar may be true for **nuclear magnetic resonance** when insulinomas were proved in low or high percentage of the patients (Liessi et al., 1992). In a recent study the sensitivity of preoperative CT and nuclear magnetic resonance was 62 and 82 %, respectively (Varma et al., 2011). **Octreoscan** based on the binding of isotope-labelled somatostatin with its receptors placed on the cell membrane of neuroendocrine tumor was repeatedly used to visualize the localization of insulinoma. However, differences were found between the cells possessing somatostatin receptors. About 50 % or less cases of insulinoma can be proved by octreoscan whereas more than 70 % positive cases with gastrinoma have been found (Krenning et al., 1994, Proye et al., 1998, Zimmer et al., 1996) by using this technique. Octreoscan does not seem to be reliable method detecting localization of insulinoma.

Better results have been obtained with **endoscopic ultrasonography**, sensitivity of which was described in 77 till 94% (Glover et al., 1992, Roesch et al., 1992, Varma et al., 2011). Insulinoma localized in the head and body of the pancreas can be preferably proved by this technique whereas tumors of the tail remain often not discovered. More invasive examination is **arteriography** visualizing vasculature of the pancreas. Finding of pathologic imaging during parenchymal phase may support diagnosis of insulinoma (Fig.1). Positive results have been found in 40 to 60 % in different centres (Pasieka et al., 1992, Vinik et al., 1991). Combining arteriography and CT is superior to single arteriography or CT (Li et al., 2010). In case of successful fine needle aspiration the tumor can be verified with cytopathology examination or by immunocytochemistry (Fig. 2)

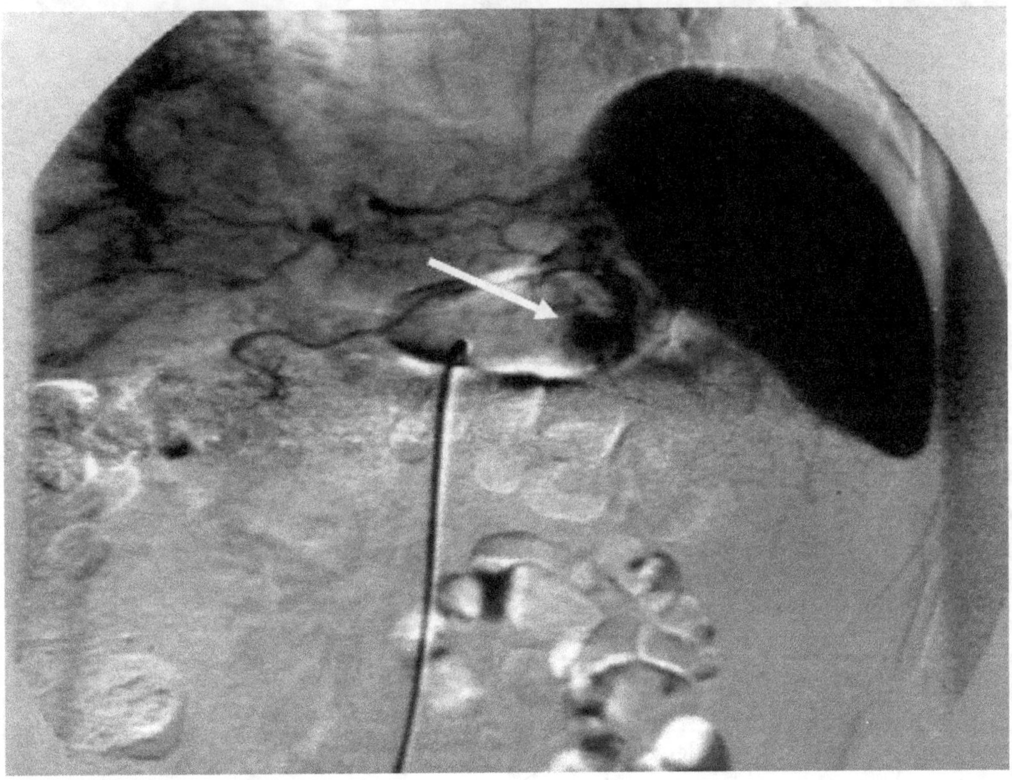

Fig. 1. Digital subtraction angiography of splenic artery with insulinoma localized in the tail of pancreas (arrow)

Some centres use **transhepatic cathetrisation of the portal system** when blood samples drawn by catheter from different parts of portal vein are tested for insulin concentration (Vinik et al., 1991). The main goal of this examination is to differentiate between head, body and tail of the pancreas as a source of measured insulin gradient. The results may be strenghten when calcium is selectively infused into different arteries (superior mesenteric artery, splenic artery or gastroduodenal artery) and blood is taken from the portal system (Doppman et al., 1995). Few centres received very positive results (Vinik et al., 1991).

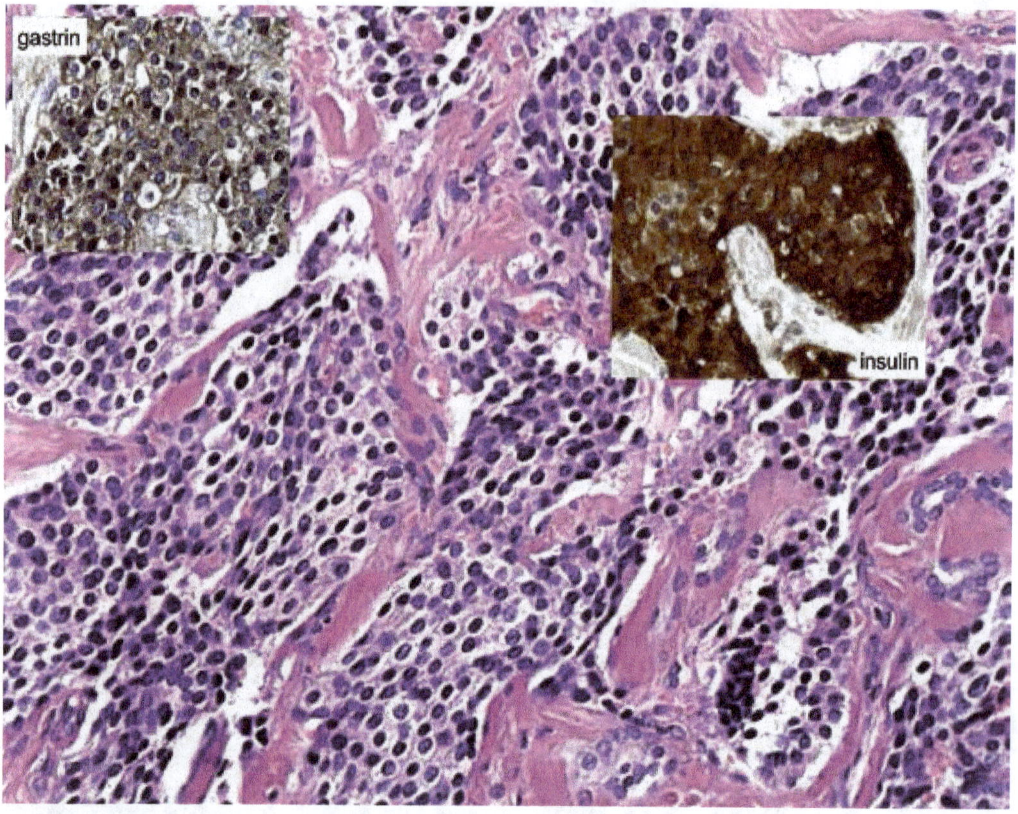

Fig. 2. Histological picture of insulinoma. Immunohistochemical examination found strong positivity of insulin and weak positivity of gastrin.

Our own results of localization of insulinoma are shown in Table 3. In 72 of 103 operated patients (70 %) the topographical localization of the tumor was only done before surgical treatment by combining different techniques when evaluating patients from the whole period of three decades.

Method	Imagine techniques (before surgery)		Surgical finding in preoperatively detected insulinoma		
	Detected	Undetected	Agreement	Other placement	Undiscovered
US	4 (8 %)	47 (92 %)	2	-	2
EU	40 (83%)	8 (17%)	33	5	2
CT	20 (24%)	65 (76%)	15	5	-
AG	39 (43%)	52 (57%)	25	8	6

Table 3. Preoperative localization of insulinoma and surgical finding by preoperatively localized tumors

The transabdominal ultrasonography was tested at our department between 1980-1995 but positive results were extremely rare. This method is not more used in diagnostic algorithm. The quality of CT has been significantly improved during the past twenty years and present

results are better then three decades ago (nearly 50 % positive cases in the last decade). However, when evaluating all patients together, positive results are low (see Table 3). Localization of insulinoma was confirmed in only 75 % of patients with positive CT scan. Angiography brought positive results in more than 40 % but the agreement with localization of the tumor during operation was done in only 64 % of positive findings. Method of choice seems to be endoscopic ultrasonography which detected more than 83 % of tumors and their localization was confirmed in the same proportion (82,5 %).
The results of imaging techniques depend on both size and properties of the insulinoma related to surrounding tissue as well as on the experience of examining staff. Best results have been observed by combining CT with endoscopic ultrasonography. In 2001-2010 we examined 51 patients with insulinoma and positive results of imaging techniques were obtained in 38 of them (75 %).

3. Differential diagnosis

Diagnosis of insulinoma has to be evaluated in consideration of all causes associated with hypoglycemia. Several classifications of hypoglycemic states exist but for clinical purposes combination of two of them is reliable. Firstly, association with ingestion of the meals can differentiate two main groups: a) hypoglycemia developing in the fasting state, typically after an overnight fast, and, b) postprandial hypoglycemia. Secondly, hypoglycemia can be classified according to pathogenesis when balance between glucose influx into blood stream and its removal would be impaired. Both classifications can be combined and diagnosis in the respective patient may be based on detailed analysis of history and symptoms (Table 4).
Evaluation of history of hypoglycemic episodes can disclose when symptoms have developed. It is the basis of clinical classification if hypoglycemia could be found either by healthy person or by ill patient already treated for some disease (Service, 1995). Specific case may be arised when first hypoglycemia episode develops during the stay at hospital.

3.1 Hypoglycemia manifesting predominantly in the fasting state

Hypoglycemia manifesting after an overnight fast needs carefull analysis because it demonstrates that the patient cannot maintain spontaneously plasma glucose concentration within the normal ranges. This condition is frequently caused by certain disease which needs to be elucidated or confirmed. Some clinical diagnoses may be a signal of serious prognosis and their knowledge and intensive treatment is therefore necessary. Both impaired glucose production and accelerated glucose utilization may participate on development of mild or severe hypoglycemic episodes (Table 4).

i.	Fasting hypoglycemia
	States with diminished glucose production
-	lack of contrainsular hormones
-	enzyme defects
-	liver disease
-	renal failure
-	impaired nutrition
-	alcohol consumption

ii. Fasting and postprandial hypoglycemia
States with accelerated glucose utilization
Exogenously caused hyperinsulinism
- diabetes treated with insulin - diabetes treated with oral agents - hypoglycemia factitia
Endogenous hyperinsulinism
- insulinoma - hyperinsulinemic hypoglycemia in infants - autoimmune syndromes causing hypoglycemia - extrapancreatic tumors - defects in oxidation of free fatty acids - drugs other then primary oral hypoglycemic agents - other conditions
iii. Reactive (postprandial) hypoglycemia
- alimentary, postoperative - functional - prediabetes - inborn errors of metabolism (enzyme defects) - newborn of diabetic mother

Table 4. Classification of hypoglycemic states according to the relationship with fasting and with underproduction or overutilization of glucose

Hypoglycemia due to diminished glucose production

Plasma glucose concentration depends on permanent glucose supply into the blood stream and removal by the cells using glucose as a simple source of energy. Glucose can be relased from glycogen or it is produced by gluconeogenesis. The glycogen stores cover the needs for few hours only whereas gluconeogenesis provided mainly by the liver and kidney depends both on substrate delivery and on metabolic pathways. Each failure may contribute to impaired glucose metabolism and consequently to lower plasma glucose concentration. Defects in glucose production may be caused either by some chronic diseases (chronic liver and kidney diseases etc.) or by exogenous factors like alcohol or drugs.

Lack of contraregulatory hormones like glucagon, catecholamines, growth hormone and cortisol manifesting by development of insufficiency in the respective organ is associated with mild hypoglycemia in the fasting state. Inborn **hypopituitarism** is characterized by fasting hypoglycemia, low plasma insulin levels, increased insulin sensitivity in the peripheral tissues, diminished responsiveness on hypoglycemia and lowered mobilization of free fatty acids. Similar features have been found in aquired hypopituitarism as well (Samaan, 1989). **Adrenal insufficiency** is associated with impaired mineral metabolism, low blood pressure, weakness and mild hypoglycemia. Untreated **hypothyroidism** develops impaired gluconeogenesis when mild hypoglycemia develops.

Inborn errors of metabolism characterized by enzyme defects are associated with fasting hypoglycemia. This group contains glycogen storing disease, galactosemia and hereditary fructose intolerance (Talente et al., 1994, Tsalikian & Haymond, 1983).

Severe **acute hepatitis** needs intensive treatment with glucose whereas **chronic liver disease** frequently develops mild hypoglycemia. Multiple metastases may be associated with low plasma glucose because both diminished glucose production and accelerated glucose consumption by the tumor may contribute to impaired glucose balance (Eastman et al., 1992). **Renal failure** is associated with mild hypoglycemia and diminished gluconeogenesis in the kidneys was proved (Garber et al., 1974). Severe hypoglycemia may be developed in **malnutrition** by kwashiorkor or anorexia nervosa and hypoglycemic coma may cause death in advanced cases (Ratcliffe & Bevan, 1982).

Special care in differential diagnosis of insulinoma needs to be done to **alcohol induced hypoglycemic episodes**. Alcohol consumption in the evening without substantial meals may be followed by unconsciousness in the morning. Profound hypoglycemia below 2.0 mmol/l may be found in a consequence of diminished glucose production in the liver when glycogen stores were exhausted. Ethanol is oxidized to acetaldehyde which blocks gluconeogenesis. Severe hypoglycemia is then falsely recognized like insulinoma. However, taken history may simply disclose the right cause of this hypoglycemic state. We evaluated several cases of alcohol induced hypoglycemia which was previously diagnosed as suspicion on insulinoma.

Diagnosis of certain disease associated with fasting hypoglycemia needs to be always confirmed because it is of great importance for proper treatment.

3.2 Hypoglycemia manifesting in fasting and postprandial state

The most of hypoglycemic episodes comes both in the fasting and postprandial conditions, typically in diabetic patients. They are caused by overutilization of glucose in the target tissues by increased insulin action.

Hypoglycemia due to accelerated glucose utilization

The most frequent hypoglycemic states are caused by hypoglycemic drugs in diabetic patients. Insulin, sulphonylurea or different combinations of antidiabetic drugs may contribute to hypoglycemia, especially when the patient is intensivelly treated to target values of diabetes control. This issue is specific chapter in diabetes books and it is not analyzed here. Confirmation of drug treatment in diabetic patients may exclude the majority of cases from consideration on insulinoma. However, newly developed repeated hypoglycemic episodes in Type 2 diabetic patient without any evidence on drug involvement have been described and insulinoma was later confirmed (Škrha et al., 1990).

Special attention needs to be done to hypoglycemia in infancy when different types of „persistent hyperinsulinemic hypoglycemia in infancy" (PHHI) have been described (Stanley, 1997). Congenital hyperinsulinism is a life threatening state in a newborn and sometimes only pancreatectomy may resolve this serious condition (De Lonley-Debeney et al., 1999). In other cases hypoglycemia develops later and more frequently it may be induced by fasting or it occurs between breast feeding (Thornton et al., 1998). Such latent hypoglycemia may be dangerous for development of the central nervous system manifesting by mental retardation. The early diagnosis and effective treatment are therefore absolutely necessary. Diagnosis is supported by hyperinsulinemia and increased plasma C-peptide concentration in hypoglycemic state together with low free fatty acids and beta-hydroxybutyrate (Cresto et al., 1998). In some children hyperammonemia was proven (Kitaura et al., 1999, Stanley et al., 1998). Persistent hyperinsulinemic hypoglycemia in infancy was subdivided into three types (Stanley, 1997).

Rapid development of severe hypoglycemia in a newborn just after delivery is typical by **autosomal recessive form** of congenital hyperinsulinism which is caused by gene mutation for sulphonylurea receptor (SUR1) associated with potassium channel in the beta-cells (Thomas, et al., 1995, Nestorowicz et al., 1996). Persistent insulin hypersecretion is due to closed K_{ATP}- channel and opened calcium channel. Histological picture disclosed two forms - diffuse and focal. Diffuse form called nesidioblastosis has all islets hyperactive whereas the other one is caused by focal hyperplastic adenomatosis (Sempoux et al., 1998). Partial pancreatectomy is sufficient for treatment of focal form but diffuse nesidioblastosis needs to be treated by total pancreatectomy.

Autosomal dominant form is usually manifested later following months or even years and clinical symptoms may be induced by fasting (Thornton et al., 1998). Drug treatment with diazoxide is often effective. Glucokinase gene mutation was found in this form (Glaser et al., 1998) and it is evident that recessive and dominant forms are totally different not only by gene determination but by treatment as well.

Hyperinsulinemic hypoglycemia with hyperammonaemia is the third form characterized by gene mutation of mitochondrial glutamate dehydrogenase. Increased alpha-ketoglutarate production stimulate insulin secretion whereas ammonium detoxification by lowered glutamate supply into liver causes hyperammonaemia (Zammarchi et al., 1996, Stanley et al., 1998, Kitaura et al., 1999).

Modern polypills treatment contributes to drug interactions. It may be therefore important to summarize which drugs accelerate the hypoglycemic effects of sulphonylurea drugs in Type 2 diabetes (Table 5).

a.	Sulphonylurea release from the binding with albumin - salicylic acid, acetylsalicylic acid - nonsteroid antiflogistics - sulphonylamides - trimetoprim - fibrates
b.	Competitive inhibitors of sulphonylurea metabolism - alcohol - H_2 - blockers - sulphonylamides - anticoagulant drugs - pyrazolon derivatives - allopurinol - inhibitors of monoaminooxidase
c.	Inhibitors of sulphonylurea excretion - probenecide - acetylsalicylic acid - nonsteroid antiflogistics - allopurinol - sulphonylamides

Table 5. Drugs accelerating the effects of sulphonylurea derivatives with possible hypoglycemia development

Arteficially induced hypoglycemia by using hypoglycemic agents, especially insulin or sulphonylurea derivatives, are clasified as **hypoglycemia factitia**. Severe hypoglycemia with neuroglycopenic symptoms may develop and clinical picture is fully comparable with insulinoma, mainly when hypoglycemia would be detected in fasting state. Clinical symptoms associated with profound hypoglycemia and hyperinsulinemia may be summarized as insulinoma and because no tumor localization is done, an exploratory laparotomy is indicated. The cause of hypoglycemic drug administration in non-diabetic subjects may be undiscovered but sometimes mental or psychiatric problems are present. Health care personel (nurses, physicians etc.) between this drug abuse has been repeatedly found.
Insulin administration may decrease endogenous secretion of both insulin and C-peptide. Finding of increased serum insulin concentration together with decreased C-peptide levels may support suspicion on hypoglycemia factitia. More difficulties bring sulphonylurea derivatives because no suppresion of C-peptide is present and low drug plasma or urine concentration is often missed. In such cases, proinsulin may be used to exclude diagnosis of hypoglycemia factitia because its plasma concentration in this case is within the normal limits whereas it is increased in insulinoma patients (Table 6).
We examined five patients with hypoglycemia factitia sent to our department as a suspition on insulinoma. One of them was nine times admitted to the hospital and twice indicated for exploratory laparotomy before the Münchhausen syndrome was confirmed.

Laboratory variable	**Insulinoma**	**Hypoglycemia factitia caused by insulin**	**Hypoglycemia factitia caused by sulphonylurea**
Plasma glucose	↓↓↓	↓↓↓	↓↓↓
Plasma insulin	↑ - ↑↑↑	↑↑↑	↑↑↑
Serum C-peptide	↑ - ↑↑	↓ - ↓↓	↑ - ↑↑
Plasma proinsulin	↑ - ↑↑	↔	↔
Sulphonylurea (urine)	negative	Negative	positive

Table 6. Laboratory variables compared in insulinoma patients with hypoglycemia factitia subjects

Other conditions may contribute to increased glucose removal from the blood stream but they are rare and single patients have been reported like case reports. Insulin antibodies or insulin receptor antibodies were rarely associated with hypoglycemia (Redmon et al., 1992, Service 1995, Walters et al., 1987). Extrapancreatic (non-islet cells) tumors like leiomyosarcoma, fibrosarcoma, mezotelioma, hepatoma and different cancers may be associated with hypoglycemia but with normal or low insulin concentration. In some of them increased plasma concentration of IGF-2 or „big-IGF-2" has been observed. High insulin levels were found in fibrosarcoma, bronchial carcinoid, neurofibrosarcoma and small cell cervical carcinoma. In such cases insulinoma is considered until ectopic insulin production would be confirmed. Different clinical picture and progression of malignant disease may differentiate these patients from those with insulinoma.
Rare carnitine deficiency is associated with impaired beta-oxidation of fatty acids. In such situation the organism cannot yield energy from fatty acids and alternative substrate like glucose is then utilized. Substrate deficit caused by blocked beta-oxidation creates consuption of glucose with severe hypoglycemia (McGarry & Foster, 1980).

Hypoglycemia may be caused by other drugs which stimulate insulin secretion (chinin) or decrease glucose production (beta-blockers, salicylates) or induce complex of not fully discovered mechanisms (haloperidol, disopyramide, pentamidine). Glucose consumption by Plasmodium falciparum was observed in malaria.

3.3 Reactive hypoglycemia

Reactive or postprandial hypoglycemia is a common diagnosis associated with weakness and other neurogenic (adrenergic) symptoms. The patient thinks on a serious disease and asks for help. Correct diagnosis and simple recommendation of reliable regimen including dietary councelling may totally remove the symptoms. In patients after gastric surgery when the meals containing saccharides quickly stimulate insulin secretion, glycemia drops down in 30 to 60 min. Sweating, tachycardia a weakness develop and only omitting of sweets may significantly improve the patient´s clinical state. Similar symptoms caused by sweets ingested in the morning develop mainly in some young women who do not eat typical breakfast. No previous operation on gut has been done by them before. They frequently do not take breakfast but after coming to their office they eat sweets like chocolate with coffee or tea. Chocolate without substantial meal induces insulin hypersecretion with small decrease of plasma glucose. Similar pattern may be obtained during oral glucose tolerance test (oGTT) with decreased plasma glucose to 2.9-3.3 mmol/l in 120 or 180 min (Brun et al., 1995). Such condition improves only after dietary recommendation when sweets are omitted. Analysis of symptoms can usually confirm this diagnosis.

Reactive hypoglycemia is frequently considered as insulinoma. In majority of patients neuroglycopenic symptoms are lacking. Hypoglycemia is not confirmed in some patients and the term „pseudohypoglycemia" is then used. If changes in dietary regimen would not be successful, fasting test is recommended to exclude uncertain cause of the weakness and other adrenergic symptoms. The patient with reactive hypoglycemia has normal glycemia without any significant decrease during the test.

4. Treatment

Recurrent profound hypoglycemia due to insulinoma or autonomous hyperplasia of the beta cells is dangerous to the patients because it may cause acute accidents like stroke or arrythmias, and consequently sudden death, especially with increasing age. They may also initiate chronic deterioration of intelectual function when they are present for a long time. The proper treatment strategy is therefore necessary and individual assessment of the risk has to be evaluated. The causal treatment involves surgical removal of the insulinoma or diffuse hyperplastic beta cell tissue (in case of „microadenomatosis"). When surgery is unsuccessful or the risk of operation is too high in old and polymorbid patient then dietary regimen and drug treatment have to be used (Škrha et al., 2009).

4.1 Surgical treatment

Selective removal of the tumor in case of solitary insulinoma is a method of choice. Enucleation of insulinoma maximally preserving the surrounding pancreatic tissue is now prefered against blind resection (Škrha, 2001) . It needs to have accurate localization of the tumor which enables to decide if laparoscopic technique or classical laparotomy may be introduced. The latter is started by gentle manual palpation of the pancreas, confirming the place with tumor and compares this finding with the results of preoperative imaging.

Perioperative ultrasound may sometimes help in confirming the tumor (Norton et al., 1988). If localization of the tumor would not make possible enucleation due to close proximity of the vessels, resection is decided. Blind resection is no more recommended although in patients with serious hypoglycemias and high hormonal activity it has to be suggested when no localization of the tumor has been done both before or during the operation. Small tumor with diameter below 5 mm may be overlooked and when neither serious symptoms nor high hormonal activity are present it can be better to operate for the second time than to make blind resection. Both types of operations may be subsequently associated with complications. Following resection, subfrenic inflammation causing localized abscess, sepsis or fistulae may be developed (Geoghegan et al., 1994). Fistulae develop sometimes after enucleation as well (Pasieka et al., 1992).

Insulinoma may be localized within the whole pancreatic tissue. However, results from different centres bring various finding (Rothmund et al., 1990). It may be partly influenced by the number of evaluated patients. Some authors describe the predominance of insulinoma within the head of pancreas, the others found regular distribution between all three parts of pancreas. In our group of 103 operated patients we found 93 solitary insulinoma distributed in 30 % in the head, 28 % in the body and 42 % in the tail (Fig. 3). Other two patients had diffuse microadenomatosis, two patients with not proven insulinoma during the first operation were successfully reoperated. Removal of insulinoma is followed by hyperglycemia developing in a consequence of suppressed beta-cell function by insulinoma. Its manifestation in the next day after the operation usually confirms surgical success. In case that hypoglycemia persists postoperatively in spite of removed insulinoma, multiple tumor may be present. In patients with diffuse hyperplasia the total pancreatectomy may sometimes be necessary with subsequent substitution of both exocrine and endocrine functions.

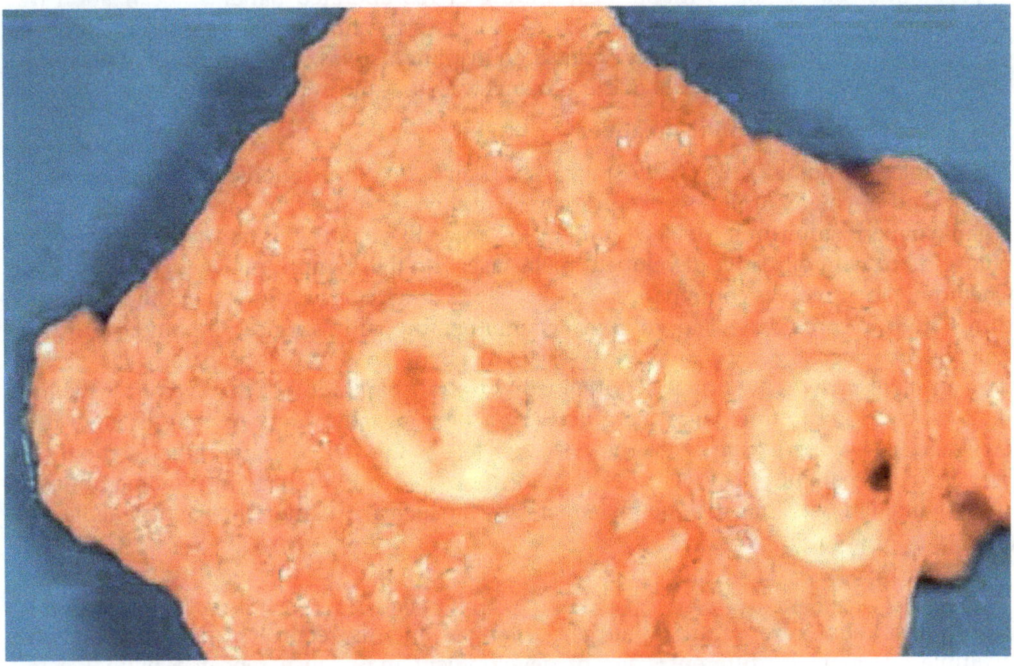

Fig. 3. Insulinoma localized in cut head of the pancreas.

4.2 Conservative treatment

Insulinoma can be operated in every age and therefore high age is not a contraindication. In case of advanced ischemic heart disease with chronic heart failure or clustering with other risks the operation cannot be recommended and the patients are treated conservatively. Diabetic diet excluding free sugars which may induce hypoglycemic attacks is recommended because it does not stimulate insulin secretion like free diet containing sugars. Several doses of meals mainly in the night are sometimes necessary when severe hyperinsulinism has been developed. Free sugars are used during hypoglycemic attack but not in its prevention. Dietary regimen is often combined with the insulin secretion blocking agent (Fajans & Vinik, 1989).

Diazoxide, a thiazide derivative, or somatostatin analogues decrease insulin levels and then hypoglycemic attacks develop less frequently or they are much less severe. Diazoxide acts as potassium channel opener and thus calcium channel is subsequently closed. This blockade of calcium movement in the beta cell lowers insulin secretion. Doses of 3 to 8 mg/kg daily are recommended but in some cases only 100 mg is sufficient to relief the clinical symptoms. Somatostatin treatment uses the presence of its receptors on beta cells which are less frequent than in other neuroendocrine tumors. Such therapy is therefore not so successful as in patients with gastrinoma. Not all patients respond on both drug therapy and then dietary regimen remains as the only one option.

From our group of 113 patients with organic hyperinsulinism total of 103 were operated and remaining 10 were primarily treated conservatively during 10-22 years. Additional 8 patients without removal of insulinoma during the operation have been treated conservatively as well. Interesting information was done when preoperative localization was compared with the finding in surgery. Operation could confirm localization in 80 % (54 of 68) of preoperatively found insulinoma when CT scan, angiography and endoscopic ultrasonography could be combined to visualize the tumors. When analyzing the results of localization of the tumors with surgical finding in 103 operated patients, localization was done in 68 (66 %) preoperatively, in 27 (26 %) cases the tumor was found and removed during the operation and in 8 (8 %) patients no insulinoma was found during the operation. Operation was successful in 92 % of our patients with organic hyperinsulinism.

Malignant insulinoma and its treatment

Malignant insulinoma (ICD-08151/3) occurs in 5-10 % of all insulinoma cases. It grows very slowly and develops typical neuroglycopenic symptoms. When diagnosed and confirmed organic hyperinsulinism it may be found by CT scans like solitary tumor in the pancreas but not seldom with already developed metastases in the lymph nodes or in the liver. Chemotherapy involves combination of streptozotocin with 5-fluorouracil or other cytostatic drugs. It is recommended to combine chemotherapy with surgical treatment with the removal of primary tumor or metastases in the liver. In one of our patient (56 yrs old woman) total pancreatectomy was combined with transplantation of the liver after the liver removal because multiple large metastases have been present. Consequently isolated islets of Langerhans were injected into the portal system using transhepatic cathetrization. One year later the patient does not suffer from any problems. Malignant insulinoma although successfully removed may develop late metastases which are no more hormonaly active.

5. Prognosis

Benign insulinoma are cured by surgical removal and its recurrency is extremely rare. Multiple adenoma in different stage of development may cause repeated hypoglycemia when only one tumor was removed. Conservative treatment with diazoxide may be successful many years, e.g. in patient with microadenomatosis. The patients after total pancreatectomy have sometimes problems with diabetes and sufficient enzyme substitution has to be added as well. Malignant insulinoma has poor prognosis because of high mortality and the patients die after several years with dissemination of the process.

6. Algorithm of diagnosis and treatment

Our own experience is the background to suggest algorithm of diagnosis and treatment in patients with endogenous hyperinsulinemia (Fig. 4). Analysis of clinical symptoms and biochemical finding of hypoglycemia in the fasting state in patients without any serious disease may serve as the basis for diagnosis of insulinoma. When the diagnosis is confirmed by fasting test the localization of the tumor has to be done. Surgical treatment is a method of choice whereas conservative treatment is followed after unsuccessful operation or in severly polymorbid patients when operation brings high risk.

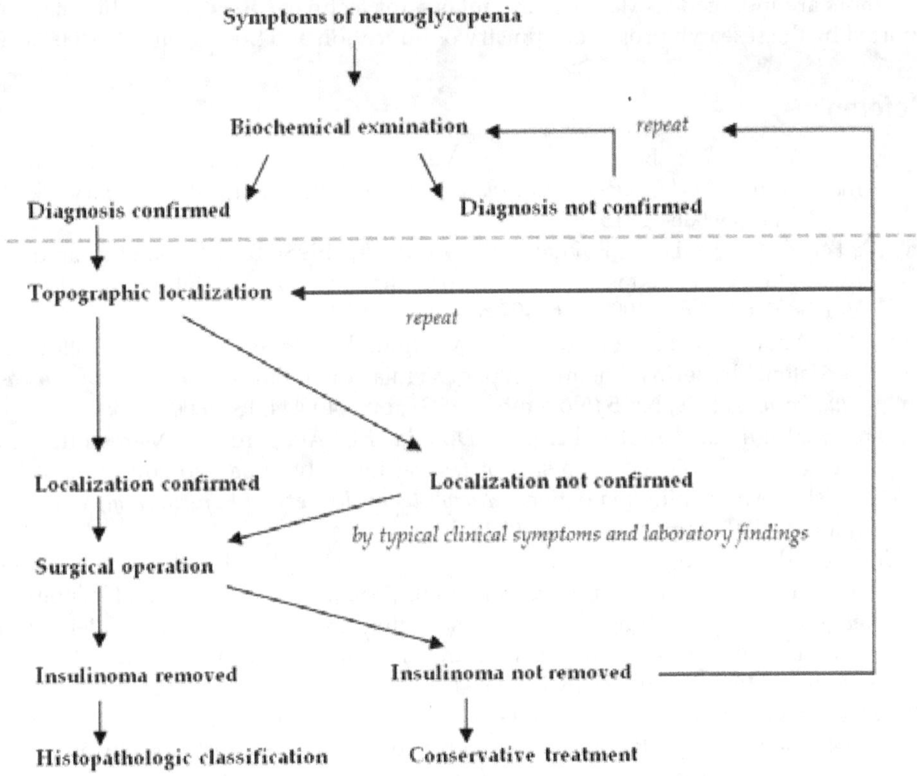

Fig. 4. Algorithm of diagnosis and treatment in patients with suspicion on insulinoma.

The dotted line expresses the level where diagnosis of endogenous hyperinsulinism need to be established and where the operation has to be decided

7. Conclusions

Insulinoma is a rare endocrine disease. Its diagnosis may be sometimes overlooked because clinical symptoms of hypoglycemia may resemble different disease. Better knowledge of neuroglycopenic symptoms may strongly improve diagnostic process and initiate further examinations. When any doubts on clinical picture exist, detailed differential diagnosis should be performed. Localization of the tumor is recommended just after confirmation that endogenous hyperinsulinism is a source of fasting hypoglycemia. Although the imaging techniques have significantly improved localization of the tumors in the past decade, some tumors have not been localized and exploration by laparotomy has to be done. Primary surgical treatment is a method of choice whereas conservative treatment may be suggested when operation was failed or poor clinical state could bring difficulties to surgical treatment. Follow-up of insulinoma patients is recommended but recurrent tumors are very rare. It may be important especially in cases with signs of perineural invasion or angioinvasion when cytostatic drugs should be decided. Close collaboration with oncological department is then necessary.

8. Acknowledgment

The authors are indebted to Marcela Jarolímková for technical assistance. This chapter was supported by the research project of Ministry of Education and Sports, Nr. MSM0021620807.

9. References

Bottger, T.C., Weber, W., Beyer, J. (1990). Value of tumor localization in patients with insulinoma. *World Journal of Surgery*, Vol. 14, Nr. 1 (January-February 1990), pp. 107-112, ISSN 0364-2313

Brun, J.F., Fédou, C., Bouix, O., Raynaud, E., Orsetti, A. (1995). Evaluation of a standardized hyperglucidic breakfast test in postprandial reactive hypoglycemia. *Diabetologia*, Vol. 38, Nr.4 (April 1995), pp. 494-501, ISSN 0012-186X

Cresto, J.C., Abdenur, J.P., Bergada, I. & Martino, R. (1998). Long term follow up of persistent hyperinsulinemic hypoglycemia of infancy. *Archives of Disease in Childhood*, Vol. 79, Nr. 5 (November 1998) , pp. 440-444, ISSN 0003-9888

Del Prato, S., Vigili de Kreutzenberg, S., Dorella, M., Avogaro, A., Marescotti, M.C. & Tiengo, A. (1993). Mechanisms of fasting hypoglycemia and concomitant insulin resistance in insulinoma patients. *Metabolism-Clinical and Experimental*, Vol. 42, Nr. 1 (January 1993), pp. 24-29, ISSN 0026-0495

Del Sindaco, P., Casucci, G., Pampanelli, S, Polonsky, K., Fanelli, C., Torlone, E., Santeusiano, F., Brunetti, P. & Bolli, G.B. (1997). Late post-prandial hypoglycemia as the sole presenting feature of secreting pancreatic beta-cell adenoma in a subtotally gastrectomised patient. *European Journal of Endocrinology*, Vol. 136, Nr. 1 (January 1997), pp. 96-99, ISSN 0804-4643

De Kreutzenberg, S.V., Riccio, A., Dorella, M., Avogaro, A., Marescotti, M.C., Tiengo, A. & Del Prato, S. (1995). Surgical removal of insulinoma restores glucose recovery from hypoglycemia but does not normalize insulin action. *European Journal of Clinical Investigation*, Vol. 25, Nr. 5 (May 1995), pp. 360-367, ISSN 0014-2972

De Lonley-Debeney, P., Travert, F.P., Fournet, J.C., Sempoux, C., Vici, C.D., Brunelle,F., Touati, G., Rahier, J., Junien C., Nihoul-Fekete, C., Robert, J.J., Saudubray, J.M. (1999). Clinical features of 52 neonates with hyperinsulinism. *New England Journal of Medicine*, Vol. 340, Nr. 15 (April 1999) , pp. 1169-1175, ISSN 0028-4793

Demeure, M.J., Klonnoff, D.C., Karam, J.H., Duh., O. & Clark, O.H. (1991). Insulinomas associated with multiple endocrine neoplasia type I: the neded for a different surgical approach. *Surgery*, Vol. 110, Nr. 6 (December 1991), pp. 998-1005, ISSN 0039-6060

Dizon, A.M., Kowalyk, S., Hoogwerf, B.J. (1999). Neuroglycopenic and other symptoms in patients with insulinoma. *American Journal of Medicine*, Vol. 106, Nr. 3 (March 1999), pp.307-310, ISSN 0002-9343

Doppman, J.L., Chang, R., Fraker, D.L., Norton, J.A., Alexander, H.R., Miller, D.L., Collier, E., Skarulis, M.C. & Gorden, P. (1995). Localization of insulinomas to regions of the pancreas by intra-arterial stimulation with calcium. *Annals of Internal Medicine*, Vol. 123, Nr. 4, pp. 269-273, ISSN 0003-4819

Eastman, R.C., Carson, R.E., Orloff, D.G., Cochran, C.S., Perdue,J.F., Rechler, M.M., Lanau, F., Roberts, C.T., Shapiro, J., Roth, J. & Leroith, D. (1992). Glucose utilization in a patient with hepatoma and hypoglycemia. Assessment by a positron emission tomography. *Journal of Clinical Investigation*, Vol. 89, Nr. 6 (June 1992), pp. 1958-1963, ISSN 0021-9738

Fabbri, H.C., de Mello, M.P., Soardi, F.C., et al. (2010). Long-term follow-up of an 8-year-old boy with insulinoma as the first manifestation of a familial form of multiple endocrine neoplasia type 1. *Arquivos Brasileiros de Endocrinologia e Metabologia*, Vol. 54, Nr. 8 (November 2010), pp. 754-760, ISSN 0004-2730

Fajans, S.S. & Vinik, A.I. (1989). Insulin-producing islet cell tumors. *Endocrinology and Metabolism Clinics of North America*, Vol. 18, Nr. 1 (March 1989), pp. 45-74, ISSN 0889-8529

Garber, A.J., Bier, D.M., Cryer, P.E., Pagliara, A.S. (1974). Hypoglycemia in compensated chronic renal insufficiency. *Diabetes*, Vol. 23, Nr. 12, pp. 982-986, ISSN 0012-1797

Geoghegan, J.G., Jackson, J.E., Lewis, M.P.N. Owen, E.R.T.C., Bloom, S.R., Lynn, J.A. & Williamson,R.C.N. (1994). Localization and surgical management of insulinoma. *British Journal of Surgery*, Vol. 81, Nr. 7 (July 1994), pp. 1025-1028, ISSN 0007-1323

Gin, H., Brottie, E., Dupuy, B., Guillaume, D., Ponzo, J. & Aubertin, J. (1987). Use of the glucose clamp technique for confirmation of insulinoma autonomous hyperinsulinism. *Archives of Internal Medicine*, Vol. 147, Nr. 5 (May 1987), pp. 985-987, ISSN 0003-9926

Gin, H., Catargi, B., Rigalleau, V., Rullier, E., Roger, P. & Tabarin, A. (1998). Experience with the Biostator for diagnosis and assisted surgery of 21 insulinomas. *European Journal of Endocrinology*, Vol. 139, Nr. 4 (October 1998), pp. 371-377, ISSN 0804-4643

Glaser, B., Kesavan, P., Heyman, M., Davis, E., Cuesta, A., Buchs, A., Stanley, C.A., Thornton, P.S., Permutt, M.A., Matchinsky, F.M. & Herold, K.C. (1998). Familial hyperinsulinism caused by an activating glucokinase mutation. *New England Journal of Medicine*, Vol. 338, Nr. 4 (January 1998), pp. 226-230, ISSN 0028-4793

Glover, J.R., Shorvon, P.J., Lees, W.R. (1992). Endoscopic ultrasound for localization of islet cell tumors. *Gut*, Vol. 33, Nr. 1 (January 1992), pp. 108-110, ISSN 0017-5749

Harrison, T.S., Fajans, S.S., Floyd, J.C., Thompson, N.W., Rasbach, D.A., Santen, R.J. & Cohen, C. (1984). Prevalence of diffuse pancreatic beta islet cell disease with hyperinsulinism: problems in recognition and management. *World Journal of Surgery*, Vol. 8, Nr. 4 , pp. 583-589, ISSN 0364-2313

Jordan, R.M. & Kammer, H. (1976). An insulinoma without fasting hypoglycemia. *American Journal of Medical Sciences*, Vol. 272, Nr. 2, pp. 205-209, ISSN 0002-9629

Kitaura, J., Miki, Y., Kato, H., Sakakihara, Y. & Yanagisawa, M. (1999). Hyperinsulinemic hypoglycemia associated with persistent hyperammonaemia. *European Journal of Pediatrics*,Vol. 158, Nr. 5 (May 1999), pp. 410-413, ISSN 0340-6199

Krenning, E.P., Kwekkeboom, D.J., Oei, H.Y., Dejong, R.J.B., Dop, F.J., Reubi, J.C. & Lamberts, S.W.J. (1994). Somatostatin receptor scintigraphy in gastroenteropancreatic tumors: an overview of European results. *Annals of the New York Academy of Sciences*, Vol. 733, pp. 416-424, ISSN 0077-8923

Li, X.H., Zhang, J.L. & Liu, Y.F. (2010). Localization of small sized insulinoma by mean of combining arteriography with CT: a case report and review of the literature. *Hepatogastroenterology,* Vol. 58, Nr. 104 (November 2010), pp. 1579-1583, ISSN 0172-6390

Liessi, G., Pasquali, C., D´Andrea A.A., Scandellari, C. & Pedrazzoli, S. (1992). MRI in insulinomas: preliminary findings. *European Journal of Radiology,* Vol. 14, Nr. 1 (January-February 1992) , pp. 46-51, ISSN 0720-048X

McGarry, J.D. & Foster, D.W. (1980). Systemic carnitine deficiency. *New England Journal of Medicine,* Vol. 303, Nr. 24, pp. 1413-1415, ISSN 0028-4793

Mitrakou, A., Fanelli, C., Veneman, T., Perriello, G., Calderone, S., Platanisiotis, D., Rambotts, A., Raptis, S., Brunetti, P., Cryer, P., Gerich, J. & Bolli, G. (1993), Reversibility of unawareness of hypoglycemia in patients with insulinoma. *New England Journal of Medicine,*Vol. 329, Nr. 12 (September 1993), pp. 834-839, ISSN 0028-4793

Morgello, S., Schwartz, E., Horwith, M., King, M.E., Gorden, P. & Alonso, D.R. (1988). Ectopic insulin production by a primary ovarian carcinoid. *Cancer,* Vol. 61, Nr.4 (February 1988) , pp. 800-805, ISSN 0008-543X

Nankervis, A., Proietto, J., Aitken, P. & Alford, F. (1985). Hyperinsulinemia and insulin insensitivity: studies in subjects with insulinoma. *Diabetologia,* Vol. 28, Nr. 7 (July 1985), pp. 427-431, ISSN 0012-186X

Nauck, M., Stöckman, F. & Creutzfeld, W. (1990). Evaluation of a euglycemic clamp procedure as a diagnostic test in insulinoma patients. *European Journal of Clinical Investigation,* Vol. 20, Nr. 1 (February 1990), pp. 15-28, ISSN 0014-2972

Nestorowicz, A., Wilson, B.A., Schoor, K.P., Inoue, H., Glaser, B., Landau, H., Stanley, C,.A., Thornton, P.S., Clement, J.P., Bryan, J., Aguilarbryan, L. & Permutt, M.A. (1996). Mutations in the sulfonylurea receptor gene are associated with familial hyperinsulinism in Ashkenazi Jews. *Human Molecular Genetics,* Vol. 5, Nr. 11 (November 1996), pp. 1813-1822, ISSN 0964-6906

Norton, J.A., Cromack, D.T., Shawker, T.H., Doppman, J.L., Comi, R., Gorden, P., Maton, P.N., Gardner, J.D. & Jensen, R.T. (1988). Intraoperative ultrasonographic localization of islet cell tumors. A prospective comparison to palpation. *Annals of Surgery,* Vol. 207, Nr. 2 (February 1988), pp. 160-168, ISSN 0003-4932

Ouyang, D., Dhall, D., Yu, R. (2011). Pathologic pancreatic endocrine cell hyperplasia. *World Journal of Gastroenterology,* Vol. 17, Nr.2 , pp. 137-143, ISSN 1007-9327

Pasieka, J.L., McLeod, M.K., Thompson, N.W. & Burney, R.E. (1992). Surgical approach to insulinomas. *Archives of Surgery,* Vol. 127, Nr. 4 (April 1992) , pp. 442-447, ISSN 0004-0010

Perry, R.R. & Vinik, A.I. (1995). Diagnosis and management of functioning islet cell tumors. *Journal of Clinical Endocrinology and Metabolism,* Vol. 80, Nr. 8 (August 1995), pp.2273-2278, ISSN 0021-972X

Proye, Ch., Malvaux, P., Carnaille, B., Pattou, F., Godchaux, J.M., Mannoury, V., Filoche, B., Pans, J.C., Huglo, D. & Lefbvre, J. (1998). Noninvasice imaging of insulinomas and gastrinomas with endoscopic and somatostatin receptor scintigraphy. *British Journal of Surgery,* Vol. 85, Nr. 9 (September 1998) , pp. 1304-1304, ISSN 0007-1323

Ratcliffe, P.J. & Bevan, (1985). Severe hypoglycemia and sudden death in anorexia nervosa. *Psychological Medicine,* Vol. 15, Nr. 3, pp. 679-681, ISSN 0033-2917

Redmon, B., Pyzdrowski, K.L., Elson, M.K., Kay, N.E., Dalmasso, A.P. & Nuttall, F.Q. (1992). Hypoglycemia due to a monoclonal insulin-binding antibody in multiple myeloma. *New England Journal of Medicine,* Vol. 326, Nr. 15 (April 1992), pp. 994-998, ISSN 0028-4793

Rosch, T., Lightdale, C.J., Botet, J.F., Boyce, G.A., Sivak, M.V., Yasuda, K., Heyder, N., Palazzo, L., Dancygier, H., Schusdziarra, V. & Classen, M. (1992). Localization of pancreatic endorcine tumors by endoscopic ultrasonography. *New England Journal of Medicine,* Vol. 326, Nr. 26 (June 1992), pp. 1721-1726, ISSN 0028-4793

Rothmund, M., Angelini, L., Brunt, M., et al. (1990). Surgery for benign insulinoma: an international review. *World Journal of Surgery,* Vol. 14, Nr. 3 (May-June 1990), pp. 393-399, ISSN 0364-2313

Samaan, N.A. (1989). Hypoglycemia secondary to endocrine deficiencies. *Endocrinology and Metabolism Clinics of North America,* Vol. 18, Nr. 1 (March 1989), pp. 145-154, ISSN 0889-8529

Sempoux, C., Guiot, Y., Lefevre, A., Nihoul-Fekete, C., Jaubert, F., Saudubray, J.M. & Rahier, J. (1998). Neonatal hyperinsulinemic hypoglycemia: heterogeneity of the syndrome and keys for differential diagnosis. *Journal of Clinical Endocrinology and Metabolism,* Vol. 83, Nr. 5 (May 1998) , pp. 1455-1461, ISSN 0021-972X

Service, F.J., McMahon, M.M., O´Brien, P. & Ballard, D.J. (1991). Functioning insulinoma - incidence, reccurence, and long-term survival of patients: a 60-year study. *Mayo Clinics Proceedings,* Vol. 66, Nr. 7 (July 1991), pp. 711-719, ISSN 0025-6196

Service , F.J., O´Brien, P.CV., Kao, P.C., & Young, W.F. (1992). C-peptide suppression test: effects of gender, age, and body mass index: implications for the diagnosis of insulinoma. *Journal of Clinical Endocrinology and Metabolism,* Vol. 74, Nr. 1 (January 1992), pp. 204-210, ISSN 0021-972X

Service, F.J. (1995). Hypoglycemic disorders. *New England Journal of Medicine,* Vol. 332, Nr. 17 (April 1995), pp. 1144-1152, ISSN 0028-4793

Service, F.J., Natt, N., Thompson, G.B., Grant, C.S., van Heerden, J.A., Andrews, J.C., Lorenz, E., Terzic, A. & Lloyd,R,V. (1999). Noninsulinoma pacreatogenous hypoglycemia: a novel syndrome of hyperinsulinemic hypoglycemia in adults independent of mutations in Kir6.2 and SUR1 genes. *Journal of Clinical Endocrinology and Metabolism,* Vol. 84, Nr. 5 (May 1999), pp. 1582-1589, ISSN 0021-972X

Stanley, C.A. (1997). Hyperinsulinism in infants and children. *Pediatric Clinics of North America,* Vol. 44, Nr. 2 (April 1997), pp. 363-374, ISSN 0031-3955

Stanley, C.A., Lieu, Y.K., Hsu, B.Y.L., Burlina, A.B., Greenberg, C.R., Hopwood, N.J., Perlman, K., Rich, B.H., Zammarchi, E & Ponz, M. (1998). Hyperinsulinismus and hyperammonaemia in infants with regulatory mutations of the glutamate dehydrogenase gene. *New England Journal of Medicine,* Vol. 338, Nr. 19 (May 1998) , pp. 1352-1357, ISSN 0028-4793

Stefanini, P., Carboni, M., Patrassi, N. & Basoli, A. (1974). Hypoglycemia and insular hyperplasia: review of 148 cases. *Annals of Surgery,* Vol. 180, Nr. 1, pp. 130-135, ISSN 0003-4932

Stefanini, P., Carboni, M., Patrassi, N. & Basoli, A. (1974). Beta islet cell tumors of the pancreas: results of a study on 1067 cases. *Surgery,* Vol. 75, Nr. 4, pp. 597-609, ISSN 0039-6060

Škrha, J., Svačina, Š., Šrámková, J. & Páv, J. (1989). Use of euglycemic clamping in evaluation of diazoxide treatment of insulinoma. *European Journal of Clinical Pharmacology,* Vol. 36, Nr. 2, pp. 199-201, ISSN 0031-6970

Škrha, J., Páv, J., Svačina, Š., Šrámková, J. & Hilgertová, J. (1990). Glucose metabolism in a patient with insulinoma complicated by hyperosmolar non-ketotic state. *Diabetic Medicine,* Vol. 7, Nr. 4 (May 1992), pp. 361-363, ISSN 0742-3071

Škrha, J., Hilgertová, J. & Justová, V. (1993). Insulin action in patients with insulinoma influenced by pharmacological and surgical therapy. *Experimental and Clinical Endocrinology,* Vol. 101, Nr. 6, pp. 360-364, ISSN 0232-7384

Škrha, J., Šindelka, G., Haas, T., Hilgertová, J. & Justová, V. (1996). Comparison of insulin sensitivity in patients with insulinoma and obese Type 2 diabetes mellitus. *Hormone and Metabolic Research*, Vol. 28, Nr. 11 (November 1996) , pp. 582-585, ISSN 0018-5043

Škrha, J. (2001). *Hypoglycemic syndrome*, Grada Publishing, ISBN 80-7169-992-6, Prague, Czech Republic (in Czech)

Škrha, J., Šváb, J., Krušina, L., Dušková, J., Hilgertová, J. & Keil, R. (2009). Diagnostics and treatment of organic hyperinsulinism - experience in 105 cases. *Časopis Lékařů Českých*, Vol. 148, Nr. 8 , pp. 389-394, ISSN 0008-7335

Talente, G.M., Coleman, R.A., Alter, C., et al. (1994). Glycogen storage disease in adults. *Annals of Internal Medicine*, Vol. 120, Nr. 3 (February 1994), pp. 218-226, ISSN 0003-4819

Thomas, P.M., Cote, G.J., Wohllk, N., Haddad, B., Mathew, P.M., Rabl, W., Aguilarbryan, L., Gagel, R.F. & Bryan, J. , (1995). Mutations in the sulphonylurea receptor gene in familial persistent hyperinsulinemic hypoglycemia in infancy. *Science*, Vol. 268, Nr 5209 (April 1995), pp. 426-429, ISSN 0036-8075

Thornton, P.S., Satin-Smith, M.S., Herold, K., Glaser, B., Chiu, K.C., Nestorowicz, A., Permutt, M.A., Baker, L. & Stanley, C.A. (1998). Familial hyperinsulinism with apparent autosomal dominant inheritance: clinical and genetic differences from the autosomal recessive variant. *Journal of Pediatrics*, Vol. 132, Nr. 1 (January 1998) , pp. 9-14, ISSN 0022-3476

Tsalikian, E. & Haymond. M.W. (1983). Hypoglycemia in infants and children. In: Service, F.J. (Ed.), 35-71, *Hypoglycemic disorders: pathogenesis, diagnosis, and treatment*. G.K.Hall, Boston, USA

Varma, V., Tariciotti, L., Coldham, C., Taniere, P., Buckels, J.A. & Bramhall, S.R. (2011). Preoperative localization and surgical management of insulinoma: single centre experience. *Digestive Surgery*, Vol. 28, Nr. 1, pp. 63-73, ISSN 0253-4886

Vinik, A.I., Delbridge, L., Moattari, R., Cho, K. & Thompson, N. (1991). Transhepatic portal vein cathetrization for localization of insulinomas. *Surgery*, Vol.109, Nr. 1 (January 1991), pp. 1-11, ISSN 00349-6060

Walters, E.G., Tavare, J.M., Denton R.M. & Walters, G. (1987). Hypoglycemia due to an insulin-receptor antibody in Hodgkin´s disease. *Lancet*, Vol. 1, Nr. 8534 (March 1987), pp. 241-243, ISSN 0140-6736

Weinstock, G., Margulies, P., Kahn, E., Susin, M. & Abrams, G. (1986). Islet cell hyperplasia: an unusual cause of hypoglycemia in an adult. *Metabolism-Clinical and Experimental*, Vol. 35, Nr. 2 (February 1986), pp. 110-117, ISSN 0026-0495

Yki-Järvinen, H., Pelkonen, R. & Koivisto, V.A. (1985). Failure to suppress C-peptide secretion by euglycemic hyperinsulinemia: a new diagnostic test for insulinoma? *Clinical Endocrinology*, Vol. 23, Nr. 4, pp. 461-466, ISSN 0300-0664

Zammarchi, E., Filippi, L., Novembre, E. & Donati, M.A. (1996). Biochemical evaluation of a patient with a familial form of leucine-sensitive hypoglycemia and concomitant hyperammonaemia. *Metabolism-Clinical and Experimental*, Vol. 45, Nr. 8 (August 1996) , pp. 957-960, ISSN 0026-0495

Zimmer, T., Stolzel, U., Baeder, M., Koppenhagen, K., Hamm, B., Buhr, H., Riecken E.O. & Wiedenmann, B. (1996). Endoscopic ultrasonography and somatostatin receptor scintigraphy in the preoperative localization of insulinomas and gastrinomas. *Gut*, Vol. 39, Nr. 4 (October 1996), pp. 562-568, ISSN 0017-5749

12

Pancreatic Beta Cell Tumors

M. Isabel del Olmo[1], J. Francisco Merino-Torres[1],
J. Luis Ponce[2] and Angel Moya[2]
[1]*University Hospital La Fe-Valencia*
Department of Endocrinology and Nutrition
[2]*Department of Surgery*
Spain

1. Introduction

Hypoglycemia is a common syndrome. The manifestations of hypoglycemia are nonspecific, vary among individuals and may change from time to time in the same individual. They are also typically episodic. Thus, although the clinical history is of fundamental importance in suggesting the possibility of hypoglycemia, the diagnosis cannot be made solely on the basis of symptoms and signs.

The vast majority of instances hypoglycemia is secondary to treatment of diabetes. Only a minority of the cases are due to other relatively unfrequent causes. In practice, the most common initial questions are whether the patient truly has hypoglycemia, and if it is likely to be reactive or whether there are grounds for considering insulinoma or islet hyperplasia.

The clinical and physiopathological features, diagnosis and treatment of pancreatic beta cell tumors will be discussed in the following chapter.

2. Historical data

Low blood glucose concentrations were first described in the 19th century as a feature of several diseases. The islets of Langerhans were discovered in 1869 and were named after the German pathologist Paul Langerhans who discovered regions within the pancreas that produced hormones. Nicholls first described in the findings of an autopsy an islet cell tumor in 1902. In 1922 Banting and Best discovered insulin; however, it was not until insulin became available for the treatment of diabetes mellitus in the early 1920s that clinical events similar to those arising from overtreatment with insulin were identified in nondiabetic patients. In 1923, Campbell and Fletcher were the first to describe the hypoglycemic complex due to an insulin excess in non-diabetic patients.

The first resection of an insulinoma was performed in 1927, when WJ Mayo removed an insulin-secreting tumor from a physician and injected it into rabbits that developed subsequently hypoglycemia. In 1938, Whipple reported a triad, considered pathognomonic for insulinoma: blood glucose levels less than 50 mg/dL, neurologic symptoms of hypoglycemia and immediate alleviation of symptoms after glucose ingestion. In 1954, Wermer described a family with a syndrome often associated with pancreatic and other neuroendocrine tumors, the multiple endocrine neoplasia type 1 (MEN1). In 1993,

Gagner et al. reported the first successful laparoscopic distal pancreatectomy and pancreatoduodenectomy. The first successful laparoscopic resection for pancreatic insulinoma was made in 1996.

3. Clinical spectrum of pancreatic beta cell tumors

Pancreatogenous hypoglycemia is a syndrome characterized by endogenous hyperinsulinemic hypoglycemia that comes from a pancreatic beta-cell malfunction. This malfunction can exist as a tumoral mass or a hyperplasia.

Pancreatic beta-cell tumors usually appear as a well-defined mass producing insulin named insulinoma. Commonly insulinomas are sporadic although a low percentage of them are associated with inherited diseases. Another small percentage are not tumoral, but a hyperplasia of beta cells or nesidioblastosis which develop a similar syndrome to insulinomas but with different pathological appearance and therapeutic management.

3.1 Sporadic insulinoma

Insulinomas are so rare that few institutions have accrued enough experience to provide meaningful data regarding epidemiological or demographic characteristics. The estimated incidence of insulinomas in the general population is estimated 1-4 per 1,000,000 yearly. However, the incidence has been reported higher in autopsy studies (0.8-10%), suggesting that these tumors frequently remain undiagnosed. The mean age of patients at presentation is between 47-50 years, patients with MEN 1 are usually younger. In most series, females show a discrete predominance over men (ratio 1.5-1:1).

Insulinomas comprise 70% to 80% of all functional neuroendocrine pancreatic tumors. The majority are solitary, benign lesions occurring in a sporadic setting; they are also single , small and hypervascular, with 90% measuring less than 2 cm and 30% measuring less than 1 cm in diameter; approximately 10% are multiple.

Malignant insulinomas represent about 10% of all insulinomas. Contrary to benign ones, malignant are more frequent in men.

Insulinomas have a lower malignancy rate than other islet cell tumors such as gastrinomas and glucagonomas. It is very difficult to distinguish between malignant and benign insulinomas since endocrine tumors show frequently mild nuclear and structural atypia. Moreover, malignant insulinomas are usually diagnosed intrasurgically or by an image evidencing liver metastases, regional nodes or local invasion.

However, malignant insulinomas, which are solitary and have no evidence of metastases, usually have a better prognosis. Several studies have been performed to investigate the mean survival of a metastatic insulinoma that has been established in 2.6 years since diagnosis (1.6-7.5) (Starke et al., 2005).

3.2 Multiple endocrine neoplasia type 1

Multiple endocrine neoplasia type 1 is an autosomal dominant predisposition to tumors of the parathyroid glands, pancreatic islet cells and anterior pituitary; hence the mnemonic device of the "3 Ps". However, the clinical spectrum of this disorder has been expanded.

A consensus statement from an international group of endocrinologists recommends that MEN1 is defined as the presence of two of the three main MEN1 tumor types (parathyroid, entero-pancreatic endocrine adenomas, and pituitary adenomas). Familial MEN 1 is defined as an index MEN1 case with at least one relative who has one of the three main MEN1 tumors. (Brandi, ML et al, 2001)

Effective treatment is usually available for hyperparathyroidism and pituitary disease; the malignant potential of pancreatic endocrine tumors is the primary life-threatening manifestation of MEN1. Functioning pancreatic islet cell or gastrointestinal endocrine cell tumors become clinically apparent in approximately one third of patients with MEN1. The most common cause of symptomatic disease is the Zollinger-Ellison (gastrinoma) syndrome (ZES), leading to multiple peptic ulcers. Symptomatic insulinomas also occur with moderate frequency, while VIPomas and glucagonomas are rare.

Insulin-producing pancreatic islet cell adenomas in MEN1 represent about 10% of the totality of insulinomas. They are often small, may be multiple, and may be associated with the simultaneous presence of other islet cell tumors. The diagnosis of insulinoma depends, as in nonfamilial causes, upon the documentation of hypoglycemia with characteristic symptoms that are rapidly reversed by the administration of glucose, and inappropriately high serum insulin concentrations.

Approximately 4 to 10 percent of patients with insulinoma have MEN1, and in most of them the MEN1 is known or suspected. Treatment is complicated in these patients by the possible presence of multiple insulinomas, the likelihood that preoperative or intraoperative location techniques may miss small tumors and the continuing risk of recurrence of pancreatic tumors after surgery. As a result, some experienced surgeons recommend local excision of any tumors found in the head of the pancreas plus a distal subtotal pancreatectomy. This approach differs from that in patients with sporadic insulinomas, who typically have a solitary tumor and in whom the localization and local excision alone are usually successful.

In a cohort study of therapeutical response, patients who required additional surgical treatment because of failed initial surgery or recurrence of insulinoma over the period 1927 to 1986 had an increased prevalence of MEN 1 with multiple tumors (25 %) and malignant insulinomas (13 %).(Service, FJ, et al. 1991)

The inheritance of classical MEN1 follows an autosomal dominant pattern. Genetic linkage analysis implicated a region on the long arm of chromosome 11 (11q13) as the site of "MEN1 gene" in 1988. In 1997 the candidate gene was found, the MEN 1 gene, whose protein product is termed "menin" was mutated in 14 of 15 families with MEN1.

Much has been learned about the biochemical and cellular functions of menin, but the precise way in which these functions relate with the tumorigenesis is still not well established. However, it is clear that most of the MEN1 gene mutations found in MEN1 patients would be expected to inactivate or disrupt menin function.

3.3 Noninsulinoma pacreatogenous hypoglycemia or nesidioblastosis

Noninsulinoma pancreatogenous hypoglycemia or nesidioblastosis is a syndrome characterized by endogenous hyperinsulinemic hypoglycemia that is not caused by an insulinoma which accounts for most cases of hyperinsulinemic hypoglycemia. Nesidioblastosis is the name given to the presence of islets in intimate association with ducts, leading to the formation of so-called ductulo-insular complexes.

Nesidioblastosis has mainly been described in neonates. Since Harness et al first described nesidioblastosis in adults, it has been reported in association with other diseases, such as Zollinger-Ellison syndrome, multiple endocrine adenomatosis, β-cell adenomatosis,

Lindau's disease, bariatric surgery, cystic fibrosis, insulinomas, pancreatic transplantation, orbital lymphoma with hypopituitarism and adrenal insufficiency, familial adenomatous polyposis, hypergastrinemia, and pancreatic polypeptidemia.(Abellán, P., et al. 2008).
Sporadic hyperinsulinemic hypoglycemia is the main clinical feature of nesidioblastosis and the diagnostic proceedings are the same as those of insulinoma. However, therapeutic management differs as the extension of the disease in the pancreatic gland may be diffuse.

4. Pathogenesis

Insulinomas are the most frequent functioning endocrine pancreatic tumors. The etiology of these kinds of tumors is poorly understood until the moment. Some tumors may harbor MEN 1 gene mutations, the susceptibility gene of the MEN 1 syndrome, but most cases show wild type MEN 1. While those tumors originated in the exocrine pancreas have been attributed to environmental risk factors and certain mutations, in those from the endocrine pancreas the evidence is quite limited.
In order to improve the diagnosis, prognosis and therapy of insulinoma patients, it is important to increase our understanding of the molecular processes underlying tumor development and progression. During tumorigenesis in general an alteration in the cell physiology takes place as a result of an accumulation of genetic alterations which lead to an uncontrolled cell growth, tissue invasion and metastatic spread. The knowledge of these molecular alterations permits us a focused molecular treatment in these tumors, especially in those with a greater malignant potential.
Therefore, a brief revision of the possible alterations which lead to tumorigenesis in the sporadic insulinoma will be discussed. The altered cellular phenotype in these tumors may involve different genes and mutations which participate in self-sufficiency growth signals, insensitivity to growth-inhibitory signals, evasion of programmed cell death (apoptosis), unlimited replicative potential, sustained angiogenesis and tissue invasion. It is also important to consider that the mechanisms involving MEN 1 insulinoma development and sporadic insulinoma are not the same (Jonkers, JMH et al. 2007) (figure 1).

4.1 Menin molecular interactions

The MEN 1 gene was the first gene described as a candidate gene implicated in insulinoma tumorigenesis. Several studies have been performed which suggest a minor role for MEN 1 inactivation by mutation in human sporadic insulinomas. Menin, the 610 aminoacid protein encoded by MEN1 has been found to partner in vitro with a variety of proteins that comprise transcription factors, DNA processing factors, DNA repair proteins and cytoskeletal proteins. The role of menin inactivation in tumorigenesis, which takes place in the MEN type 1, is diverse participating in mechanisms of failure in DNA repair (via FANCD2), transcription and proliferation (via p27/p18), switching growth suppression to growth proliferation (via JunD), functional stimulation of S-phase kinase and essential component for the S-phase entry, transcriptional activation of NFKB which inhibits apoptosis and stimulates cell growth or neutralizing cell growth inhibition through SMAD3.
Although this inactivation only occurs rarely in sporadic insulinomas, studies which focus on the molecular alterations of menin interacting proteins should be developed.

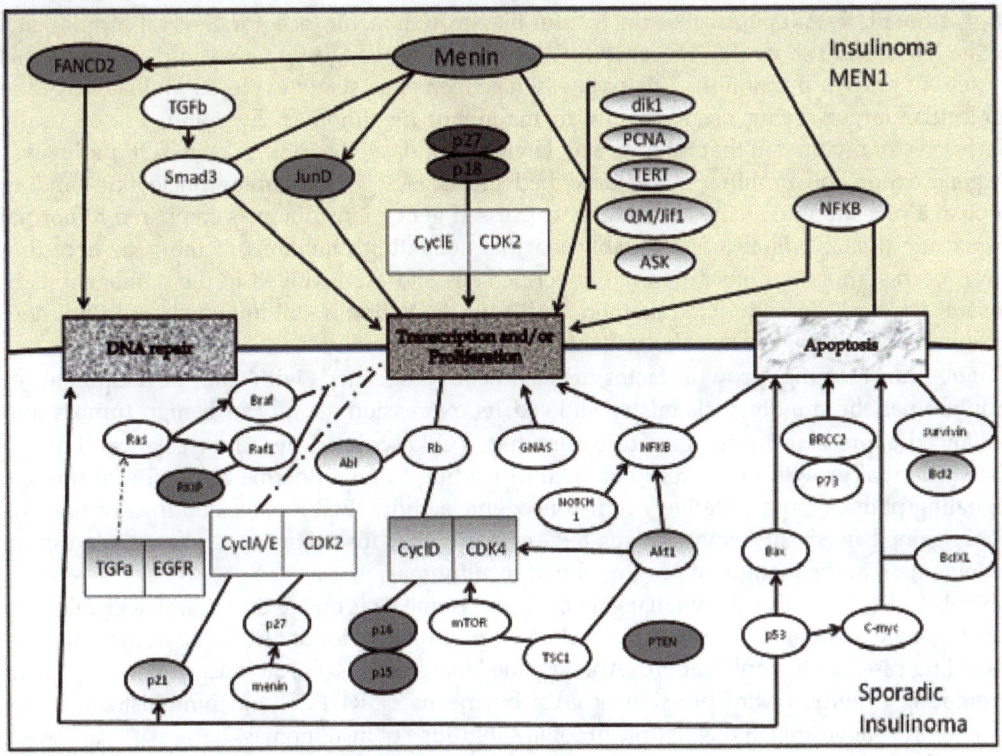

Fig. 1. Signaling molecules and paths that may be involved in insulinoma tumorigenesis. The upper part (shaded in grey) represents those which participate in MEN 1 and the lower part (white) those in sporadic insulinoma. Those whose role have been suggested but not confirmed are in white, those with a loss of function are in grey and those with a gain are shaded. (Adapted from Jonkers, YMH. et al. 2007)

4.2 Self-sufficiency in growth signals

Cell cycle deregulation is one of the defining features of cancer. The roles of several proteins have been suggested to stimulate cell proliferation in insulinomas.

Cyclin dependent kinase 4 (CDK4) together with its regulatory subunit cyclin D governs cell cycle progression through G1 phase. The deregulation of this complex has been studied in islet β-cell proliferation. Several studies show that knock-in mice with an homozygous CDK4 mutation develop multiple neoplasia, most commonly endocrine tumors, including benign insulinomas. However, CDK4 mutations have not been detected in sporadic human insulinomas neither a significantly altered expression of CDK4. On the other hand, overexpression of cyclin D1 has been observed in benign insulinomas compared to normal pancreatic islets, suggesting that this oncogene is involved at least in the tumorigenesis in a certain subgroup of these tumors.

The Akt 1 gene has also been described to induce β-cell proliferation via CDK4 by increasing cyclin D1 and D2 levels. Transgenic mice which overexpress a constitutively active form of Akt 1 in islet beta cells exhibit striking increases in β-cell mass, proliferation, cell mass and malignant tumor formation. The Akt 1 gene is located on a region which has often found to be gained in insulinomas of malignant behavior. One of the growth factors which seems to trigger the PI3K/Akt pathway is the insulin-like growth factor receptor. Several components of the IGF system show differences in mRNA expression suggesting a prominent role of this system in growth promotion. This pathway has been extensively explored and is one of the molecular targets being used recently in malignant insulinomas. Everolimus is an orally derivative of rapamycin that inhibits Ser/Thyrosine kinase, the PI3k/Akt/mTOR pathway.

A gene expression profiling study described the GNAS gene (guanine nucleotide binding protein alpha subunit) as the most highly expressed gene in insulinomas compared to normal pancreatic tissue. It is also well established that activating mutations of the gene encoding GNAS can stimulate proliferation of endocrine cells and are involved in the pathogenesis of several tumors. The underlying method of this up regulation is still unknown and until now no mutations of this gene have been identified in human insulinomas.

TGFα (transforming growth factor α) has been associated with the development of insulinomas. Immunohistochemistry showed its expression already in benign tumors and enhanced expression in malignant insulinomas. TGFα secreted by tumor cells can bind to the epidermal growth factor receptor (EGFR) leading to an autocrine activation of the Ras signaling pathway and putatively to its oncogenic activity. EGFR is located in chromosome 7p12, gained in 8% of benign versus 89% of malignant insulinomas, thus, speculating an involvement in the malignant progression of insulinomas.

Recent studies have also shown that gain of chromosome 9q is one of the earliest aberrations in insulinoma development. FISH analysis showed multiple copies of cAbl gene in these tumors including cases with amplification. cAbl tyrosine kinase gene is a proto-oncogene with growth promoting activity. Overexpression of cAbl by means of RT-PCR and inmuhistochemistry were found suggesting and early role in some subgroups of insulinomas.

In conclusion, several proteins involved in self-sufficiency cell growth, including cyclin D, Akt 1, GNAS, TNFα and cAbl have been suggested to stimulate cell proliferation in insulinomas, although their individual roles still remain elusive.

4.3 Insensitivity to anti-growth signals

Within a normal tissue, multiple antiproliferative signals operate to maintain cellular quiescence and tissue homeostasis. Cancer cells must evade these anti-proliferative signals if they are to prosper.

At the molecular level, many antiproliferative routes are controlled by the retinoblastoma protein (pRb). In tumors with pRb inactivation as the basis of pathology somatic loss of one Rb allele commonly accompanies a point mutation or micro-deletion of the other allele. Deletion of Rb gene has so far been detected only in one human insulinoma. However, other mechanisms of inactivations of pRb are phosphorylation, but studies done until the moment conclude that pRB may not be strictly involved in de initiation of insulinomas.

CDKN2 locus on chromosome 9p21 harbors tumor suppressor genes which restrain cell growth by affecting the function of pRb and p53. Downregulation of expression of CDKN2A/p16, CDKN2B/p15 and CDKN2D/p14 have been studied. Absence of expression of p15 was detected in 33% of benign insulinomas. On the other hand, a low frequency of alterations were detected in p16 but a down-regulation of p16 protein was detected and it is likely to be involved in insulinoma tumorigenesis. Two other inhibitors of CDK2, p21 and p27 have been studied. P27 was expressed in 88% of insulinomas, including malignant tumors but was also expressed in normal pancreatic islet cells. The strong expression of p21 and p27 may explain the slow growth in a subset of tumors and suggests differences in tumorigenesis between MEN1-associated and sporadic insulinomas.

The Raf-1 kinase inhibitory peptide (RKIP) binds to Raf-1 and MEK in vivo and in vitro, thus interfering with the activation of the ERK signaling pathway, and plays an important role in the inhibition and beta-cell proliferation. Expression of RKIP was studied in insulinomas showing an absence of expression in comparison with normal islet cells.
PTEN (phosphatase with tensin homology) is a potent negative regulator of the PI3K/Akt signaling pathway. The PTEN gene is located on chromosome 10q23 a region which is often lost in malignant insulinomas. Loss of PTEN has been associated with malignancy of insulinomas, as it was not observed in benign insulinomas.
In conclusion, evading antiproliferative signals, for example through inactivation of pRb, p15, p16 and/or PTEN may be important features involved in the development of insulinomas.

4.4 Evading apoptosis

The ability of tumor cell population to expand is not only determined by the rate of proliferation but also by the rate of cell death or apoptosis. Acquired resistance toward programmed cell death (apoptosis) is a hallmark of most types of cancer.
Certain apoptotic factors such as Bcl-2 have been studied, and are frequently expressed in gastroenteropancreatic neuroendocrine tumors which are usually slow-growing and less aggressive tumors, suggesting that in these tumors Bcl-2 expression leads to indolent tumor growth. Another factor such as c-Myc has also been demonstrated to induce highly malignant beta-cell tumors in mouse models. All this evidence suggests that suppression of apoptosis may contribute also to the initiation of these tumors.
Survivin, a member of another family of apoptosis inhibitors is a protein that can suppress apoptosis and regulate cell division. The gene encoding this protein, BIRC5, is located in chromosome 17q25 a region gained in one third of malignant insulinomas versus none of the benign insulinomas.
The P73 gene, encodes a protein with similar function to p53, and might be an interesting candidate for insulinoma progression. It is located on chromosome 1p36, a region that is deleted in 44% of malignant insulinomas and associated with metastasic disease.
In conclusion, due to the overall low proliferation rate in insulinomas, it is tempting to speculate that evasion of apoptosis is more important in their development instead of increased proliferation.

4.5 Unrestricted replicative potential

Human cells carry a cell-autonomous program that limits their multiplication. This program is independent from of the cell to cell signaling pathways. The progressive erosion of telomers during successive cycles of replication eventually causes cells to lose their ability to protect the ends of chromosomal DNA, which results letal to them.
Telomere maintenance is evident in virtually all types of malignant cells. For this purpose the malignant cells up-regulate the expression of telomerase enzymatic activity. Also stem cells do have a high telomerase activity. Because pancreatic stem cells are suggested as the clonal origin of insulinomas, telomerase activity may be expected in these tumors. This fact has not been demonstrated in sporadic insulinomas, however, in MEN1-associated insulinomas may play an important role.
On the other hand, telomeric loss has been shown by array to be associated with malignant behavior of insulinomas. In insulinomas with uncertain behavior telomeric losses were more

frequently observed than chromosomal instability. This suggests that telomeric loss occurs prior to and is causative of chromosomal instability during insulinoma tumorigenesis. These data indicate that escape from replicative senescence, which is expected to occur as a result of telomeric loss, is the basis of tumor progression.
Therefore telomeric loss and chromosomal instability seem to accumulate during tumor progression and it is tempting to speculate that p16 down regulation and telomerase activity in addition ensure unrestricted replicative potential. Inactivation of menin may trigger activation of telomerase earlier in tumor development (MEN1).

4.6 Sustained angiogenesis

Tumorigenesis in general is critically dependent on the development of vascular supply. The fact that endocrine tumors are highly vascular in nature renders analysis of angiogenesis as a prognostic factor highly pertinent. However, in contrast to other cancers, a high vessel density in endocrine pancreatic tumors was found to correlate with good prognosis as well as with hormone production.
Endocrine pancreatic tumor cells overproduce the angiogenic peptide vascular endothelial growth factor (VEGF), which is likely to play an important role in the angiogenic process associated with endocrine tumorigenesis but they seem to lose this expression during tumor progression. In conclusion, although activation of angiogenesis is not indicated in tumor progression, it will be necessary to study additional angiogenic factors that may substitute loss of blood supply in insulinomas.

4.7 Markers to predict metastasic disease and clinical outcome in insulinomas

Certain markers such as CK-19 are associated with malignancy. Immunostaining of CK19 has resulted a reliable indicator of tumor-specific death in insulinomas. Also, chromosomal instability indentified by array has been detected as an optimal predictor of metastasic disease. Ki-67 $\geq$ 2% and p53 overexpression were found to be associated with malignancy in a few individual insulinoma cases.

5. Histopathology

Insulinomas exhibit four main histological patterns including: solid, trabecular, gland-like (tubular or acinar) and mixed forms. Larger tumors are encapsulated but the capsule is usually incomplete. Smaller tumors and microadenomas are rarely encapsulated. Tumor cells frequently exhibit a bland cytology and cells with large pleomorphic nuclei are rare. If present, these features are not predictive of malignant behavior. A relatively uncommon, but characteristic finding in insulinomas is the deposite of amyloid. Its major component is islet amyloid polypeptide or amylin that can be visualized by immunohistochemistry. Calcifications and intracytoplasmatic pigment may unfrequently be seen in insulinomas. (Figure 2)
The majority of insulinomas exhibit immunoreactivity for insulin and proinsulin. Insulinomas without any positive staining for insulin are also found indicating that the produced insulin is not stored inside the cells, but immediately released. In such cases, proinsulin staining or insulin messenger RNA in situ hybridization are valuable alternatives, but rarely used and more costly.
The byosinthesis of insulin takes place usually in the endoplasmic reticulum. In normal pancreatic beta-cells, proinsulin-insulin conversion occurs in acidic immature secretory

granules of the trans-Golgi apparatus. In contrast to beta-cells, the proinsulin-insulin conversion in insulinomas occurs already in the Golgi apparatus, but remains incomplete, resulting in the formation of secretory granules containing both proinsulin and insulin.. The distribution pattern of proinsulin and insulin has been investigated and no correlation was found between a particular staining pattern, histological type, multihormonality or the degree of malignancy of insulinoma. (De Lellis, et al.2004).

Approximately 10-15% of insulinomas are classified as malignant on the basis of the presence of organ and/or lymph node infiltration or distant metastases. The most common sites of metastases for insulinomas are the peripancreatic lymph nodes with occasional hepatic metastases.

According to the WHO criteria histopathologically pancreatic neuroendocrine tumors (including insulinomas) should be classified into four groups (Komminoth, P. et al, 2004):

- Well differentiated endocrine pancreatic tumors in the absence of all adverse criteria
- Well differentiated endocrine pancreatic tumors of uncertain behavior: tumor diameter > 2cm, >2 mitosis/10 high power fields, angioinvasion or a proliferative index Ki-67 > 2%.
- Well differentiated endocrine pancreatic carcinomas: gross local invasion or metastases.
- Poorly differentiated pancreatic endocrine carcinomas: > 10 mitosis/ 10 high power field

Because these criteria are not always reliable, markers have to be detected to predict a possible malignant outcome of insulinomas in an earlier stage.

In the case of nesidioblastosis, the morphological criteria for establishing its diagnosis are the presence of differently-sized islets often with somewhat irregular outline, and irregularly sized and poorly defined endocrine cell clusters scattered in the acinar parenchyma and often intimately connected with small or large ducts (ductulo-insular complexes). Another feature is a distinct islet cell hypertrophy with nuclear enlargement, often resulting in the presence of giant and bizarre nuclei. Nesidioblastosis is classified into focal and diffuse types characterized by different clinical outcomes. Focal nesidioblastosis exhibits nodular hyperplasia of islet-like cell clusters, including ductuloinsular complexes and hypertrophied insulin cells with giant nuclei. In contrast, diffuse nesidioblastosis involves the entire pancreas with irregularly sized islets. (Figure 2)

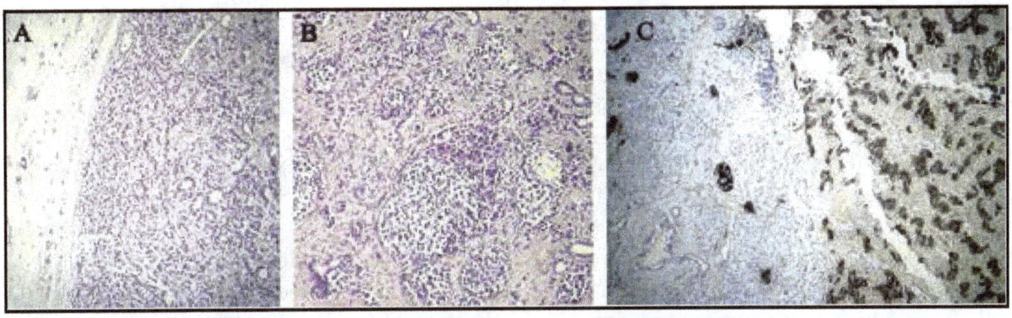

Fig. 2. Histopathological characteristics of insulinoma and nesidioblastosis. A. Insulinoma with peripancreatic fat. Haematoxylin and eosin (100x). B. Nesidioblastosis. Cluster of islets of varied size and shape in apposition to pancreatic ductules. Haematoxylin and eosin (250x). C. Insulin immunostaining showin insulinoma (right) with pancreatic tissue (100 x).

6. Clinical features

Insulinoma patients characteristically present at diagnosis with symptoms of hypoglycemia, especially neuroglycopenic symptoms that may or may not be preceded by symptoms due to sympathetic overdrive. The leading symptoms establishing the diagnosis of endogenous hyperinsulinism are comprised in the Whipple's triad. The neuroglycopenic symptoms of insulinomas include confusion, visual change, and unusual behavior. Neuroglycopenic symptoms are the direct result of central nervous system neuronal glucose deprivation. Neurogenic symptoms are the result of the perception of physiologic changes caused by the autonomic nervous system discharge triggered by hypoglycemia. Sympathoadrenal symptoms may include palpitations, diaphoresis and tremulousness. Amnesia for hypoglycemia is common in these patients. (Table 1)

This common clinical manifestation takes place usually in a fasting state. However, postprandial hypoglycemia may be a feature or even the sole manifestation of hypoglycemia in some patients. In retrospective reviews done to patients with confirmed insulinoma, 21% reported fasting and postprandial symptoms and 6% reported only postprandial symptoms (Placzkowski, KA, et al. 2009). The hypoglycemia in patients with insulinoma is primarily due to reduced hepatic glucose output rather than increased glucose utilization.

The mean duration of these symptoms before the diagnosis is established is less than 1.5 years. However, a few patients can be symptomatic for decades and can be misdiagnosed with a neurologic or psychiatric disorder. Clinical manifestations of an insulinoma can mimick central nervous system disorders, like epilepsy.

Adrenergic symptomatology	Neuroglucopenic syptomatology
Tremulousness Palpitations Anxiety Hunger Parestesias Hyperhidrosis/sweat	Confusion Letargy Headache Visual manifestations Fatigue, dizziness Difficulty to talk Unusual behavior Seizures Coma Death

Table 1. Hypoglycemic symptomatology.

7. Diagnosis

Neuroendocrine tumors (NETS) are rare, slow growing neoplasms characterized by their ability to store and secrete different peptides and neuroamines. Some of these substances cause specific clinical syndromes, whereas others may have elevated plasma or urine levels that are not associated with specific syndromes or symptom complexes.

The biochemical markers are those hormones or amines secreted by the neuroendocrine cells from which these tumors are derived. In the case of the insulinoma, derived from the beta pancreatic cells, the biochemical marker secreted is insulin which leads in excess, to an hypoglycemic syndrome.

The Whipple's triad is the cornerstone for the suspicion of an insulinoma, although other causes must be ruled out.

WHIPPLE'S TRIAD	
1. Hypoglycemia symptoms induced by fasting	
2. Blood glucose	< 50 mg/dL + symptoms < 40 mg/dL regardless of symptoms
3. Relief of symptoms when glucose is raised to normal	

Fig. 3. Whipple's triad

Clinical syndrome is therefore the first step that leads to the suspicion of an insulinoma.

7.1 Laboratory confirmation

The diagnosis of an insulinoma can be established by determining plasma proinsulin, insulin, c-peptide and glucose levels, which are usually performed during a 72-hour fast. It is important to realize that insulin levels are increasingly being determined by immunochemiluminiscent assays or specific immunoradiometric assays that do not cross-react with proinsulin and give lower values than that obtained with most insulin radioimmunoassay, which can affect the proposed criteria listed in many reviews for diagnosis, which were based on radioimmunoassay results.

There are six main criteria for the diagnosis of insulinoma: documented blood glucose levels of 45 mg/dL or less (2.2 mmol/L), concomitant insulin levels of 6 μU/mL or greater (≥ 36 pmol/L; ≥ 3 μU/mL), c-peptide levels 200 pmol/L or greater, proinsulin levels 5 pmol/L or greater, β–hydroxybutyrate levels 2.7 mmol/L or less and absence of sulfonylurea (metabolites) in the plasma and/or urine. (Table 2)

Biochemical tests	Confirmation of insulinoma
Plasma glucose	<45 mg/dL
Insulin	≥ 3 μU/mL
C-peptide	≥ 200 pmol/L
Proinsulin	≥ 5 pmol/L
β–hydroxybutyrate	< 2.7 mmol/L

Table 2. Main criteria for the diagnosis of insulinoma

Further controlled testing under supervision includes the 72-hour fast, which is the gold-standard criterion for establishing the diagnosis of insulinoma. Actually, 98% of the patients with insulinoma will develop symptomatic hypoglycemia within 72 hours. When the patient develops symptoms and the blood glucose levels are < 40(45) mg/dL or less (<2.2 mmol/L), blood should also be drawn for c-peptide, proinsulin and insulin, and the fast should be stopped. Failure in appropriate insulin suppression in the presence of hypoglycemia substantiates an autonomously secreting insulinoma.

7.1.1 How to perform a fast test

The 72-h fast test can be initiated at any hour and may be prolonged until 72-hours. It is important to date the onset of fast as well as the last ingestion of calories. During the whole test, the patient may only be allowed to drink calorie and caffeine free beverages. It is important to ensure that the patient is active during waking hours and in some cases some exercise can be recommended at the end of the fast if it resulted negative.

In the basal state with the initiation of the fast state a 6mL extraction for glucose, insulin and c-peptide will be done. These measurements should be repeated every 12 hours with a previous measurement of capillary glucose at 12, 24, 36, 48, 60 and 72 hours and after exercise if it takes place.

The end of the fast will be when the patient presents signs and symptoms of hypoglycemia and plasma glucose is <40 mg/dL. In this moment blood glucose will be drawn as well as insulin and c-peptide. Hypoglycemia will not be reversed until the central laboratory confirms the glucose value or the patient is unconscious and has fits. The reversal of the hypoglycemia will be with the administrations of oral glucose or intravenous if needed (dextrose 40% 250mL).

At the end of the fast, a measurement of glucose, insulin, c-peptide and sulphonylurea screen (blood and urine spot), should be done. If the patient presents no symptoms during the fast, it can be finished with a 15-30 min exercise (for example brisk walk) around the hospital and re-measuring.

7.1.2 Interpretation of a fast test

90% of insulinomas will present hypoglycemia before 72 hour fast and insulin will be inappropriately high in relation with glucose levels.(Figure 4)

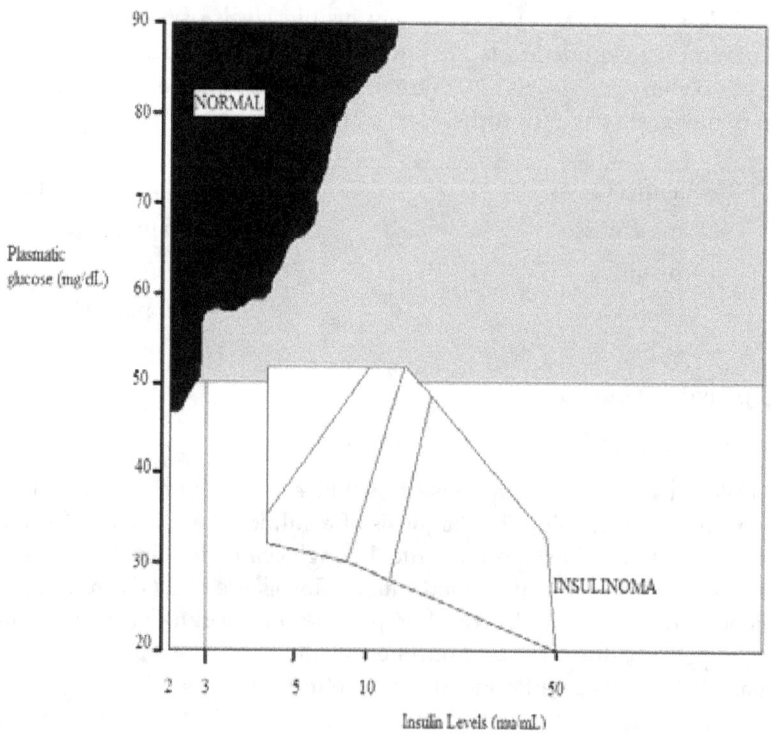

Fig. 4. Plasmatic insulin and glucose limits after a fast in normal subjects and patients affected of an insulinoma. The black area represents the normal response to hypoglycemia. The striped area represents the usual response in patients affected of an insulinoma. (Redrawn from Service, FJ. et al, 1999).

Rare disorders, in which the biochemical findings simulate those of an insulinoma because they are also associated with endogenous hyperinsulinemia include administration of exogenous insulin or sulphonylureas and insulin autoimmune hypoglycemia.
The fast test permits us to differ between insulinoma, exogenous administration of insulin and sulphonylureas administration. If this last is suspected, urine and plasma collection of sulphonylureas should be performed. (Table 3)

	Insulin	C-peptide	Proinsulin	Sulphonylureas
Exogenous administration of insulin	↑	↓	↓	NEGATIVE
Insulinoma	↑	↑	↑	NEGATIVE
Exogenous administration of sulphonylureas	↑	↑	↑	POSITIVE

Table 3. Differential diagnosis determined by the results of a fast test.

Insulin autoimmune hypoglycemia occurs in patients who have antibodies directed to endogenous insulin or to the insulin receptor. Symptoms can occur postprandially, fasting, or in both states. In patients with insulin autoantibodies, insulin secreted in response to a meal binds to the antibody and then disassociates in an unregulated fashion causing hyperinsulinemia and hypoglycemia. In patients with antibodies to the insulin receptor, hypoglycemia occurs as a result of antibody activation of the receptor. The presence of insulin or insulin receptor antibodies can distinguish insulin autoimmune hypoglycemia from insulinoma. The antibodies do not have to be measured during an episode of hypoglycemia.

7.1.3 48 hour versus 72 hour fast

It has been proposed that the sensitivity of the 48h fasting test is between 94.5 and 95.7% and should be enough for the diagnosis of insulinoma instead of the 72-hour fast. In a series of 127 patients with insulinoma, the fast was ended due to hypoglycemia in 42.5% in 12 hours, 66.9% by 24 hours and 94.5% in 48 hours (Hirshberg, et al. 2000).

7.1.4 Other laboratory tests

7.1.4.1 Intravenous secretin test for insulinoma

In patients harboring and insulinoma, insulin production by normal pancreatic beta cells is significantly suppressed. Following intravenous injection of secretin (2 units/kg of body weight), plasma insulin rises more than 200% in normal individuals, whereas in patients with insulinoma, the secretin stimulation test does not cause a rise in plasma insulin due to the unresponsiveness of insulinoma cells to secretin. (Imamura, M., et al. 1990)

7.1.4.2 C-peptide inhibition test with hog insulin

After proinsulin cleavage, insulin and c-peptide are secreted. Infusion of hog insulin for 1 hour leads to the decrease of plasma c-peptide levels in healthy subjects, but no such decrease is observed in insulinoma patients. Insulin release from insulinoma cells is not inhibited by the administration of exogenous insulin, whereas insulin secretion from normal beta-cells is inhibited by the increased plasma insulin. (Service, FJ., et al. 1992)

7.2 Diagnostic imaging

The diagnostic suspicion of an insulinoma is based on symptoms, and laboratory techniques usually confirm the diagnosis. The treatment, on the other hand, is usually surgery of the tumoral mass as complete as possible, including the primary tumor and metastases if present. Imaging of the primary tumor location and the extent of the disease is needed for all phases of management of pancreatic neuroendocrine tumors. It is needed to determine whether the surgical resection for possible cure or possible cytoreductive surgery is needed and whether treatment for advanced metastatic disease is appropriate and during follow-up to assess the effects of any antitumor treatment as well as the need for deciding whether additional treatments are indicated. Imaging plays also a pivotal role in differentiating these tumors from adenocarcinomas of the pancreas. As a result, a fundamental part in the process of the diagnosis and treatment of an insulinoma will be the localization with imaging techniques.

Insulinomas are often of a small size and localization may be difficult. A number of different imaging modalities have been widely used including conventional imaging studies (CT, MRI, ultrasound, angiography), endoscopic ultrasound, functional localization studies measuring hormonal gradients, intraoperative methods particularly intraoperative ultrasound and recently PET preoperatively.

7.2.1 Abdominal ultrasound

Abdominal ultrasound has the advantages of being a non-invasive technique, free of radiation, anatomically precise, low-cost and world-wide used. On the other hand, key major drawbacks include its dependence on the operator expertise and on the limitations based on the patient's habitus that is usually unfavorable since many insulinoma patients are overweight or obese.

Regular ultrasound investigation of the pancreas is rarely helpful in the localization of an insulinoma. The sensibility reported with this technique to detect insulinoma is low, about 9%. However, it is done routinely to exclude the presence of liver metastases before surgery. Commonly, it is the first imaging technique to detect liver metastases and therefore leading to the performance of more precise techniques which detect the malign insulinoma.

7.2.2 Endoscopic ultrasonography (EUS) of the pancreas

EUS is a relatively new technique. It is remarkably accurate locating pancreatic neuroendocrine tumors, especially those located in the pancreatic tail (Figure 5). EUS requires the availability of expensive echoendosonographic and processing equipment. Such equipment is found only in large hospitals or endoscopy units.

Most gastroenterologists now consider EUS to be the most accurate, least expensive preoperative method of locating neuroendocrine pancreatic tumors. The technical advantage of EUS imaging over transabdominal ultrasonography is due to the close proximity of the transducer to the target. This permits the use of high scanning frequencies, which provide much greater spatial resolution. Rosch et al. prospectively compared the accuracy of EUS and ultrasonography, computed tomography, and endoscopic retrograde cholangiopancreatography in the detection of pancreatic tumors.22 The sensitivity and specificity of EUS in localizing pancreatic tumors is 99 and 100%, respectively, compared with ultrasonography (67 and 40%, respectively) and computed tomography (77 and 53%, respectively) and is equal to endoscopic retrograde cholangiopancreatography (sensitivity of 90%).

In a recent multicenter study, EUS was shown to be the most sensitive localization modality in accurate detection of pancreatic tumors (sensitivity of 82 versus 27%) and had a specificity of 95%. EUS accurately defines the size of tumors to within 2 mm of the excised lesion.

EUS is a valuable method of localizing insulinomas. The technique requires specialized endoscopic skill, but it is both safe and effective in experienced hands. EUS should prove to be very helpful for localization of insulinomas undetectable by transabdominal ultrasonography or computed tomography, but it is not a satisfactory method for evaluating the liver in patients suspected to have metastatic disease. (Andersen, A., et al, 2004)

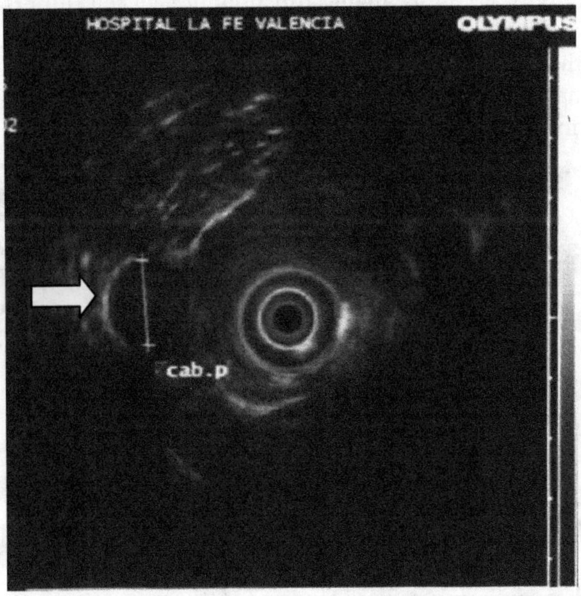

Fig. 5. Endoscopic ultrasonography of a bening insulinoma. The arrow points the tumoral mass.

7.2.3 Computed tomography (CT)

Although in recent years gadolinium-enhanced MR imaging, somatostatin-receptor imaging, and endosonography have emerged as potentially competing or complementary techniques to CT, dual-phase helical CT, particularly with technical improvements afforded by multidetector CT, remains the dominant imaging modality for the diagnosis of all pancreatic neoplasms, including islet cell tumors. In expert hands, helical CT can detect about two-thirds of the insulinomas.

Because of their rich vascular supply, insulinomas classically are hyperattenuating compared with the surrounding pancreatic parenchyma on contrast-enhanced CT. Capturing the vascular blush is essential for the diagnosis of small tumors, which often do not distort the contour of the pancreas. This is particularly true in the investigation of functioning insulinomas because these are often small, with 50% measuring less than 1.3 cm. The classic and most common enhancement pattern of islet cell tumors is that of a hyperattenuating lesion in the arterial and venous phases. Many small lesions enhance more prominently and thus are easier to detect in the arterial phase or become inconspicuous in the venous phase. In a series of 11 cases of functioning islet cell tumors reported by Van Hoe et al., most lesions were hyperattenuating and two were more conspicuous on arterial phase imaging. Helical CT is not only useful for the detection of the insulinoma but also in the staging of malignant insulinoma on dual-phase CT. Three-dimensional CT reconstructions exquisitely show local extension and encasement of the major peripancreatic arteries and veins for surgical planning. The liver and regional lymph nodes are the most common sites for metastases. Like the primary tumor, liver metastases are hypervascular. Arterial phase images show the number and size of the hepatic lesions better than images acquired in the venous phase, particularly for small metastases. Spread to regional lymph nodes also is more conspicuous in the arterial phase.

The reported sensitivity of CT in localizing functioning islet cell tumors varies from 71% to 82% because small tumors are more frequently missed. Small hyperattenuating islet cell tumors located in the pancreatic neck or body can be confused with adjacent vascular structures; multiplanar reconstruction is helpful in separating the lesion from surrounding vessels, thus improving diagnostic confidence. (Sheth, S., et al, 2002).

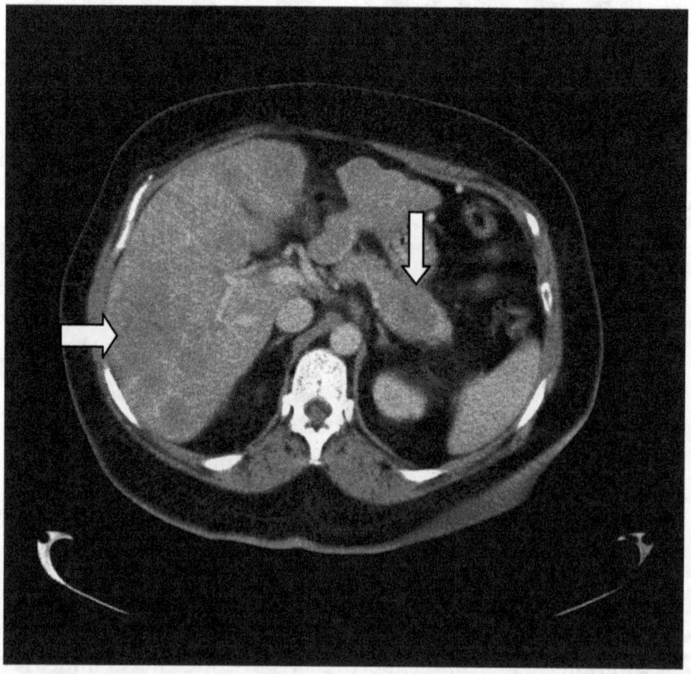

Fig. 6. CT scan of malignant insulinoma (no contrast). Hypointense solid irregular mass of 2 x 3 cm in the tail of the pancreatic gland. Hepatomegaly with multiple metastases, solid and hypointense, of different sizes, the bigger one of 5.5cm.

7.2.4 Magnetic resonance imaging

Recent reports have suggested an important role for MRI in the detection of pancreatic NET, in particular with the use of fast spin echo and fat saturation techniques. MRI has presented excellent results, its sensitivity ranges from 85-95% in the detection of insulinomas (including those with less than 1.5 cm in diameter) and the determination of the presence of metastases.
Using conventional sequences, small insulinomas usually have a low signal on T1-weighted sequences and a high signal on T2-weighted sequences. Some insulinomas containing fibrous tissue may show low signal intensity on both T1 and T2 weighted images.
An improvement in MRI techniques is the use of diffusion weighted MRI. Fat suppressed T_1 weighted sequences have been reported to be particularly useful in imaging pancreatic lesions, especially islet cell tumours. The normal pancreas is of relatively high signal intensity on fat saturated T_1 weighted images. Islet cell tumors are of lower signal intensity than normal pancreatic tissue. This increased contrast between tumors and pancreas explains the greater detection rate with fat suppressed T_1 weighted images. (Semelka, RC., et al, 2000)

7.2.5 Angiography and arterial stimulation of the pancreas

Although most insulinomas are small, they have been successfully detected by computed tomography and magnetic resonance imaging recently. However, preoperative localization of the insulinomas by arterial stimulation with venous sampling is crucial when they show atypical findings on these imaging modalities.
That is, it is difficult to determine whether the tumor is benign or malignant, whether it is a nonfunctioning tumor accompanying an extra or undetectable pancreatic insulinoma, or whether it is one of the multiple insulinomas. Morphological imaging modalities do not reflect hormonal functions; however, the addition of angiography and arterial stimulation helps regionalize a tumor by verifying the hormonal function. This procedure enhances a more accurate surgical approach in clinical exploration and can prevent a possible resurgery. Thus, for atypical insulinomas, preoperative localization of insulinomas by angiography and arterial stimulation may be particularly important.
Mesenteric angiography is a well established invasive technique in which pancreatic endocrine tumors appear as a well circumscribed blush, usually four to eight seconds after the contrast injection. The reported sensitivity for the detection of primary tumors ranges between 28 and 70 percent. The accuracy for diagnosing hepatic metastases is higher (sensitivity 62 to 78 percent).
Arterial stimulation venous sampling involves selective injections into arteries supplying the pancreas of a stimulating secretagogue. Insulin production is measured in the pancreatic gland by a catheterization of the main arteries (superior mesenteric artery, gastroduodenal artery, hepatic artery and splenic artery). Insulin secretion is stimulated by an injection in each of these arteries of calcium (0.025 mEq/kg) diluted in a 5 mL injection. Plasma extractions are done at 0, 30, 60, 90 and 120 seconds after the injection. The test is considered positive if there is an increase of insulin two-fold greater the basal between 30 and 120 seconds. This technique permits de location of the tumor in the portion of the pancreas which is irrigated by one of these arteries.
Results with this technique are encouraging. One report evaluated 24 patients with proven hyperinsulinemia. Seven of these patients had negative imaging technique and in all of them calcium infusion permitted localization of the source of insulin secretion. Although helpful, angiography and arterial stimulation is an invasive and costly technique that should be reserved for atypical insulinomas or when nesidioblastosis is suspected.

7.2.6 Scintigraphy with octeotride

The absence of somatostatin receptors in half of insulinomas and the lack of spatial discrimination with nuclear scanning are detractions to the routine use of this new localization test.

In addition, scintigraphic imaging with Octreoscan has been introduced in an attempt to improve topographic assessment of insulinomas. The results were disappointing, since Octreoscan scintigraphy with planar imaging led to detection of only 20–50% of insulinomas

7.2.7 Positron emission tomography PET

The results of 18-fluordeoxyglucose (18-FDG) PET imaging for insulinomas are not very promising, maybe due to the low proliferative potential of these tumor cells. Positive results have been shown using 11 C-5-hydroxi-L-tryptophan, 18-3, 4-Dihydroxy-6-fluoro-DL-phenylalanine and 67-Ga-DOTA-DPhe 1-Tyr 3-octeotride due to selective uptake in tumor tissue compared to surrounding tissue. These techniques produce very good tumor visibility and can be used for the examination of both the thorax and abdomen. However, the lack of general availability of PET scanning and high cost, limits its use.

7.2.8 PET/TC

The 18-fluorine-18-fluoro-2-deoxyglucose Positron Emission Tomography coupled with computed tomography is a non invasive exploration. Several studies have shown that PET-CT has superior efficacy over conventional imaging techniques in distinguishing a benign pancreatic tumor from a malignant one. It contributes to the diagnosis of cancer in patients with a doubtful mass, much more in case of chronic pancreatitis.

7.2.9 Intraoperative localization techniques

Intraoperative ultrasonography allows high resolution examination of the pancreas. When combined with palpation of the organ, the sensitivity for tumor detection ranges 83 to 100 percent. Intraoperative transillumination has equivalent efficacy (sensitivity of 83 percent). Neither of these tests should replace preoperative imaging; they are used as adjuncts to intraoperative palpation. (Figure 7)

Diagnostic algorithm for insulinomas

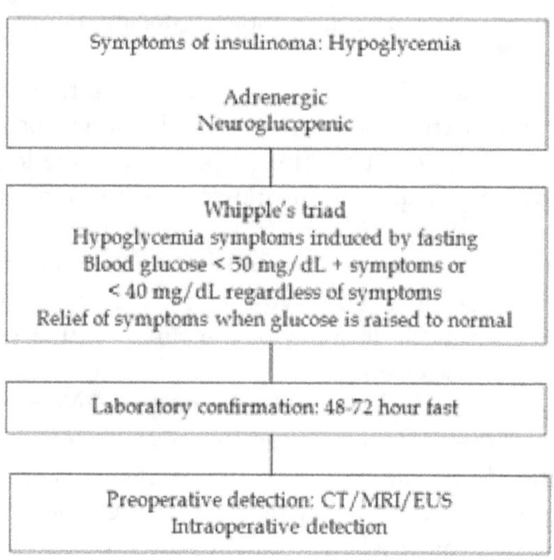

8. Staging of insulinoma tumors

After the performance of imaging techniques, insulinomas which are the most frequent neuroendocrine pancreatic tumors, must be classified. The classification proposed by AJCC (American Joint Committee on Cancer) ENETS (European Neuroendocrine Tumor Society) for neuroendocrine pancreatic tumors is the following (Table 4):

AJCC	ENETS
Primary Tumor (T)	**Primary Tumor (T)**
TX Primary tumor cannot be assessed T0 No evidence of primary tumor T1 Tumor limited to the pancreas, <2 cm in greatest dimension T2 Tumor limited to the pancreas, >2 cm in greatest dimension T3 Tumor extends beyond the pancreas but without involvement of the celiac axis or the superior mesenteric artery T4 Tumor involves the celiac axis or the superior mesenteric artery (unresectable primary tumor)	TX Primary tumor cannot be assessed T0 No evidence of primary tumor T1 Tumor limited to the pancreas and size<2 cm T2 Tumor limited to the pancreas and size 2- 4 cm T3 Tumor limited to the pancreas and size > 4 cm or invading duodenum or bile duct T4 Tumor invading adjacent organs (stomach, spleen, colon, adrenal gland) or the wall of large vessels (celiac axis or superior mesenteric artery)
Regional lymph nodes (N)	**Regional lymph nodes (N)**
NX Regional lymph node(s) cannot be assessed N0 No regional lymph node metastasis N1 Regional lymph node metastasis	NX Regional lymph nodes cannot be assessed N0 No regional lymph node metastasis N1 Regional lymph node metastasis
Distant metastases (M)	**Distant metastases (M)**
M0 No distant metastasis M1 Distant metastasis	MX Distant metastasis cannot be assessed M0 No distant metastasis M1 Distant metastasis
Endocrine and Exocrine pancreas	**Endocrine and Exocrine pancreas**
Stage T N M	Stage T N M
0 T0 N0 M0	
IA T1 N0 M0	I T1 N0 M0
IB T2 N0 M0	
IIA T3 N0 M0	IIa T2 N0 M0
IIB T1 N1 M0 T2 N1 M0 T3 N1 M0	IIb T3 N0 M0
III T4 Any N M0	IIIa T4 N0 M0 IIIb Any T N1 M0
IV Any T Any N M1	IV Any T Any N M1

Table 4. Staging of TNEs of the pancreas according to AJCC and ENETs

The WHO has an alternative classification and staging for pancreatic neuroendocrine tumors, which considers also certain anatomopathological findings. The proliferative rate has been repeatedly shown to provide significant prognostic infromation for NETs. The proliferatice rate can be assessed as the number of mitosis per unit area of tumor (usually expressed as mitosis per 10 high power microscopic fields or 2mm) or as the percentage of neoplastic cells immunolabeling for the proliferation marker Ki-67. The use between mitotic count and Ki-67 is controversial. When the amount of tumor tissue is limited, it may not be able to perform an accurate mitotic count. In these cases Ki 67 staining provides a more accurate assessment of proliferative rate, and it is particularly helpful to separate well-differentiated tumors from poorly differentiated neuroendocrine carcinomas, which usually have dramatically different Ki 67 labelling rates. However, when adequate tissue is present to perform an accurate mitotic count, there are no data to demonstrate that the Ki67 labeling index adds important information, and in some cases, the two measures of proliferative rate may provide conflicting information about grading.(Table 5)

Grade (WHO)	Biological behavior	M1	Histology	Angio invasion	Primary tumor (cm)	Ki-67%	Mitotic count
1	Benign	-	Good differentiation	-	< 2	<2	<2
1	Undefined	-	Good differentiation	+/-	>2	2-5	<2
2	Malignancy low grade	+	Good differentiation	+	>3	5-15	2-10
3	Malignancy high grade	+	Poor differentiation	+	whatever	>15	>10

Table 5. WHO staging for pancreatic neuroendocrine tumors

9. Medical management of insulinoma related to hormone hypersecretion

Benign insulinomas, as well as malignant, usually produce high concentrations of insulin secretion developing the well-known hypoglycemic syndrome. Independently of their surgical possibilities, hypoglycemia must be controlled.

With insulinomas, dietary modification with frequent small feedings may help control hypoglycemia. Sometimes endovenous glucose infusion may be needed to maintain acceptable glucose levels usually in the preopreatory or when it is a high secreting malignant insulinoma. Glucose infusion must be done with care as patients may develop in rare cases acidosis secondary to large volumes of glucose infusion (Ramos,A., et al., 2010).

When diet modification does not control the symptoms, pharmacological treatment must be used. There are several pharmacological treatments the most frequently used is diazoxide followed by somatostatin analogues. (Hirshberg, B., et al 2005)

9.1 Diazoxide

Administration of diazoxide (200-600 mg/day) successfully controls hypoglycemia in 50 to 60 % of the patients. The most common side effect reported with diazoxide is hirsutism as well as nausea at higher dose administration. Also, diazoxide frequently leads to fluid

retention requiring diuretics such as triclormetiazide which not only counteracts this side-effect but has also a hyperglycemic effect.
Diazoxide enables the control of the hypoglycemia by two mechanisms: it inhibits insulin secretion by beta-cell pancreatic cells and it has a peripheral effect stimulating glucogenolisis. Treatment with diazoxide has proven to be efficient, including cases with nesidioblastosis in which surgery seemed to be a very radical option. In advanced metastatic disease in which surgery is not an option, diazoxide has demonstrated in some studies to be more effective in the symptomatic control at short-time.

9.2 Calcium antagonists and others

Calcium antagonists may also be useful controlling hypoglycemia because they inhibit insulin secretion by the blockage of the calcium receptor. There are some works on advanced metastatic disease that describe a better symptomatic control with verapamil added to the long-acting somatostatin analogues. On the other hand, the data of their use is limited, therefore limiting their use to cases with advanced disease in which other treatments are uneffective.
Other options to control hypoglycemia may be beta blockers, that can be useful, although they might be used with precaution as they can mask hypoglycemia symptoms. Other pharmacological treatments include phenytoin or glucagon. Glucocorticoids increase gluconeogenesis and create insulin resistance, so they can also be useful. The recommended dose is of 1mg/kg of prednisone.

9.3 Somatostatin analogues

Long-acting somatostatin analogues have proved to be a novel and very useful treatment in the control of hypoglycemia.
Lately the presence of somatostatin in pancreas islets and other areas of the digestive tract, as well as its inhibitory effect of the secretion of other hormones, such as insulin, its role as neurotransmisor or neuromodulator and cytostatic effect have been recognized. Somatostatin was therefore considered as a possible treatment for those endocrinological syndromes caused by excess hormone production. However, human somatostatin has a very short half-life effect, which made the development of what today we know as the long-acting somatostatin analogues.
Their main indication is in the preoperatory phase, or in cases of recurrence and malignancy. Also, although it is not their main indication, cases of complete resolution in benign insulinomas have been reported. These analogues function predominantly over subtype 2 somatostatin receptor and less over subtype 5, controlling therefore about 50% of the hypoglycemic events caused by insulinomas. The somatostatin subtype 5 receptor has been involved in insulin secretion and seems to be related with a more aggressive tumoral behavior. New somatostatin analogues are being developed with a greater affinity to this and other receptors such as BIM23244 and SOM230.An important aspect before starting the treatment of an insulinoma with somatostatin analogues is to analyze the possible efficacy by the performance of an Octreoscan or by demonstrating an improvement on glucose and insulin levels with short-acting somatostatin analogues. This is important because their use in tumors which do not express subtype 2 may worse the hypoglycemia by the inhibition of the contrarregulatory response of glucagon and growth hormone without affecting insulin secretion. Another possible problem when long-acting somatostatin analogues are used long-

term, is a desensibilization of the tumor by a decrease in the expression of the somatostatinreceptors. Initially this can be overwhelmed by increasing the dose of the analogue or decreasing the interval administration, but can cause at the end a therapeutic fail.

9.4 New agents to control hypoglycemia

Recent studies in small numbers of patients show that mTOR inhibitors, such as rapamycin or everolimus, may control hypoglycemia in patients with metastasic insulinomas.
Everolimus is an orally derivative of rapamycin that inhibits Ser/Thyrosine kinase mTOR. The PI3k/Akt/mTOR pathway has an important role in pancreatic cancer biology. It has demonstrated to have an antitumor activity, but its effects on pancreatic beta cells remains unclear. Data suggest that functional insulin receptors are present on beta cells and mediate insulin stimulated insulin production and release and that mTOR inhibition downstream of insulin receptors may decrease insulin production and release. It is also possible that everolimus induces insulin resistance peripherically.
Recent case series have reported malignant insulinomas with severe hypoglycemic syndrome who were able to cease, or significantly reduce symptoms after the introduction of everolimus.

MEDICAL THERAPY FOR UNCONTROLLED HYPOGLYCEMIA			
DRUG	CLASS	SYMPTOM CONTROL	ADVERSE EFFECTS
Diazoxide	Alpha adrenergic agonist	50-60% of patients	peripheral edema, nausea, hirsutism
Octeotride	Somatostatin analog	40-60% of patients	bloating, abdominal cramping, malabsorption, cholelithiasis
Verapamil	Calcium channel blocker	unknown	constipation, peripheral edema, nausea
Propranolol	Beta-blocker	unknown	bradycardia, depression, may potentiate hypoglycemia
Phenytoin	Anticonvulsivant	unknown	hypertrichosis, gingival, hypertrophy, peripheral neuropathy
Prednisone	Glucocorticoids	unknown	Cushingsyndrome
Glucagon	Glucagon	palliation	risk of rebound hypoglycemia

Table 6. Medical Therapy for Uncontrolled hypoglycemia

10. Surgical treatment of benign insulinoma or primary tumor

All experts agree that surgical resection of an insulinoma either benign or malignant should be considered whenever possible. Local resection or enucleation of the insulinoma is generally recommended, and more advanced surgical resections such as Whipple resections

are not routinely recommended and should be considered only in carefully selected patients. (Figure 7 and 8)
Generally pancreatic neuroendocrine tumors are surgically approached by a laparotomy to allow an extensive exploration of the entire abdomen and search for lymph node metastases. Insulinomas in non-MEN 1 with benign characteristics are increasingly being treated with a laparoscopic approach; in 85% of patients, there are single tumors, they are invariably intrapancreatic, and if they can be localized preoperatively, they can be cured in 70% to 100% using laparoscopic approach. At the present surgical cure rates for benign insulinomas approach 100%.

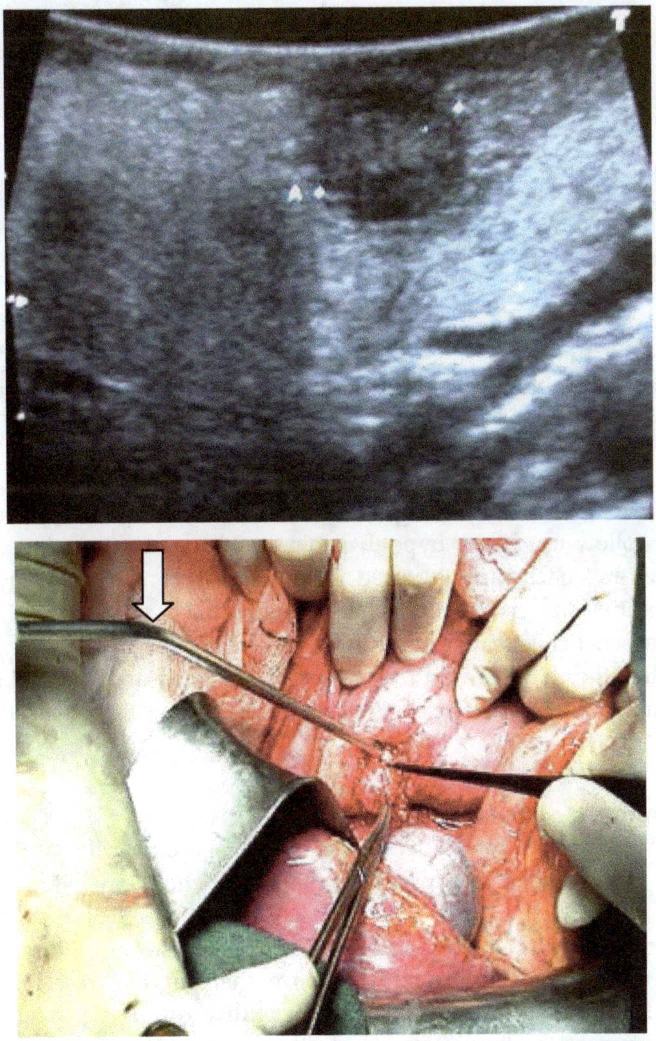

Fig. 7. Bening insulinoma. .Upper image:. Intraoperatory ultrasonography. .Lower image:. Enucleation of the same tumoral mass.

When clinical examinations including angiography stimulation suggest nesidioblastosis, a partial pancreatectomy is usually performed. Even if a frozen biopsy confirms the diagnosis of nesidioblastosis, the extent of pancreatic resection remains questionable. A distal pancreatectomy which can control the symptoms of the majority of patients, is well tolerated, and does not induce endocrine or exocrine insufficiency. Recovery after a partial pancreatectomy can remove enough abnormal proliferative tissue to achieve normoglycemia. However, some investigators recommend an initial near-total pancreatectomy. Such extensive resections lead to an increased risk of post-surgical diabetes and pancreatic insufficiency. It seems that the best recommendation is a 70%-80% pancreatectomy, administration of diazoxide when hypoglycemia persists post-operatively, and a more extensive resection when previous measures fail.

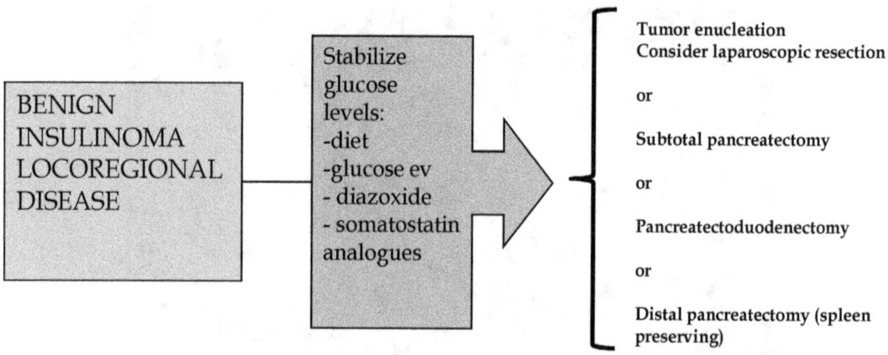

Fig. 8. Therapeutical algorithm for benign insulinoma or primary located disease

11. Additional management in advanced insulinomas

Malignant insulinomas, although unfrequent, may require multiple managements involving a mutidisciplinar follow-up. Firstly hypoglycemic syndrome must be adequately controlled. Secondly, surgical approach must be used if possible, to control metastasic and primary disease. When curative surgery is not possible, usually due to metastasic disease, debulking surgery is often a beneficial treatment for local (intestinal obstructions, etc.) and endocrine symptoms. On the other hand, when the disease is extended and surgical approach is not possible, other therapeutic options can be used depending on the organ affected.(Figure 9 and 10).

11.1 Surgical approach of metastasic disease

Hepatic resection is indicated for the treatment of metastasic liver disease in the absence of diffuse bilobar involvement, compromised liver function or extensive extrahepatic metastases.

However, the role of cytoreductive surgery in these cases is controversial. Whereas numerous uncontrolled studies provide evidence that surgical resection may improve symptom control and perhaps extend survival, neither result is proven at the present. Nevertheless, because of the low efficacies of other tumor treatments, most conclude that surgical resection should be attempted in any patient with a malignant insulinoma if it is thought that at least 90% of the visible tumor could be removed. Unfortunately, surgical resection of at least 90% of all visible tumor is possible only in 5% to 15% of patients with insulinoma and metastasic disease.

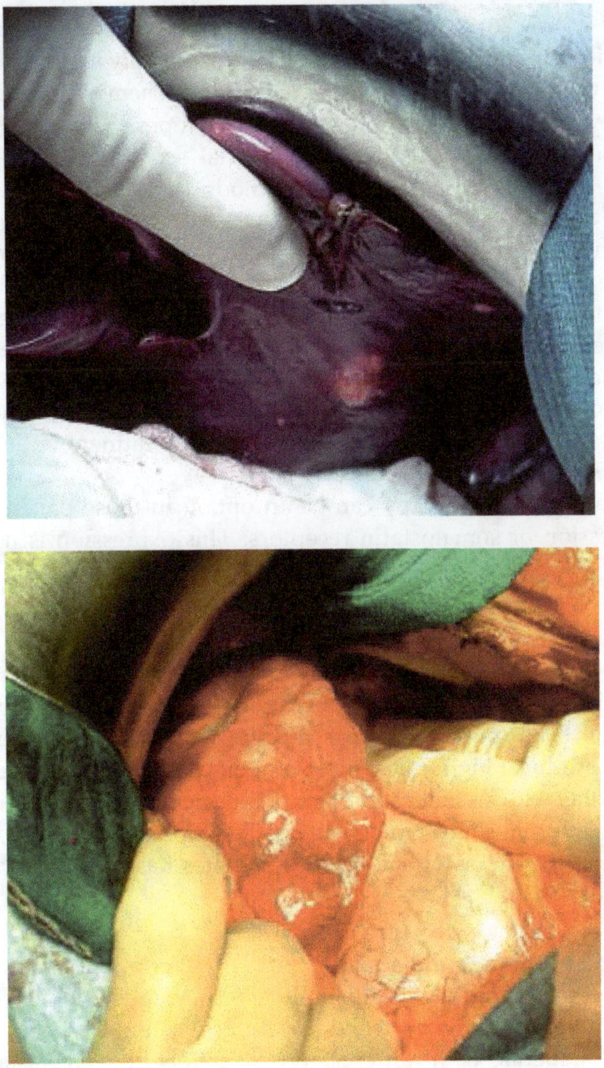

Fig. 9. Metastasic disease of insulinoma.Upper image: single hepatic metastases. Lower image: multiple hepatic metastases.

Transplantation for metastasic disease has been proposed for the occasional, younger patient with a metastasic insulinoma that is unresectable and limited to the liver, especially if it is symptomatic and cannot be controlled by other available therapies, that liver transplantation remains an option that should be considered.

11.2 Other invasive therapies

Hepatic artery embolization is recommended as a palliative option in patients with hepatic metastases who are not candidates for surgical resection, have an otherwise preserved performance status, have disease primarily confined to the liver, and have a patent portal vein. The response rates associated with embolizations, as measured either by decrease in hormonal secretion or by radiographic regression are generally greater than 50%. Improved

techniques have, in recent years, reduced the incidence complications related to embolization, making embolization an important and generally safe treatment. A number of techniques can be used and include bland embolization, chemoembolization, embolization with chemotherapy and embolization using radioisotopes. These techniques should be considered especially for a patient with a functional secreting insulinoma in which the hormone excess cannot be controlled by other methods. (O'Toole, D., et al 2005)
Other approaches to the treatment of hepatic metastases in a patient with malignant insulinoma include the use of radiofrequency and crioablation, either alone or in conjuction with cytoreductive surgery. These approaches can be performed using a percutaneous or laparoscopic approach. Although they seem to be less morbid than either hepatic resection or hepatic artery embolization, the clinical benefit of these approaches in patients with asymptomatic, small volume disease has not been clearly established. Similarly, these approaches may not be applicable in patients with large-volume hepatic metastases. Ablative techniques should therefore be considered as a treatment option only in carefully selected patients. (Steinmuller, T., et al 2008)
Peptide receptor radionuclide therapy can be an option in those pancreatic tumors which have an overexpression of somatostatin receptors. This expression is not frequent within insulinomas.

11.3 Radiotherapy

Experience with external beam radiotherapy in the management if islet tumor cells is limited. Although pancreatic neuroendocrine carcinomas were previously considered to be radioresistant, data from published case reports and small case series suggest that radiotherapy can produce high rates of symptom palliation and freedom from local progression in patients who are not candidates for surgical resection. There are no specifical data on the rate of symptom control in patients with symptomatic insulinomas.
However, radiotherapy with or without biphosphonates has proven to be highly useful in patients with painful bony metastases.

11.4 Traditional chemotherapeutic agents

A number of chemotherapeutic agents either alone or in combination have been reported to have sufficient antitumor activity to be clinically useful. Systemic chemotherapy is recommended for patients with unresectable liver or lung metastases. Trials using chemotherapeutic drugs including doxorubicin, streptoxocin, 5-FU, temozolamide, and dacarbazine have established cytotoxic effects in pancreatic tumors. The combination of doxorubicin and streptozocin has a reported 69% objective response rate in the treatment of patients with advances islet cell carcinoma. A retrospective review from the MD Anderson Center reported an objective response rate of 39% with the combination of 5FU, doxorubicin and streptozocin. Fine et al have reported on the synergy between capecitabine and temozolamide for the induction of apoptosis in neuroendocrine cell lines. Recently, an oral regimen using temozolamide and thalidomide was found to be useful in a number of neuroendocrine malignancies. (Kouvaraki, M., et al. 2004)

11.5 Newer agents

11.5.1 Biotherapy: Somatostatin analogues and interferon

Somatostatin analogues have a double purpose in the treatment of insulinomas, firstly they can control hypoglycemia and secondly they are used in those patients with advanced disease for their possible effect on tumor growth. The clinical benefit of the direct antineoplasic effects of somatostatin analogues either with or without interferon remains uncertain, although recent studies suggest they have a cytostatic effect in 40 to 70% of patients and cause a tumor reduction of less than 15% with both agents. This tumoristatic effect can be long lasting especially in those with low proliferative rate. (Plockinger, U., et al. 2007)

11.5.2 Anti-angiogenic treatments

Recent studies using vascular endothelial growth factor (VEGF) pathway inhibitors such as bevacizumab have suggested that these agents may have a modest antitumor activity in patients with malignant pancreatic tumors. Actually there are several active studies combining chemotherapy and bevacizumab in adavanced pancreatic NETs. However the recruited patients are small, and for the moment there are no specifical results for malignant insulinomas.

Sunitinib inhibits celular signaling by targeting multiple receptor tyrosine kinases. These include all receptors for platelet-derived growth factor (PDGF-Rs) and VEGF receptors, which play a role in both tumor angiogenesis and tumor cell proliferation. The simultaneous inhibition of these targets therefore leads to both reduced tumor vascularization and cancer cell death, and ultimately tumor shrinkage. In phase 1 and 2 trials, sunitinib showed antitumor activity in patients with pancreatic neuroendocrine tumors. A phase 3 has been recently conducted in well-differentiated pancretic neuroendocrine tumors in which the results were promising causing a discontinuation of the study. Median progression-free survival was 11.4 months in the sunitinib group as compared with 5.5 months in the placebo group (hazard ratio for progression or death, 0.42; 95% confidence interval [CI], 0.26 to 0.66; $P<0.001$). There are no results for the moment specifical in malignant insulinomas. (Raymond, E., et al 2011)

11.5.3 Inhibiton of m-TOR

Everolimus, an inhibitor of mTOR has also being study recently not only from the antihipoglycemic but also from the antitumoral point of view. Its efficacy has been studied combined with somatostatin analogues in neuroendocrine tumors. Considering insulinomas, the mean survival without progression was estimated in 63 weeks. (Yao et al., 2008). Considering other studies with pancreatic NETs in general, everolimus (at a dose of 10 mg/day) caused a 65% reduction in the estimated risk of progression (progression-free survival of 11 months with everolimus versus 4.6 months with placebo, $p< 0.001$). Confirmatory studies of these promising results are being performed.

12. Posttreatment surveillance

After the complete removal of the tumor, a patient with a benign insulinoma is cured, but periodic follow-up is necessary in those with metastasic insulinoma or multiple endocrine neoplasia type 1 (MEN1).

12.1 MEN 1

All patients with MEN 1 syndrome should be followed with every 3-6 months during the first year after resection with physical examination, tumoral markers and calcium levels as appropriate and with imaging studies such as CT/MRI. The follow-up tests must be repeated every 6 months, 1-3 years after surgery and annually thereafter.

All close family members of patients with MEN 1 should be genetically counseled and genetic testing should be considered.

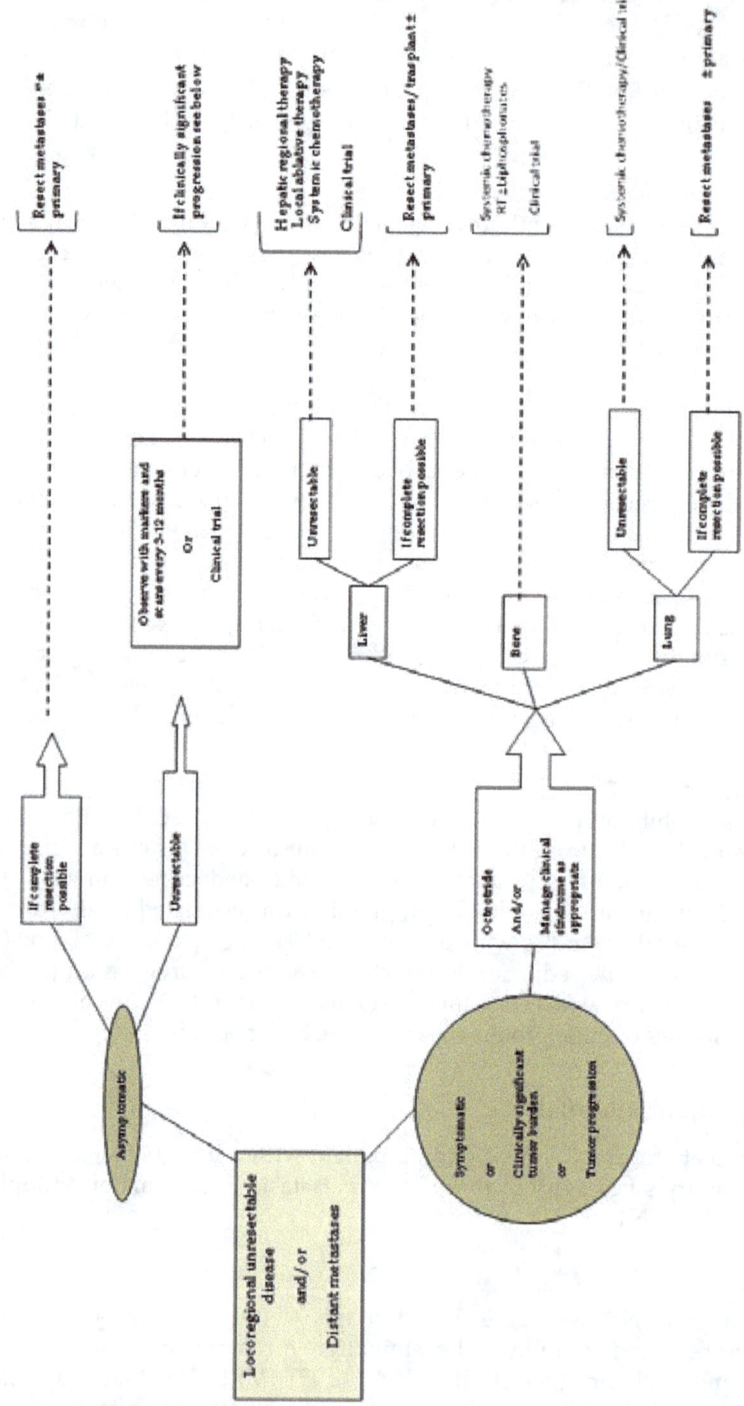

Fig. 10. Therapeutic algorithm of malignant insulinoma. Adapted from National Comprehensive Cancer Network, 2010.

12.2 Malignant insulinoma

There are no evidence-based guidelines for follow-up after resection of a malignant insulinoma. Consensus derived guidelines from the National Cancer Network following treatment of an islet cell tumor include the following:

- Three and six months postresection: history and physical examination, tumor markers (insulin) and CT/MRI.
- Long-term: history and physical examination with tumor markers every 6-12 months for years 1 to 3. Imaging studies are recommended only if clinically indicated.

13. Conclusions

Pancreatic beta cell tumors are a relatively rare cause of hypoglycemia. The suspicion of a probable insulinoma by the physician is important as the diagnosis of these tumors may be delayed up to 1-2 years and may be confused with other diseases such as neurological or psychiatric.

The diagnostic suspicion of an insulinoma is based on symptoms, and laboratory techniques usually confirm the diagnosis. The treatment, on the other hand, is usually surgery of the tumoral mass as complete as possible, including the primary tumor and metastases if present and possible. Imaging of the primary tumor location and the extent of the disease is needed for all phases of management of insulinomas, especially if they are malignant.

The development of new treatments based upon a better knowledge of the molecular pathways involved in tumorigenesis make the therapeutic future of these tumors promising, leading to a better prognosis in those with a more aggressive behavior.

On the other hand, the low incidence of these tumors makes especially important their management in specialized centers with experience and modern imaging and diagnostic techniques.

14. Acknowledgement

The authors want to thank Dr. Alberola and Dr.Rayon for the histological images lended.

15. References

Abellán, P., Cámara, R., Merino-Torres, JF., Pérez-Lázaro, A., del Olmo, MI., Ponce, JL., Rayón, JM., & Piñón, F. Severe hypoglycemia after gastric bypass surgery for morbid obesisty. *Diabetes Research and Clinical Practice,* Vol. 79, No.1, (January 2008), pp. e7-e9, 0168-8227.

Anderson, M., Carpenter, S., Thompson, NW., Nostrant, T., Elta, G., & Scheimann, JM. Endoscopic ultrasound is highly accurate and directs management in patients with neuroendocrine tumors of the pancreas. *The American Journal of Gastroenterology,* Vol.95, No.9, (April 2000), pp. 2271-2277, 0002-9270.

Arnold, A. (2009). Pathogenesis of Endocrine Tumors, In: *Williams Textbook of Endocrinology,* Kronenberg, H., Melmed, S., Polonsky, K., & Larsen, R., pp. 1713-1720, Elsevier Saunders, 978-1-4160-2911-3, United States.

Assalia, A., & Gagner, M. Laparoscopic pancreatic surgery for islet cell tumors of the pancreas. *World Journal Surgery,* Vol. 28, No.12, (December 2004), pp.1239-1247, 0364-2313.

Brandi, ML., Gagel, R., Angeli, A., Bilezikian, JP., Beck-Peccoz, P. Bordi, C., Conte-Devolx, B., Falchetti, A., Gheri, RG., Libroia, A., Lips, CJ., Lombardi, G., Mannelli, M., Pacini, F., Ponder, BA., Raue, F., Skogseid, B., Tamburrano, G., Thakker, RV., Thompson, NW., Tomassetti, P., Tonelli, F., Wells, SA., & Marx, SJ., Guidelines for diagnosis and therapy of MEN type 1 and type 2. *The Journal of Clinical Endocrinology & Metabolism,* (August, 2001), Vol.86, No. 12, pp. 56-58, 0021-972X.

Cryer, P. (2009). Glucose Homeostasis and Hypoglycemia, In: *Williams Textbook of Endocrinology,* Kronenberg, H., Melmed, S., Polonsky, K., & Larsen, R., pp. 1519-1550, Elsevier Saunders, 978-1-4160-2911-3, United States.

Gagel, R., & Marx, S. (2009). Multiple Endocrine Neoplasia, In: *Williams Textbook of Endocrinology,* Kronenberg, H., Melmed, S., Polonsky, K., & Larsen, R., pp. 1721-1762, Elsevier Saunders, 978-1-4160-2911-3, United States.

Gomez, JM., & Soler, J.(2002) Prueba de ayuno, In: *Manual de Pruebas Funcionales de Endocrinología,* Gomez, JM & Soler, J, pp.107-109, Septem Ediciones, 84-95687-37-2, Spain.

Hirshberg, B., Livi, A., Batlett, DL., Libutti, SK.., Alexander, HR., Doppman, MC., Skarulis, MC., & Gorden, P. Forty-Eight-Hour Fast: The Diagnostic Test for Insulinoma. *The Journal of Clinical Endocrinology & Metabolism,* Vol.85, No.9, (June 2000), pp.3222-3226, 0021-972X.

Hirshberg, B., Cochran, C., Skarulis, MC., Libutti, SK., Alexander, HR., Wood, BJ., Hang, R., Kleiner, DE., & Gorden, P. Malignant insulinoma: spectrum of unusual clinical features. *Cancer,* Vol. 104, No.2, (2005), pp.264-272, 1097-0142.

Imamura, M., Hattori, Y., Nishida, O., Honda, T., Shimada, Y., & Miyahara, T. Unresponsiveness of insulinoma cells to secretin: significance of the secretin test in patients with insulinoma. *The Journal of Clinical Endocrinology and Metabolism.* Vol. 74, (1992), pp.467-473, 0021-972X.

Jensen, R.(2002), Tumores endocrinos del tubo digestive y del páncreas, In: *Harrison: Principios de Medicina Interna,* Braunwald, E., Fauci, A., Kasper, D., Hauser, D., Longo, D., & Jameson, L., pp.701-714, Mc Graw Hill, 84-486-0665-5, Spain.

Jonkers, YMH., Ramaekers, FCS., & Speel, EJM. Molecular alterations during insulinoma tumorigenesis. *Biochimica et Biophysica Acta,* 1775, (May 2007), pp 313-332, 0167-4838, 0378-1119.

Marazuela, M., Martin-Perez, E., Larrañaga, E., Caniego, JL., Lopez-Iglesias, M., & Gómez-Pan, A. Diagnóstico y tratamiento del insulinoma: nuestra experiencia en 10 casos. *Endocrinología y Nutrición,* Vol.52, No.7, pp.338-343, 1575-0922

Klimstra, D., Modlin, I., Coppola, D., Lloyd, R., & Suster, S. The pathologic classification of Neuroendocrine tumors: A review of Nomenclature, Grading and Staging Systems. *Pancreas,* Vol.39, No.6, (August 2010), pp.707-712, 0885-3177.

Komminoth, P., Perren, A., Öberg, A., Rindi G., Heitz, U., & Klöppel G. (2004). Insulinoma, In: *World Health Classification of Tumours. Pathology and genetics of tumours of endocrine organs,* DeLellis, RA., Lloyd, RV., & Heitz, PU., pp.183-187, IARC press, 92 832 2416 7, Lyon.

Koopmans, K., Neels, O., Kema, I., Elsinga, P., Sluiter, W., Vanghillewe, K., Brouwers, A., Jager, P., & de Vries, E. Improved Staging of Patients with carcinoid and islet cell tumors with 18F-dihydroxy-phenyl-alanine and 11C-5-hydroxy-tryptophan positron emission tomography. *Journal of Clinical Oncology,* Vol.26, No.9, (March 2008), pp. 1489-1495, 0732-183X.

Kouvaraki, M., Ajani, J., Hoff, P., Wolff, R., Evans, DB., Lozano R., & Yao, C. Fluouracil, doxorubicin and streptozocin in the treatment of patients with locally advanced and metastatic pancreatic endocrine carcinomas. *Journal of Clinical Oncology.* Vol. 22, No.23, (December 2004), pp.4762-4771, 0732-183X.

Kouvaraki, MA., Shapiro, SE., Cote, GJ, Lee, JE., Yao, JC., Waguespack, SG., Gagel, RF., Evans, DB., & Perrier, ND. Management of pancreatic endocrine tumors in multiple endocrine neoplasia type 1. *World Journal Surgery,* Vol.30, No 5, (April 2006), pp.643-653, 0364-2313.

Kulke, M., Anthony, L., Bushnell, D., de Herder, W., Goldsmith, S., Klimstra, D., Marx, S., Pasieka, J., Pommier, R., Yao, J., & Jensen, R. NANETS Treatment Guidelines: Well-differentiated Neuroendocrine Tumors of the Stomach and Pancreas. *Pancreas,* Vol. 39, No.6, (August 2010), pp. 735-752, 0885-3177.

National Comprehensive Cancer Network (NHHN, 2010). NCCN Clinical Practice Guidelines in Oncology: Neuroendocrine Tumors. V.I.2010.

Placzkoski, KA., Vella, A., Thompson, GB., Grant, CS., Reading, CC., Charboneau, JW., Andrews, JC., Lloyd, RV., & Service, FJ. Secular Trends in the presentation and management of functioning insulinoma at the Mayo Clinic, 1987-2007. *The Journal of Clinical Endocrinology and Metabolism,* Vol. 94, No.4, (April 2009), pp. 1069-1073, 0021-972X.

Plockinger, U., Wiedenmann, B. Neuroendocrine tumors. Biotherapy. *Best Practice & Research: Clinical Endocrinology & Metabolism.*Vol.21, No.1, (March 2007), pp. 145-162,1521-690X

Ramos-Prol, A., del Olmo-Garcia, MI., Pérez-Lázaro, A., Caballero-Soto, M., Argente-Pla, A., León de Zayas, B., & Merino-Torres, JF. Metabolic acidosis as a complication of intravenous dextrose administration in a patient with insulinoma. *Endocrine,* Vol 38, (October 2010), pp.402-405, 0969-711X.

Raymond, E., Dahan, L., Raoul, JL., Bang, YJ., Borbath, I., Lombard-Bohas, C., Valle, J., Metrakos, P., Smith, D., Vinik, A., Chen, JS., Hörsch, D., Hammel, P., Wiedenmann, B., Van Custem, E., Patyna, S., Ray Lu, D., Blanckmeister, C., Chao, R., & Ruszeniewski, P. Sunitinib Malate for the Treatment of Pancreatic Neuroendocrine Tumors. *The New England Journal of Medicine,* Vol. 364, No.6, (February 2011), pp. 501-513, 0028-4793.

Rockall, AG., & Reznek, RH. Imaging of neuroendocrine tumours (CT/MR/US). *Best Practice & Research: Clinical Endocrinology & Metabolism.*Vol.21,No.1, (March 2007), pp. 141-148,1521-690X

Semelka, RC., Custodio,CM., CemBalci, BN., & Woosly, JC. Neuroendocrine tumors of the pancreas: spectrum of appearances on MRI. *Journal of Magnetic Resonance Imaging.* Vol.11, No.2, (February 2000), pp.141-148, 1053-1807.

Service, FJ., McMahon, MM., O'Brien, PC., & Ballard, DJ., Functioning insulinoma: incidence, recurrence, and long term survival of patients: a 60-year study. *Mayo Clinic Proceedings,* Vol.66, (July 1991), pp. 711-719, 0025-6196.

Service, FJ., O'Brien, PC., Kao, PC., & Young, WF. C-peptide suppression test: effects of gender, age and body mass index; implications for the diagnosis of insulinoma. *The Journal of Clinical Endocrinology and Metabolism.* Vol,74, (1992), pp.204-210, 0021-972X.

Service, FJ. Diagnostic approach to adults with hypoglycemic disorders. *Endocrinology and metabolism clinics of North America.* Vol. 28, No.3, (September 1999), pp. 519-532, 0889-8529.

Sherman, S., Gagel, R. (2002). Trastornos que afectan a sistemas endocrinos múltiples, In: *Harrison: Principios de Medicina Interna,* Braunwald, E., Fauci, A., Kasper, D., Hauser, D., Longo, D., & Jameson, L., pp.2555-2563, Mc Graw Hill, 84-486-0665-5, Spain.

Sheth, S., Hruban, R., & Fishman, E. Helical CT of islet cell tumors of the pancreas: Typical and Atypical Manifestations. *American Journal of Roetgenology.* Vol. 179, N0.3, (September, 2002), pp. 725-730, 0361-803X.

Starke, A., Saddig, C., Mansfeld, L., Koester, R., Tschahargane, C., Czygan, P., & Goretzki, P. Malignant metastasic insulinoma: postoperative treatment and follow-up. *World Journal of Surgery.* Vol. 29, (May 2005), pp. 789-793, 0364-2313.

Steinmuller, T., Kianmanesh, R., Falconi, M., Scarpa, A., Taal, B., Kwekkeboom, D., Lopes, JM., Perren, A., Nikou, G., Yao, J., Delle Fave, GF., O'Toole, D., & other Frascati Conference Participants. Consensus guidelines for the management of patients with liver metastases from digestive (neuro)endocrine tumors: foregut, midgut, hindgut, and unknown primary. *Neuroendocrinology,* Vol. 87, (November 2008), pp.47-62, 1423-0194.

O' Toole, D., Ruszniewski, P. Chemoembolization and other ablative therapies for liver metastases of gastrointestinal endocrine tumours. *Best Practice & Research: Clinical Endocrinology & Metabolism.*Vol.19, No.4, (August 2005), pp. 585-594,1521-690X

Thoeni, R., Mueller-Lisse, UG., Chan R., Ky Do, R., & Shyn, PB. Detection of small, functional islet cell tumors in the pancreas: selection of MR imaging sequences for optimal sensitivity. *Radiology,* 214, (February 2000), pp. 483-490, 0033-8419.

Thompson, GB., Service, FJ., Andrews, JC., Lloyd, RV., Natt, N., van Heerden, JA., & Grant, CS. Noninsulinoma pacreatogenous hypoglycemia syndrome: an uptake in 10 surgically treated patients. *Surgery,* Vol. 128, No.6, pp.937-944, ISSN.

Vaidakis, D., Karoubalis, J., Pappa, T., Piaditis, G., & Zografos, G. Pancreatic insulinoma: current issues and trends. *Hepatobiliary & Pancreatic Diseases International,* Vol.9, No.3, (June 2010), 1499-3872.

Vinik, A., Woltering, E., Warner, R., Caplin, M., O'Dorisio, T., Wiseman, G., Coppola, D., & Go, VL. NANETS Consensus Guidelines for the diagnosis of Neuroendocrine Tumor. *Pancreas,* Vol.39, No.6, (August 2010), pp. 713- 734, ISSN 0885-3177.

Virgolini, I., Traub-Weidinger, T., Decristoforo C. Nuclear medicine in the detection and management of pancreatic Islet-cell tumours. *Best Practice & Research: Clinical Endocrinology & Metabolism.*Vol.19,No.2, (June 2005), pp. *213-227,*1521-690X

Yao, J., Phan, A., Chang, D., Wolff, R., Hess, K., Gupta, S., Jacobs, C., Mares, J., Landgraf, A., Rashid, A., & Meric-Bernstam, F. Efficacy of RAD001 (everolimus) and Octeotride LAR in Advanced-Low-to intermediate -Grade Neuroendocrine tumors: results of phase II study. *Journal of Clinical Oncology,* Vol.26, No.26, (September 2008), pp. 4311-4319, 0732-183X.

Part 5

Section E

13

Hypoglycemia Caused by Septicemia in Pigs

Everlon Cid Rigobelo and Fernando Antonio de Ávila
Universidade Estadual Paulista,Campus Experimental de Dracena
Faculdade de Ciências Agrárias e Veterinárias de Jaboticabal
Brazil

1. Introduction

Swine production is continuously improving the quality of its products although of your living together with carcass fat content. The strategy of industry is offers natural products as special cuts semi prepared food. Others questions are the swine importance for Human medicine is related the products that are makes from swine used in Humans. The great variety of products originated of swine and used in Human medicine and mainly the use of organs as skin, cardiac valves for transplant shall to be interpreted as result of similarly that there is between the organisms: human and swine.

The pancreas swine is an organ that itself get insulin. This hormone is essentials for diabetics. It allows the entry of glucose in the cells and also decreases its fee in the blood avoiding that way that the glucose levels becomes fatal.

Other utility of pancreas of swine for Human is in the supply of pancreatic islets for implants into diabetic peoples that haven´t. These implants will let the diabetics free of injections of insulin for many years. Actually the insulin is also made by genetic engineering through bacterial multiplication.

The pituitary gland of swine is used for get of ACTH. This hormone is used in human medicine for treatment of arthritis and inflammatory diseases that causes great suffering for many peoples in worldwide.

The thyroid of swine is used for get medicaments that will be used by peoples that have thyroid glands with lower actives.

The skin of swine may to be used temporally by Human in cases of burn that causes great discontinuity of your skin.

The gut mucosa of swine is used for obtaining of a substance called Heparin. This substance has function of blood clotting and is applied in Human medicine in hemorrhagic cases.

The heart of swine is used for get the cardiac valves that will may be transplanted in adults and also into children. The swine used for provide these valves weight of 16 to 25 Kg. Theses valves are withdraw of heart and conserved in the chemical preparation and they can be preserved for five years. The cardiac valves of Human can be replaced by mechanic valves made with artificial materials. The swine valves however have advantage on this mechanics on this account are less rejected by organism and have similar structure of valves human and also resist more against infections.

Modified genetically swine can produce Human hemoglobin (blood pigment that takes the oxygen for the all the body). In current researchers were injected three embryos of swine with copy of two genes responsible for producing of human hemoglobin. The technique made with that 15% of hemoglobin found was of human type. The two hemoglobins may be after separate by difference of electric charge. This product can to be stocked by months to the contrary of normal blood that itself conserve just for one week.

By similarity among swine and Human is being possible the realization of all events cited above. Also by similarity among both our study will has as focus the monitoring of some biochemical parameters into an experimental infection caused by *Leptospira interrogans wolffi* sorovar in eight swine. The biochemical parameters were tracked during 36 days. The main parameter analyzed was the glucose fee during all occurrence of septicemia. This chapter also will discuss the relation of occurrence of hypoglycemia caused by the septicemia in pigs that collaborates with critical condition of animal leading it the die.

2. Some drawbacks of swine

The swine when are produced without hygienic conditions can represent a high risk for several diseases. The medical science considers that swine can to be host of many parasites and potential diseases. The meat of swine may content dangers toxins, vermin and latent diseases. Many theses infestations are found also in others animals, but some veterinary said that swine are more predisposed that the others animals, on this account are opportunist and highly omnivores with extensive feeding and including virtually any type of food comestible.

The swine meat contains amount of fat similar with others meat as birds and bovine and also it is responsible by nourish million of people in worldwide. Other advantage of consuming of swine meat is the great amount of protein for that the swine meat has both an economic and of public health. It is the meat further consumed in the worldwide allowed survival of many peoples.

However the swine meat also may forward many diseases as *Leptospira interrogans wolfii* sorovar.

The septicemia is an infection in the bloodstream. It appears when an infection is occurring in the people; this may be into the lungs, abdomen, and urinary routes or in the skin. The infections may also occur after a surgery in an infected area or in a body part that is colonized by many bacteria as for example the gut.

During the septicemia occurrence are found three distinct processes hence interconnected that occurs together as infectious focus hemodynamic changes and inflammatory answers local and generalized. The treatment of sick with septicemia is made with antibiotic and drugs that interfere in cardiac changes without intervene in inflammatory answers can be this reason of right mortality of patients with septic shock. Moreover still not has been established contribution of each inflammatory mediator in lethally resultant of septic shock.

3. Sepsis pathophysiology

The sepsis is defined as systemic inflammatory answers syndrome caused mainly by bacterial infections although also may be caused by fungus helminthes and virus. The infections caused by gram negatives bacteria are the further frequent, despite of last decade have been an increased of cases of sepsis due gram positive bacteria. The definition of sepsis included sepsis and also similar diseases from of causes noninfectious as trauma ischemia, burning, pancreatitis and hemorrhage.

The inflammatory response represents an important component of sepsis because elements of the response drive the physiological changes that become manifest as the systemic

inflammatory response syndrome. The inflammatory response eliminates the invading microorganism without to cause damage to issues, organs or other systems.
Abnormalities in the coagulation system resulting from systemic diseases which cause local disturbances in homeostasis and the thrombotic potential of cancer patients have been described since the time of Virchow.
Virchow´s classic triad consists of changes in coagulability endothelial cell injury and abnormal blood flow to vital organs. In septic patients, all three classic changes are present and culminate in reduced blood flow to vital organs.
Septic patients frequently have poor tissue perfusion and addition to inappropriate use of oxygen with resulting cytopathic hypoxia. The coagulation abnormalities in septic patients are profound and have led to a successful; Food and Drug Administration approved therapeutic intervention activated protein C.
The sepsis occurs when patients present hyperthermia or hypothermia, tachycardia, total white cell blood number upper of 12.000/mm^3 or below of 4.000/mm^3 or with further of 10% of immature forms. A lesion of sepsis that may arise is due the dysfunction of syndrome of multiple organs that affects approximately 30% of patients with sepsis while almost all develop dysfunction of an organ. The septic shock is characterized by high hemodynamic changes.
The clinical manifestations of sepsis are fever hypercoagulation and periferic hypotension caused by release of inflammatory mediators by immune and endothelial cells. The triggering factors cellular activation and of cascade of events of plasma are components of cell wall of this organisms lipoteichoic acid and peptidoglycan derivatives of gram positive bacterial or the lipopolysaccharide of gram negative bacterial. The lipopolysaccharide (LPS) is a molecule composed by hydrophilic polysaccharide chain divided in O antigen and core lipid A portion. The lipid A is a conserved region of toxin being responsible by your toxicity. The LPS importance in the triggering of sepsis was demonstrated after your administration in healthy Humans propagation of hemodynamic changes in patients with sepsis in experimental models.

3.1 Hyperinflammatory response

The sepsis is directly related with the high production of pro-inflammatory molecules. This problem have as result a rather simple when the inflammation is excessive. Usually this occurs in three cases. First, in septic patients with increased levels of specific mediators such as tumor necrosis factor (TNF) are at increased risk for death. Second, injection of TNF molecules at experimental animals results in widespread inflammatory changes. Third, experimental animals injected with a lethal doses of endotoxin elevated levels of the same mediators. The inhibition of these specific mediators improves survival in endotoxin shock models.
Whereas under normal conditions the endothelium exhibits antithrombotic properties by expressing tissue factor pathway inhibitors thrombomodulin surface releasing tissue factor during pathogenesis sepsis.Endothelial cells respond to LPS through toll like receptor followed by the release of pro-inflammatory cytokines such as interleukin - 6 (IL-6) and monocyte chemoattractant protein-1 and increased expression of adhesion molecules including intracellular adhesion molecule and vascular cell adhesion molecule.
The expression levels of cytokines and cell adhesion molecules are regulated by factor in inflammation.

4. Experimental models

4.1 Intravenous administration of live bacteria or bacterial components

Intravenous administration of LPS (endotoxemia) or of bacterial as *E. coli* widely used for sepsis study, as for example, the hemodynamic changes and cardiac, decrease of urine output, reduction of tissue perfusion, hyporesponsiveness vasoconstrictor agents, disseminated coagulation and production of large amount of cytokines in the circulation. Moreover is a practice model and reproducible in many species as mouse, rabbit, dogs, primate and including Humans. However the incidence of sepsis and septic shock in the clinic is due the entry of large amounts of LPS or of bacteria in the circulation same when amounts this bacterium is small. This puts in doubt effectiveness of this model.

4.2 Intraperitoenal administration of live bacteria or microbial components

This model also is very used for study of sepsis for reproduce of signs observed in diseases presented reproducibility as observed in endotoxemia model. Furthermore the administration of LPS or bacterial in the peritoneal cavity itself close of sepsis situation observed in the clinic because the process itself start from infectious focus or of dissemination of LPS administrated in the peritoneal cavity and not in the circulation. Even so, the start of process occurs rapidly and not gradually as happens in the majorly of clinic cases.

4.3 Gut injury model with consecutive release of microbial flora

The injury model with release microbial flora is the further similar to the sepsis situation in Humans, arising of traumas with perforations of gut, colitis or postoperative peritonitis. In this model after perforation of intestinal wall occurs the gradual liberation of contents causing peritonitis that may to evolve for a sepsis and septic shock.

Although this model is near the clinical and for that to be model further interesting for a study of sepsis the majority of studies in experimental sepsis is based into models where the bacterial or the LPS are administrated by IV or IP. The literature data shown that the pathogeneses of sepsis caused by LPS or bacterial IV differs those induced by an infectious focus as happens into peritonitis. The difference of results these models is due the amount of stimulus to the local and also administration form inducing the distinct kinetic of liberation of inflammatory mediators.

The biological activities of endotoxin and exotoxin are due of active of serum systems of endothelial cells and also leucocytes. Consequently the this infectious process occurs the syntheses or release of endogen mediators as cytokines, radioactive oxygen of nitrogen and lipid mediators being the activation of inflammatory cells the predominant factor for the development of sepsis.

The introduction of an object as an intravenous catheter, a urinary catheter or drainage-tube also may cause septicemia. The probability of septicemia increases with the time during the period that the object remains placed. This situation usually occurs between the people drugs dependents.

4.4 Relationship among hypoglycemia and septicemia

In septicemia the homeostasis finds itself threatened by invaders microorganisms. The body reacts to the challenge establishing a complex response: first prioritizing the supply of energy for vital organs, second, stimulating immune system and after stimulating the return of homeostasis.

When an infection occurs the cells need of glucose to synthesize defense molecules and also increases your metabolism in result of all changes physiological and morphological caused by the diseases. This result in a hypoglycemia by increase of consume of glucose by tissues. In majority of domestic animals during a septicemia occurs a hypoglycemia. This hypoglycemia caused by septicemia increases much the severity of diseases and also is the great responsible by high mortality in these situations.
Changes of hepatic gluconeogenesis and a depletion in glycogen content at liver is responsible by changes of glucose homeostasis this occurs by metabolic hallmarks in shock and sepsis. The shock and sepsis-induced glucose dyshomeostasis is characterized by an initial hyperglycemia followed by a progressive hypoglycemia.
The depletion in hepatic glycogen content following endotoxin administration is associated with an increase in glycogen phosphorylase coupled with a decrease in glycogen synthase activities.
The endotoxin-induced changes in glucose metabolism are augmented by the in vivo treatment of animals with protein kinase C (PKC) activator, PMA, while they are antagonized by PKC inhibitors, H7 and polymyxin B. The PKC plays a pivotal role in the pathogenesis of altered hepatic glucose homeostasis in shock and sepsis. Since the available information regarding the involvement of PKC in glucoregulatory disturbances in shock and sepsis derived mainly from the use of activators or inhibitors of PKC.
Previous studies demonstrated that cystolic PKC activity was inactivated during late phase of sepsis in rat liver. During the sepsis, the CLP-induced septic rat model used exhibited two metabolically distinct phases: an initial hyperglycemic and a subsequent hypoglycemic phase.
The finding some authors showed that cytosolic PKC activity was inactivated during late stage of sepsis may have a pathophysiological significance in contributing to the development of hypoglycemia during late phase of sepsis.
The kinetic analysis of the data showed by some authors indicated that the Vmax for PM Ca2+ pump was decreased by 42% while the Km value for Ca2+ remained unaffected.
The similarity in the patterns of change in the kinetics between the PKC-mediated phosphorylation of PM Ca2+- ATPase and the sepsis-induced impairment of PM Ca2+ transport strongly suggests that the impairment in Ca2+ transport by rat liver PM during late sepsis is a result of inactivation of PKC. Thus, a decrease in cytosolic PKC activity, as reported in this study, would impair PM Ca2+ transport, impede Ca2+ efflux, and hence elevating intracellular Ca2+ in hepatocytes during late phase of sepsis.

5. Hypoglycemia

The hypoglycemia is a disorder where the glucose serum concentration finds itself usually low.
Usually the organism keeps the serum glucose concentration in a range of 70 to 110 mL/deciliter of blood. In hypoglycemia the glucose concentration remains low. This results in a malfunction of brain that is sensitive the low glucose serum concentration because the glucose is the main energetic source of brain. It reacts through of nervous system and stimulates the adrenal glands to release epinephrine. This hormone stimulates the liver to release glucose for adjust the glucose concentration into the blood. When the concentration becomes very low the brain function may be damaged.
The hypoglycemia has several different causes between them the excessive secretion of insulin by pancreas an excessive dose of drugs for reduce the glucose serum concentration, an abnormality in the pituitary or of adrenal or an alteration of carbohydrate storage or into

the production of glucose by liver. Generally the hypoglycemia may be classified as related with drugs or no related. The majority of hypoglycemia cases related into diabetic people are related with drugs.

The hypoglycemia that is not related with drugs may be subdivided into fasting and reactive. In this case a reaction occurs to the carbohydrate ingested. Further frequently the hypoglycemia is caused by insulin or others drugs as sulfonylurea that are administered to the diabetic peoples for reduce the glucose serum concentration. When the dose is very high for the food ingested, the drug may cause an excessive reduction of glucose serum concentration.

The people with severe diabetics are particularly prone for the severe hypoglycemia. This occurs because the pancreatic islet cells not produce normally glucagon and the adrenal not produce normally epinephrines that are main mechanisms for combat the low glucose serum concentration. Some drugs that are not used for treatment of diabetics especially the pentamidine used for treat a type of pneumonic related with the SIDA may cause hypoglycemia.

Sometimes the hypoglycemia is observed into people with psychological disorders by administer insulin in themselves or oral hypoglycemic. The people that may present these types of behavior are those that have access to the drugs as health professional or diabetic's family.

The alcohol consumption into people that drink heavily without consuming food by long period may cause a severe hypoglycemia by stupor.

A long fasting only leads a hypoglycemia when the people are carriers of other diseases especially pituitary diseases or of adrenal or when this people consumes a large amount of alcohol. The neonates that present problems often of hypoglycemia need be investigated as to the metabolism functioning of carbohydrates or amino acids mainly when that occurs in the diseases absence diagnosed as septicemia and endotoxin. When the neonates present hypoglycemia periodically is necessary suspect of glycogen storage diseases when this clinical is accompanied of hepatomegaly, acidosis and ketosis

When the animal present hypoglycemia by result of a hydrolytic complication your probability to die increases in up to eight times in septicemia situations. The metabolic homeostasis need be maintained in neonates because the hypoglycemia may cause neurological damage when it isn´t identified

The carbohydrates reserves of liver may decrease into very low level that people cannot keep a glucose serum concentration appropriate. Some people with liver dysfunction into only some hours of fasting may cause hypoglycemia. The infants and children with an alteration of either of liver enzymatic systems that metabolize the glucose may present hypoglycemia between the meals. Others people that were submitted the certain types of gastric surgery present hypoglycemia between the meals, the alimentary hypoglycemia, a reactive hypoglycemia type. The hypoglycemia occurs because the glucose is quickly absorbed stimulating the excessive insulin production. The high insulin concentration causes a rapid drop of glucose serum concentration. Rarely the alimentary hypoglycemia occurs in people not submitted for gastric surgery.

The hypoglycemia may be due a kidney or heart failure, a cancer, malnutrition, pituitary or adrenal dysfunction or shock an infection serious.

6. Hypoglycemia in animals

Some studies realized in rats in 4 day old monitoring the glucose levels during seizures the authors reported that the metabolic cerebral balance during sustained seizures suggests that energy balance may be maintained in hyperglycemic animals and its decline occurs slowly in normoglycemia, but this not occurs while the animal have more old. The results suggest that the hypoglycemia in old animals can become critical when associated with other types or metabolic stress. The differences are reflecting in cerebral energy metabolism. In adult animals the ATP keeps whether invariable. This decline is rapid when the animals are convulsing and slower when the systemic effects of anoxia and convulsions are prevented by paralysis and oxygenation.

The hypoglycemia is characterized by low levels of blood glucose. Against the hypoglycemia in the individual is involved the release of glucagon, norepinephrine, cortisol, epinephrine and growth hormone. These elements are related with limit glucose utilization. The main stimulus for increase of glucose production is the glucagon and it is also a response to insulin induced hypoglycemia in the normal individual. When individual has diabetes its cells are more prone to low blood sugar due the abnormalities in the cell response in relation to hypoglycemia. Some studies verified using a conscious catheterized dog model that the hypoglycemia increased glucagon´s ability overcame the inhibitory effect of insulin on hepatic glucose production.

The glucagon is main defense against a low blood glucose level. The insulin exerts a great effect on glucagon´s action. The some studies have showed that the glucagon can have such a prominent role in counterregulation.

7. Leptospirose interrogans wolffi sorovar

Adolf Weil in 1882 described the diseases that He observed in two situations involved four patients in 1870. The clinical signs were similar and much private at patients. The disease was characterized by sudden appearance, high fever, splenomegaly and icterus.

In 1881 in Praga city, Weiss described the disease called "*icterus catarrhalis*" that probably will be the disease of Weil. Globig in 1890 described the "Badeepidemie" the disease that showed a great differ when compared to disease of Weil. In 1891, F. Muller described the *Schlamfieberepidemie* in chleisen the disease with symptoms much similar. Rimpau et al., described *Feldfieber* in which was the name that descrived the Leptospirose not icterus. The Lepiospirose was recognized with different names including bilious typhus by Weil others authors called it of Weil disease, icterus infectious.

The agent was isolated by first time, in Japan, in 1915 by Inada & Ito. The researchers isolated Leptospira of minas workers called *Spirochaeta icterohaemorrhagiae.*

In 1915, Uhlenhut & Fromme, showed the existence of etiologic agent, inoculating the army blood suspect of have Weil disease in guineas pigs. The animals inoculated died and Leptospira were identified microscopically, being called of *Spirochaeta icterohaemorrhagiae.* Miyajima, Ido, Hoki, Ito & Wani (1917) demonstrated that mouses were carriers of leptospira showed that 40% them were renal carriers.

8. General characteristics

The cells are flexible helical with 0.1 μm of diameter and 6-20μm of length. They are faintly stained by aniline days. The cells not cored are visible by contrast microscopy or by darkfield microscopy. The helical conformation is to right side (clock spring) existing in one or both extreme typical hook. Two perisplasmatic flagella (fibril axial and endoflagelo) occurs in each cell where is inserted in each extreme and rarely whether overrides in central region. When it is liquid medium has characteristics movements with alternated rotation to the long of axis and translation in direction from extreme without hook. In viscose medium are observed snak movements. They are aerobic its colonies are diffuse and formed surface below of medium with 1% of agar and turbid colonies at agar 2%. Optimal temperature is of 28-30ºC. The genus is chemical organotrophs using fatty acids or fatty alcohol having 15 carbonic atoms with energy source. Not use carbohydrates with energy source being necessary serum and albumin to your growth.

Leptospirose is a disease caused by bacteria of Leptospiracea family genus Leptospire that might to be found in worldwide. The infections by leptospire have been reported in human being, cattle, pigs, horses, sheep, dogs, rodents and also severe wilds animal's species in the Brazil and also worldwide. Leptospirose is disease of acute manifestation of third to tenth four day after infection. Leptospire enters the host through mucosa and broken skin, resulting in bacteremia. The spirochetes multiply in organs, most commonly the central nervous system, kidneys, and liver. They are cleared by the immune response from the blood and most tissues but persist and multiply for some time in the kidney tubules. Infective bacteria are shed in the urine. The mechanism of tissue damage is not known.

This disease might itself make chronic after this period and, in the last thirty years the pigs have been appointed as main domestic animals carriers of Leptospire being accountable by epidemics occurrences in the Human and others domestic species. Leptospire could to be considered main agent of problems related with reproductive failure in pigs.

The symptoms of chronic infection are known to induce reproductive failure in farm animals, the acute lethal form of leptospirosis is generally observed in animals. There is various serogroups of Leptospire and in farm animals; bacterins need to contain five serogroups because of variation in local epidemiological condition.

Pathogenic leptospires infect a variety of animals as has been said, but the naturally acquired clinical disease has been documented only in a limited range of mammals. Leptospirosis has been reported mainly in sheep and goats are among the domestic species which are less susceptible to the pathogenic action of leptospirores. In most cases of leptospire infection are asymptomatic, severe outbreaks do occur with a significant loss of sheep, goats and pigs.

The animals considered of high risk to leptospire infection are gravid and young animals be infected by any pathogenic serovar depending upon the specific epidemiologic situation.

The Leptospiroses are divided in further of 200 sorovar grouped in 23 serogroups. In pigs the Leptospirose is characterized by occurrence of abortions in the final third of gestation, heat repetition, fetal mummification, birth of weak piglets, and low number of piglets, vulvae discharge and embryonic death.

The pigs are might to be definitive hosts especially, *pomona, bratislava* and *tarassoli* sorovars and still accidental hosts as in cases of infection by *icterohaemorrhagie, canicola sorovars.* In first case there is a hosts parasite adaptation where the Leptospire are kept in urinary tract for long period being eliminated by urine in conditions for infect others animals. The signs are moderate being detected the infection just in pregnant female. In accidental infection when are infected by an adapted sorovar the other specie the signs of diseases are further evident but the permanence in urinary tract occurs by low time occurring the elimination of lower number of Leptospire in urine.

Although actually be available a large number of techniques for laboratorial diagnostic of routine for Leptospira this techniques still not satisfy some requirement as sensibility, specificity and practice. The antibody presence anti-Leptospire in serologic samples

collected in animals of slaughterhouse no represents adequate sampling for a study with Leptospire in pigs in a region determined. This samples also no reflect the situation grange inside. Nevertheless it allows that itself has a general basis of its occurrence and may to suggest what are the Leptospire sorovars that has large importance in region of animal origin.
Other method of detection of Leptospira is the agglutination serum, in which it is employed in suspensions of strains.
The results of serologic test applied to the diagnostic of Leptospira depends of technique employed, of antigen collections used and also variations related the farms localization year of period into that samples were performed moving of animals. The interference of these factors becomes necessary the existence of epidemiologic sanitary systems permanent that enables the monitoring of spatial distribution of sorovars of Leptospira present in different regions so to rationalize the control using the immunoprophylaxis.
In pigs the biochemical dosage in blood involved bilirubin, glucose fatty acid and plasma proteins in responses the experimental infections by leptospira are scarce in literature. The blood dosage may to assist in diagnostic, prognostic and in the treatment of animals. The bilirubin determination represent a parameter for detect acute hemolysis.
The disease caused by Leptospira is characterized by clinical stages with remissions and exacerbations.
Leptospira organisms are very thin, tightly coiled, obligate aerobic spirochetes and also are characterized by a unique flexuous type of motility.
The genus is divided into two species: the free-living leptopire L biflexa and the pathogenic leptospiras L interrogans. This leptospira is of serotypes causes of zoonotic disease.
The Humans may be accidental hosts. However the primary hosts are domestic animals and also wild. In Humans this disease may have severity from fatal to subclinical.The first case of leptospirosis, in Humans was described in 1886 as a severe icteric illness and was referred to as Weil's disease; however, most human cases of leptospirosis are nonicteric and are not life-threatening.
In contrast to the pathogenic leptospiras, serotypes of L biflexa exist in water and soil as free-living organisms.
Although L biflexa has been isolated from mammalian hosts on occasion, no pathology has been found.
The explanation of why the leptopire not occurence of infections at animals of laboratory yet not is knowledge. The widespread distribution of L biflexa in fresh water and the leptospiras has the capacity to pass through 0.45 to 0.22-µm-pore-size sterilizing filters, they have been found as contaminants of filter-sterilized media.

9. Prophylaxis

In current days the immunization by vaccination is a practice more important in cattle hygienic with results direct and an economic return of activity and warrant of excellent sanitary standard of flocks and the opening and maintain of makers. The vaccination represents the minor costs of inside of productive process and may be decisive for obtaining of good results at animal production.

10. Experimental infection

In Brazil occurs a high incidence of Leptospira interrogans *wolfii* sorovar. This data was reported after a serologic survey in pigs with historic of reproductive failure. This same study showed a possible relation between biochemical results of blood with infection induced by this sorovar. That way, the present study was realized with aims of verify itself is possible to relate biochemical parameters of blood including glucose fee with occurrence of septicemia caused by *Leptospira interrogans wolfii* sorovar. In our experiment eight, 90 days old pigs of the Wessex lineage all castrated male were used experiment divided into two groups of four animals. Biochemical alterations in the serum of the animals were analyzed in both groups during 36 days. Control (Group I) received 0.5mL of a 0.9% sterile sodium choride inoculated by intracranial vein injection; Group II animals were inoculated by the same way with 5.0mL of Brazilian "armadillo". Three days after inoculation blood was collected without anticoagulant; the same process was repeated at 72 hours intervals during eighteen days in both, control and experiments groups. Quantitative biochemical parameters were direct, indirect and total bilirubin all were observed after six days. Glucose fatty acid decreased after the third day inoculation. The increased bilirubin levels could be due to acute hemolisys, hypoglycemia, hypolypidemia that could be related to hepatic lesions and septicemia.

In the Group II has been observed an increased of direct bilirubin levels in the third day after inoculation which came back the initial values from the sixth day when compared to Group I. This increase of direct bilirubin in the third day observed in the pigs of Group II may be due the hemolysis which indicates that liver no presented any lesions and suggest efficiency in the hepatic conjugation of bilirubin with glucuronic acid. When there is hepatic lesions this cause damage in parenchymal hepatic cells difficult the conjugation.

In values of indirect bilirubin might itself to observe that between start of experiment and third day there was a decrease followed of a increase of levels in the sixth day in the inoculated animals with *wolfii* sorovar and that from ninth day has been verified a fall in levels that itself kept stables to fifteenth day similar behavior has been observed in control. However this bilirubin increased has been discrete when compared to animals inoculated. This decreased of levels of bilirubin to third day after the inoculation with serum *wolfii sorovar* has been verified by others authors. After hemolysis the indirect bilirubin is not apparent in the first hours. The marked increase of bilirubin seems to indicate a hemolysis excessive. Some endotoxins cause changes in carbohydrate metabolism of erythrocytes with a consequent decrease of ATP. That would be a possible explanation for loss of motility of contractile system of erythrocytes membrane.

That loss of motility causes changes in the morphology of erythrocytes, passing from biconcave disk to spherical shape (spherocytosis). That abnormality would result in the detection and removal of spherocytic cells by reticulum macrophage system, spleen, liver and bone marrow where would be destroyed with release of hemoglobin that would be transformed in bilirubin.

In the inoculated pigs has been observed a fall of levels of fatty acids while in control Group there was the fall then an increase, being the major value detected to twelfth day. The decrease of fatty acids in the pigs inoculated with *wolfii* sorovar caused a secondary hypoglycemia and a hypolipidemia.

The glucose levels presented a decrease to third day after inoculation then of constant increase thus to overcome the initials values in the fifteenth. In the control Group also has been verified a fall of glucose fee then an increased from third day reaching to the maximum value in the ninth day and decreased the lower values than initials between the twelfth and fifteenth day. The hypoglycemia observed occurs by increase of consumption of glucose by tissues in septicemia case. The plasma protein levels have been unchanged despite to has increased in third day in pigs of Group II after the inoculation with *wolfii* sorovar. This hypoproteinemia in inoculated animals could to be related with a hepatic lesion discrete that may have been caused by leptospire infection. In some cases of septicemia may have an increase of capillary permeability that allow the leakage of albumin for extracellular compartments which possibly could prove the septicemia have started just in the third day of experiment. The leptospirose induction model with intravenous inoculation of *wolfii* sorovar showed effective. The blood biochemical variations of pigs inoculated were hypoglycemia, suggesting a hepatic lesion and the occurrence of a bacterial septicemia and also hyperbilirubinemia, indicating with this that a main cause of toxicity of *wolfii* sorovar showed in this study is grave anemia hemolytic.

The lost of piglet ranging of 4 to 10% in childbirth, others 20% may die before weaning. The causes of die of piglet are many. The hypoglycemia may to be caused by septicemia or to be a result of all a complex evolving needs specific temperature interfering in glycogens feeding frequency and amount of colostrums that subsequently the milk ingestion.

11. Conclusion

Concluding the model of induction of leptospirose caused by intravenous inoculation of *wolfii* sorovar showed itself effective. The biochemical variations in the blood of inoculated pigs with *wolfii* sorovar were: hypoglycemia, hypolipidemia and hypoproteinemia suggesting a hepatic lesion and bacterial septicemia. The hyperbilirubinemia might to indicate that main cause of toxicity of *wolfii* sorovar is a severe hemolytic anemia. However the low glucose fee has aggravating role in the septicemia in pigs.

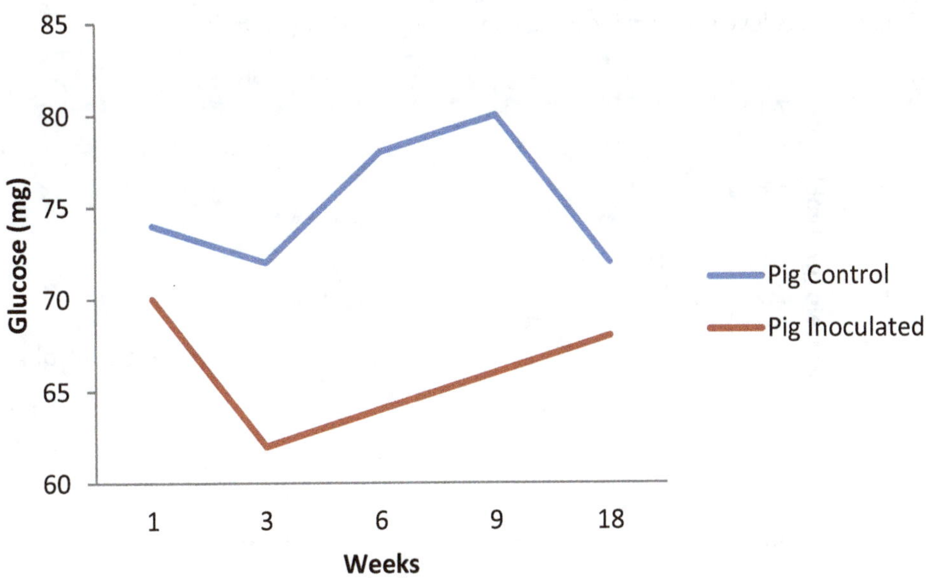

Fig. 1. Comparative of glucose level in pigs inoculated and uninoculated (control)

The figure shows the comparison of two Groups of four pigs. The Group I (pig control) the pigs received 5.0mL of a 0.9% sterile sodium chloride solution by intracranial vein injection;

Group II (pig inoculated) animals were inoculated by the same way with 5.0mL of a cell culture containing 1.0x10[8]cells mL-1 of *Leptospira interrogans sorovar wolffi*, wild strain L-10, isolated from a wild species of Brazilian.
The biochemical changes were analyzed in the serum of the animals in broth Groups during 36 days. All parameters returned to normal levels after fifteen days, in all animals tested.

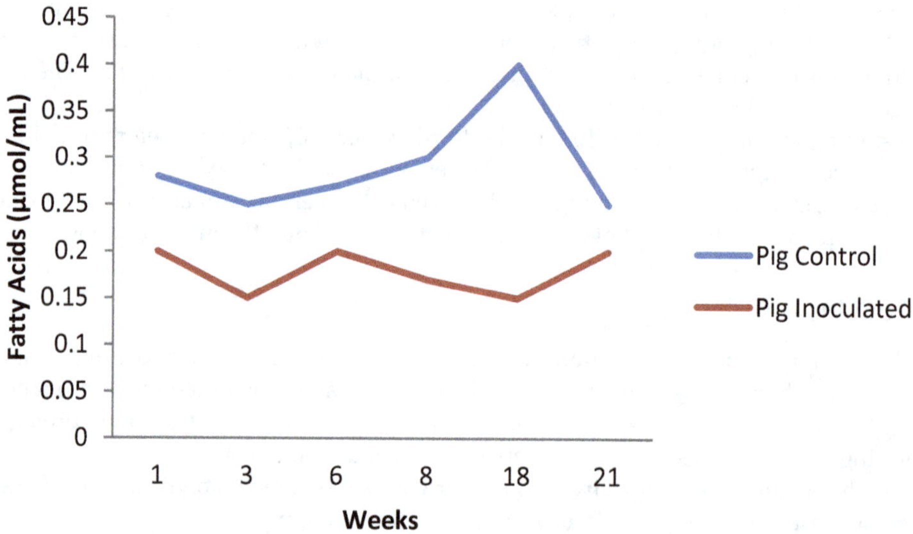

Fig. 2. Fatty acids levels in pigs inoculated and uninoculated (control).

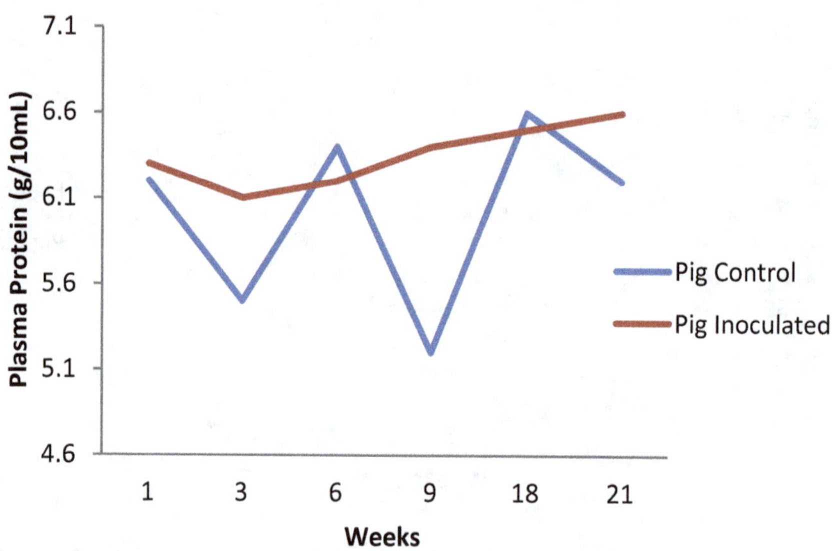

Fig. 3. Plasma protein levels of pig inoculated and pig uninoculated (control).

12. Acknowledgments

The authors thanks to Prof. Dr. José Carlos Rende by realization of these experiments.

13. References

Arino J, Guinovart JJ. (1986). Phosphorylation and inactivation of rat hepatocyte glycogen synthase by phorbol esters and mezerein. *Biochemical Biophysiology Reserch Community* Vol.134: pp.113–119.

Ávila, F.A. et al. (1977). Freqüência de aglutininas anti-leptospiras em soros de suínos de Minas Gerais. *Arquivo da Escola de Veterinária da UFMG*, Belo Horizonte, Vol.29, n.3, pp.263- 268.

Bacila, M. (2003). Bioquímica veterinária. 2.ed. São Paulo: *Robe Editorial*. pp. 583.

Bagby GJ; et al. (1991). Divergent efficacy of antibody to tumor necrosis factor-alpha in intravascular and peritonitis models of sepsis. *Journal Infect Disease* Vol.163: pp. 83-88.

Baker CC; et al. (1983). Evaluation of factors affecting mortality rate after sepsis in a murine cecal ligation and puncture model. *Surgery* Vol.94, pp. 331- 335.

Bem-Shaul V; et al. (1999). Lipopolysaccharide-induced oxidative stress in the liver: comparison between rat and rabbit. Shock Vol.12, pp. 288-293.

Bessis, M. (1973). Living blood cells and their ultrastructure. *New York: Springer Verlag*. pp.717.

Blackmore, PF, Strickland WG, Bocckino SB, Exton JH. (1986). Mechanism of hepatic glycogen synthase inactivation induced by Ca2+-mobilizing hormones. Studies using phospholipase C and phorbol myristate acetate. *Biochemical Journal* Vol.237, pp. 235–242.

Blackwell, TS & Christman JW. (1996). Sepsis and cytokines: current status. Br *Journal Anaesthesiology* Vol.77, pp. 110-117.

Blobe, GC, Stribling S, Obeid LM, Hannun YA (1996). Protein kinase C isoenzymes. Regulation and function. *Cancer Survery* Vol.27, pp. 213–248.

Bone, Rc; Grodzin Cj & Balk Ra. (1997). Sepsis: A new hypothesis for pathogenesis of the disease process. Chest. Vol.112, pp.235-243.

Brenner, A.F.; Kaufmann, et al. (1999). Further determination of DNA relatedness between serogroups and serovars in the family Leptospiraceae with a proposal for *Leptospira alexanderi* sp nov and four new *Leptospira* genomospecies, *International Journal Systemic Bacteriological.*, Vol.49, pp. 839–858.

Bretcher, G.; Bessis, M. (1972). Present status of spiculed red cell, and their relationship to the discotype-echionocyte transformation: a critical review. *Blood*, Vol.40, pp.333-344.

Burnstein, T.; BAKER, J. (1954). Lepstospirosis in swine caused by *Leptospira Pomona*. *Journal of Infectious Diseases*, New York, Vol.94, pp.52-64.

Burtis, C.A.; Ashwood, E.R. (1998). Fundamentos de química clínica. 4.ed. Rio de Janeiro: Guanabara Koogan, pp.842

Bush, B.M. (2004). Interpretação de resultados laboratoriais para clínicos de pequenos animais. São Paulo: *Roca*, pp.276.

Chan, KM, Junger KD. (1983). Calcium transport and phosphorylated intermediate of (Ca2+-Mg2+)-ATPase in plasma membranes of rat liver. *Journal Biological Chemical* Vol.258, pp.4404–4410.

Coles, E.H. (1984). Função hepática. In: COLES, E.H. Patologia clínica veterinária. 3.ed. São Paulo: *Manole*, pp.185- 219.

Crowley, Sr. (1996). The pathogenesis of septic shock. Heart Lung Vol.25, pp.124-134.

Cryer, PE, et al (2003). Hypoglycemia in diabetes. *Diabetes Care*. Vol.26, No.6, pp.1902–1912.

Cryer, PE. The prevention and correction of hypoglycemia. (2001). In: Jefferson L, ed. Handbook of Physiology: The Endocrine Pancreas and Regulation of metabolism. New York, New York, USA: *Oxford University Press*; pp.1057–1092.

Davies, Mg & Hagen, P. Systemic inflammatory response syndrome. Br. *Journal Surgery* 84: 920-935, 1997.

Dikken, H. & Kmety, E. Serological typing methods of leptospiras. (1978). In: Bergan, T & Norris, Journal Editors, *Methods in Microbiology*, Academic Press, London. pp. 259–307.

Dinarello, CA. (1997). Proinflammatory and anti-inflammatory cytokines as mediators in the pathogenesis of septic shock. *Chest* Vol.112, pp.321S-329S.

Dobbins, RL, et al. (1991). Role of glucagon in countering hypoglycemia induced by insulin infusion in dogs. *American Journal Physiology*. pp. E773–E781.

Dole, V.F.; Meinertz, H. (1960). Microdetermination of long chain fatty acids in plasma and tissues. *Journal of Biology and Chemistry*, Vol.235, pp.25-95.

Domas, B.T.; Wu, T.Y. (1991). The measurement of bilirubin fraction in serum. *Critical Reviews in Clinical Laboratory Science*, Vol.28, pp.415-445.

Echtenacher B; et al. (1990). Requirements of endogenous tumor necrosis factor/cachectin for recovery from experimental peritonitis. *Journal Immunological* Vol.145, pp. 3762-3766.

Evers C, Hugentobler G, Lester R, Gmaj P, Meier P, Murer H. (1988). ATPdependent Ca2+ uptake and Ca2+-dependent protein phosphorylation in basolateral liver plasma membrane. *Biochimical Biophysiologycal Acta* Vol.939, pp.542- 550.

Fabiato, A. (1988). Computer programs for calculating total from specified free or free from specified total ionic concentrations in aqueous solutions containing multiple metals and ligands. *Methods Enzymology* 157: 378–417, 1988.

Fain JN, Li SY, Litosch I, Wallace M. (1984). Synergistic activation of rat hepatocyte glycogen phosphorylase by A23187 and phorbol ester. *Biochemical Biophysiology Reserch Community*. Vol.119, pp. 88–94.

Faine, S. et al. (1999). Leptospira and leptospirosis (2ª Ed.), *Medisci*, Melbourne, Austrália.

Farina, R. et al. (1999). *Leptospirosis* in swine: experimental infection with serotype *bratislava*. *International Journal of Zoonosis* v.4, p.38-44.

Fisher CJ; et al. (1993). Influence of na antitumor necrosis factor monoclonal antibody on cytokine levels in patients with sepsis. *Critical Care* Medicine, Vol.21, pp. 318-327.

Florquin, S. et al. (1994). Systemic release and protective role of endogenously synthesized nitric oxide in Staphylococal enterotoxin B-induced shock in mice. *Journal Immunological* Vol.153, pp. 2618-2623.

Furukawa, KI, Tawada Y, Shigekawa M (1989). Protein kinase C activation stimulates plasma membrane Ca2+ pump in cultured vascular smooth muscle cells. *Journal Biological Chemical* Vol.264, pp.4844–4849.

Galanos, C & Freudenberg Ma (1993). Mechanism of endotoxin shock and endotoxin hypersensitivity. *Immunobiology* Vol.187, pp.346-356.

Gali RR, Pugazhenthi S, Khandelwal R.L (1993). Reciprocal effects of the protein kinase C inhibitors staurosporine and H-7 on the regulation of glycogen synthase and phosphorylase in the primary culture of hepatocytes. *Metabolism* Vol.42, pp.1475–1480.

Gérard C; et al. (1993). Interleukin 10 reduces the release of tumor necrosis factor and prevents lethality in experimental endotoxemia. *Journal Express Medicine* Vol.177, pp.547- 552.

Gerich J, et al. (1979). Hormonal mechanisms of recovery from insulin-induced hypoglycemia in man. *American Journal Physiology*. Vol.236, pp.E380–E385.

Girio, R.J.S. et al. (1998). Alterações reprodutivas e anatomopatológicas em fêmeas suínas com títulos de anticorpos contra *Leptospira* de *Ciência Veterinária*, Vol.5, No.3, p.99-103.

Hadjiminas D, et al. (1994). Enhanced survival from cecal ligation and puncture with pentoxifylline is associated with altered neutrophil trafficking and reduced interleukin-1 beta expression but not inhibition of tumor necrosis factor synthesis. *Surgery* Vol.116, pp.348-355.

Hampton Mb; Kettle Aj & Winterbourn CC. (1998). Inside the neutrophil phagosome: Oxidants, myeloperoxidase, and bacterial killing. *Blood* Vol.92, pp.3007-3017.

Hanson, L.E. et al. (1971). Leptospirosis in swine caused by serotype *grippotyphosa*. *American Journal of Veterinary Research*, Vol.32, No.6, pp.855-860.

Hinshaw LB, et al. (1992). Lethal sthaphylococcus aureus-induced shock in primates: prevention of death with anti-TNF antibody. *Journal Traumatism* Vol.33, pp.568- 573.

Hunter,P. (2004). Leptospirosis In: Coetzer J.A.W. & Tustin, RC. *Infectious Diseases of Livestock*. Oxford University Press. 2ª Ed., Vol. 3, chapter. 136, pp. 1445- 1456.

Inaba H, Araki M, Numai, T. (1993). Modulation of protein kinase C alters hemodynamics and metabolism in the isolated liver in fed and fasted rats. *Journal Hepatology* Vol.19, pp. 475–484.

Inaba H, Filkins, J.P (1991). Augmentation of endotoxin lethality and glucose dyshomeostasis by phorbol ester. *American Journal Physiology* Vol.260,pp.R494–R502.

Inaba, H, Pilkins, J.P. (1991). Antagonism of endotoxic glucose dyshomestasis by protein kinase C inhibitors. *American Journal Physiology* Vol.261, pp.R26–R31.

Inzana, T.J. et al. (1979). Experimentally induced *Leptospira interrogans* serovar *autumnalis* infections in young swine. *American Journal of Veterinary Research*, Vol.40, No.10, pp.1355-1358.

Kang YH, Mekenna T, Watson LP, Williams R, Holt M. (1988). Cytochemical changes in hepatocytes of rats with endotoxemia or sepsis: Localization of fibronectin, calcium and enzymes. *Journal Histochemical Cytochemical* Vol.36, pp.665- 678.

Kimura, S, et al. (1984). Stimulation of hepatic glycogenolysis by 12-0-tetradecanoylphorbol-13-acetate (TPA) via a calcium requiring process. *Biochemical Biophysiology Reserch Community*. Vol.122, pp. 1057–1064.

Kingscote, B.F. (1986). Leptospirosis outbreak in Piggery in Southern Alberta. *Canadian Veterinary Journal*, No.27, pp.188-190.

Lagast, H, Pozzan T, Waldvogel FA, Lew PD. (1984). Phorbol myristate acetate stimulates ATP dependent calcium transport by the plasma membrane of neutrophils. *Journal Clinical Investiment*. Vol.73, pp. 878–883.

Latimer, K.S (2003). Veterinary laboratory medicine: clinical pathology. 4.ed. Iowa: *A Blackwell*, pp.450.

Lau YT, Hwang TL, Chen MF, Liu MS (1992). Calcium transport by rat liver plasma membranes during sepsis. *Circulatory Shock* Vol.38, pp.238–244.

Levett, PN. (2001). Leptospirosis, *Clinical Microbiology Review*., Vol.24. No.14, pp. 296–326.

Li P; Ye X. et al. (1995). Mice deficient in Il- 2beta-converting enzyme are deficient in production of mature IL-1beta and resistant to endotoxic shock. *Cell* Vol.80, pp.401- 411.

Liu, J.P. (1996). Protein kinase C and its substrate. *Molecular Cell Endocrinological* Vol.116, pp.1- 29.

Liu, MS, Kang GF (1987). Liver glycogen metabolism in endotoxin shock. II.Endotoxin administration increases glycogen phosphorylase activitiesin dog liver. *Biochemical Medicine Metabologycal Biologycal* Vol.37, pp.73–80.

Liu, MS, Sharma C (1981). Glycolytic enzyme activities in normal and diabetic dog livers during endotoxic shock. *American Journal Physiology* Vol.240, pp.R10–R15.

Lowry OH, Rosebrough NJ, Farr AL, Randall R. J. (2000). Protein measurement with the Folin phenol reagent. *Journal Biological Chemical* Vol.193, pp. 265–275.

Macarthur H; et al. (2000). Inactivation of catecholamines by superoxide gives new insights on the pathogenesis of septic shock. *Proceeding National Academy Science* USA Vol.97, pp. 9753-9758.

Martineau L & Shek PN. (2000). Peritoneal cytokine concentrations and survival outcome in an experimental bacterial infusion model of peritonitis. *Critical Care Medicine* Vol.28, pp.788-794.

McGilvery, R.W (1979). Storage of glucose as glycogen. In: RW McGilvery (ed). Biochemistry, A Functional Approach. W.B. Saunders Company, Philadelphia, pp 483–510.

Mitaka, C. et al. (1997). Beneficial effect of carboxy-PTIO on hemodynamic and blood gas changes in septic shock dogs. *Critical Care* (London), Vol.1, pp.45-50.

Monteith, GR, Roufogalis, B.D (1995). The plasma membrane calcium pump - a physiological perspective on its regulation. *Cell Calcium* Vol.18, pp.459–470.

Morais, M.G. et al. (2000). Variação sazonal de bioquímica clínica de vacas aneloradas sob pastejo contínuo de Brachiara decumbens. *Arquivo de Medicina Veterinária e Zootécnica,* Vol.52, Nol.9, pp.98-104.

Murray, R.K. et al. (2000). Harper's biochemistry. 25.ed. Connecticut: *Appleton & Lauge,* pp.927.

Newton, A.C. (1995). Protein kinase C: Structure, function, and regulation. *Journal Biological Chemical* Vol.270, pp.28495–28498.

Ohlsson, K, et al. (1990). Interleukin-1 receptor antagonist reduces mortality from endotoxin shock. Nature, Vol.348, pp.550-552.

Oliveira, S.J, et al. (1994). Evidências de infecção por *Leptospira bratislava* em transtornos reprodutivos em suínos. *Ciência Rural,* Vol.24, No.2, pp.345-348.

Oliveira, S.J. (1988). Leptospirose em Suínos. *A Hora Veterinária,* Nol.41, pp.5-8.

Patel, T.B. (1987). Stimulation of hepatic glycogenolysis by phorbol 12-myristate 13-acetate. *Biochemical Journal* Vol.241, pp. 549–554.

Pavoine, C, Lotersztajn S, Mallat A, Pecker, F. (1987). The high affinity (Ca2+- Mg2+)-ATPase in liver plasma membrane is a Ca2+ pump: Reconstitution of the purified enzyme into phospholipid vesicles. *Journal Biological Chemical* Vol.262, pp.5113–5117.

Power, S.B. (1991). Diagnosing Leptospira in pigs. *Veterinary Record,* Vol.128, pp.43.

Prescott, J,F. et al. (1993). Leptospira In: Gyles, L & Thoen, CO. Pathogenesis of Bacterial Infections in Animals. Ames, *Iowa University Press* 2ª Ed., pp.287-296.

Quezado, Zmn, Banks, S.M & Natanson, C. (1995). New strategies for combatting sepsis: the magic bullets missed the mark...but the search continues. *Tibtech* Vol.13, pp.56-63.

Ramnanan, C, et al (2010). Molecular characterization of insulin-mediated suppression of hepatic glucose production in vivo. *Diabetes*. Vol.59, No.6, pp.1302–1311.

Ramos, A, et al. (1981). Inquérito sociológico de leptospirose em suínos no Estado do Rio de Janeiro e região limítrofe. *Pesquisa Veterinária Brasileira*, v.1, n.3, p.81-83.

Redl, H, et al. (1993). Interleukin-8 release in baboon septicemia is partially dependent on tumor necrosis factor. *Journal Infect Disease* Vol.167, pp.1464-1466.

Remick, D.G, et al. (2000). Comparison of the mortality and inflammatory response of two models of sepsis: lipopolysaccharide vs cecal ligation and puncture. *Shock* 13:110-116.

Rende, J.C, et al. (2007). Experimental infection by Leptospira interrogans serovar wolffi in young pigs: Determination of biochemical parameters. Ciência Rural, Vol.37, No.2, pp.458-463.

Rivera, N, et al. (2010). Insulin-induced hypoglycemia increases hepatic sensitivity to glucagon in dogs. *Journal of Clinical Investigation* Vol.120, No.12, pp.4425-4435.

Roach, P.J, Goldman, M. (1983). Modification of glycogen synthase activity in isolated rat hepatocytes by tumor-promoting phorbol esters: Evidence for differential regulation of glycogen synthase and phosphorylase. *Proceeding National Academy Sciences* USA 80, pp.7170–7172.

Rogy, M.A, et al. (1995). Human tumor necrosis factor receptor (p55) and interleukin 10 gene transfer in the mouse reduces mortality to lethal endotoxemia and also attenuates local inflammatory responses. Journal Express Medicine Vol.181, pp.2289-2293.

Rot, A. (1992). Endothelial cell binding of NAP-1/IL-8 role in neutrophil emigration. *Immunological Today* Vol.13, pp.291-294.

Rovai, L. E, et al (1998). The murine neutrophil- chemoattractant chemokines LIX, KC and MIP-2 have distinct induction kinetics, tissue distributions and tissue specific sensitivities to glucocorticoid regulation in endotoxemia. *Journal Leukocyte Biological* ,Vol.64, pp.494-502.

Sayeed, M.M. (1986). Alterations in cellular Ca2+ regulation in the liver in endotoxic shock. *American Journal Physiologycal* Vol.250, pp.R884–R891.

Schenck, J.A.P. (1976). Isolamento de leptospira do sorogrupo *hebdomadis* de tatus (*Dasypus novemcintus*) capturados no Estado de Minas Gerais. 75f. Dissertação (Mestrado em Medicina Veterinária Preventiva) - Curso de Pós-graduação em Medicina Veterinária, Universidade Federal de Minas Gerais.

Schönberg, A. et al. (2002). *Leptospira interrogans* serovar *bratislava* in pig breeding herds. In: Germany International Leptospirosis Society, 3., 2002, Bridgetown, Barbados. Proceedings Bridgetown, Barbado: *Internacioanl Leptospiros Society*, Vol.276, pp.49.

Stalheim, O.H.V. (1973). Urinary precipitate in porcine leptospirosis. *Cornell Veterinary*, Vol.64, pp.20-24.

Steiner, K.E, et al. (1990). Effects of insulin on glucagon-stimulated glucose production in the conscious dog. *Metabolism*. Vol.39, No.12, pp.1325–1333.

Suffradini, A.F, et al. (1989). The cardiovascular response of normal humans to the administration of endotoxin. *National England Journal Medicine* Vol.321, pp.280-287.

Sweet, M.J & Hume, D.A. (1996). Endotoxin signal transduction in macrophages. *Journal Leukocite Biological* Vol.60, pp. 8-26.

Tagliabue, S.; Farina, R. (1995). Inchesta sieroepidemiologica sulla diffusione delle leptospirosi tragli animali domestici Ed alcune specie selvatiche. *Selezione Veterinária*, Vol.36, pp.941-953.

Tavares-Murta, B.M. et al (1998). The intravenous administration of tumor necrosis factor alpha, interleukin 8 and macrophage-derived neutrophil chemotactic factor inhibits neutrophil migation by stimulating nitric oxide production. Br *Journal Pharmacological* Vol.124, pp.1369-1374.

Thompson, J.C.; Manktelow, B.W. (1986). Pathogenesis and red blood cell destruction in haemoglobinaemic leptospirosis. *Journal of Comparative Pathology*, Vol.96, pp.529-538.

Van, DER Poll T, et al. (1993). Tumor necrosis factoralpha: its role in the metabolic response to sepsis. *Clinical Science* Vol.84, pp.247-256.

Van Der Poll T; et al. (1996). Changes in edotoxin-induced cytokine production by whole blood after in vivo exposure of normal humans to endotoxin. *Journal Infect Diseases* Vol.174, pp.1356-1360.

Van Zee, K.J, et al. (1991). IL-8 in septic shock, endotoxemia and after IL-1 administration. *Journal Immunological* Vol.146, pp.3478-3482.

Wakabayashi, G, et al. (1991). A specific receptor antagonist for interleukin 1 prevents Escherichia coli-induced shock in rabbits. *FASEB Journal* Vol.5, pp.338-343.

Walley, K.R, et al. (1996). Balanced of inflammatory cytokines related to severity and mortality of murine sepsis. *Infect Immunity* Vol.64, pp.4733-4738.

Wanidworanun, C & Strober, W. (1993). Predominant role of tumor necrosis factor-a in human monocyte IL-10 synthesis. *Journal Immunological* Vol.151, pp. 6853-6861.

Wasterlain, C.G et al. (2010). Brain Energy Metabolism During Experimental Neonatal Seizures *Neurochemical Research.* Vol.35, pp.2193–2198.

Wichterman, K.A, Baue, A.K, Chaudry, I.H. (1980). Sepsis and septic shock – A review of laboratory models and a proposal. *Journal Surgery Reserch* Vol.29, pp.189–210.

Wichtermann, K.A, et al. (1980). Sepsis and septic shock-a review of laboratory models and a proposal. *Journal Surgery Reserch* Vol.29, pp.189-201.

Wise, B.C, Raynor, R.L, Kuo, J.F. (1982). Phospholipid-sensitive Ca2+-dependent protein kinase from heart. I. Purification and general properties. *Journal Biological Chemical* Vol.257, pp.8481–8488.

Woods, G.T, et al. (1962). Experimental infection of swine with *Leptospira ballum. Zoonoses Research*, New York, Vol.1, No.10, pp.165-184.

Wright, L.C, Chen, S, Roufogalis, B.D (1993). Regulation of the activity and phosphorylation of the plasma membrane Ca2+-ATPase by protein kinase C in intact human erythrocytes. *Archieve Biochemical Biophysiologycal* Vol.306, pp.277–284.

Wu, L.L, Tang, C, Liu, M.S (1997). Hyper and hypocardiodynamic states are associated with externalization and internalization, respectively, of a- adrenergic receptors in rat heart during sepsis. *Shock* Vol.5, pp.318–323.

Zanetti, G. et al, (1992). Cytokine production after intravenous or peritoneal gramnegative bacterial challenge in mice. *Journal Immunological* Vol.148, pp.1890- 1897.

Zantl, N, et al (1998). Essential role of gamma interferon in survival of colon ascendens stent peritonitis, a novel murine model of abdominal sepsis. *Infect Immunity* 66: 2300-2309, 1998.

Permissions

All chapters in this book were first published by InTech Open; hereby published with permission under the Creative Commons Attribution License or equivalent. Every chapter published in this book has been scrutinized by our experts. Their significance has been extensively debated. The topics covered herein carry significant findings which will fuel the growth of the discipline. They may even be implemented as practical applications or may be referred to as a beginning point for another development.

The contributors of this book come from diverse backgrounds, making this book a truly international effort. This book will bring forth new frontiers with its revolutionizing research information and detailed analysis of the nascent developments around the world.

We would like to thank all the contributing authors for lending their expertise to make the book truly unique. They have played a crucial role in the development of this book. Without their invaluable contributions this book wouldn't have been possible. They have made vital efforts to compile up to date information on the varied aspects of this subject to make this book a valuable addition to the collection of many professionals and students.

This book was conceptualized with the vision of imparting up-to-date information and advanced data in this field. To ensure the same, a matchless editorial board was set up. Every individual on the board went through rigorous rounds of assessment to prove their worth. After which they invested a large part of their time researching and compiling the most relevant data for our readers.

The editorial board has been involved in producing this book since its inception. They have spent rigorous hours researching and exploring the diverse topics which have resulted in the successful publishing of this book. They have passed on their knowledge of decades through this book. To expedite this challenging task, the publisher supported the team at every step. A small team of assistant editors was also appointed to further simplify the editing procedure and attain best results for the readers.

Apart from the editorial board, the designing team has also invested a significant amount of their time in understanding the subject and creating the most relevant covers. They scrutinized every image to scout for the most suitable representation of the subject and create an appropriate cover for the book.

The publishing team has been an ardent support to the editorial, designing and production team. Their endless efforts to recruit the best for this project, has resulted in the accomplishment of this book. They are a veteran in the field of academics and their pool of knowledge is as vast as their experience in printing. Their expertise and guidance has proved useful at every step. Their uncompromising quality standards have made this book an exceptional effort. Their encouragement from time to time has been an inspiration for everyone.

The publisher and the editorial board hope that this book will prove to be a valuable piece of knowledge for researchers, students, practitioners and scholars across the globe.

List of Contributors

Toshiyuki Kimura
National Agricultural Research Center for Tohoku Region, Japan

Tatjana Ábel
National Health Center, Hungary

Pietro Galassetti
University of California, Irvine, United States of America

Boby G. Thekadeth, P Zachariah, Zeenat Parveen, Pavan Patel, Matthew Schoeck, Andrew Mazulis, Lawrence Perlmuter and Sant P.Singh
Rosalind Franklin University of Medicine and Science VA Med Ctr, North Chicago, IL, USA

Blanca Álvarez Fernández and Irene Cuadrado Pérez
University Hospital of Getafe, Madrid, Spain

Outi Tammela and Tarja Vanhatalo
Pediatric Research Centre, University of Tampere, Finland

Praveen Kumar and Shiv Sajan Saini
Neonatal Unit, Department of Pediatrics, Postgraduate Institute of Medical Education and Research, Chandigarh, INDIA

Kristen Helms and Kristi Kelley
Auburn University, Harrison School of Pharmacy, United States

Marek Pytliak, Viola Vargová and Viola Mechírová
Medical Faculty of the University of P.J. Safarik, Košice, Slovakia

Josef Hořejš
Department of Radiology, Czech Republic

Chen-Hsen Lee, Justin Ging-Shing Won and Hsiao-Shan Tseng
Departments of Surgery, Internal Medicine and Radiology National Yang-Ming University and Taipei Veterans General Hospital, Taipei, Taiwan

Jan Škrha
Charles University, Czech Republic
Laboratory for Endocrinology and Metabolism, Czech Republic

Jaroslava Dušková
Laboratory for Endocrinology and Metabolism, Czech Republic

Jan Šváb
Department of Surgery, Czech Republic

Jiřina Hilgertová
Laboratory for Endocrinology and Metabolism, Czech Republic

Radan Keil
Faculty of Medicine, Department of Internal Medicine, Prague, Czech Republic

M. Isabel Del Olmo and J. Francisco Merino-Torres
University Hospital La Fe-Valencia Department of Endocrinology and Nutrition, Spain

J. Luis Ponce and Angel Moya
Department of Surgery, Spain

Everlon Cid Rigobelo and Fernando Antonio de Ávila
Universidade Estadual Paulista,Campus Experimental de Dracena Faculdade de Ciências Agrárias e Veterinárias de Jaboticabal, Brazil

Index

www.ingramcontent.com/pod-product-compliance
Lightning Source LLC
LaVergne TN
LVHW080634210926
848485LV00003B/264